Atlas of Primary Cleft Rhinoplasty

Percy Rossell-Perry
Editor

Atlas of Primary Cleft Rhinoplasty

Springer

Editor
Percy Rossell-Perry
Union Peruvian University (UpeU)
School of Human Medicine, Lima
Lima, Peru

ISBN 978-3-031-68011-3 ISBN 978-3-031-68012-0 (eBook)
https://doi.org/10.1007/978-3-031-68012-0

Editorial Contact: Erica de Cassia Ferraz

This Springer imprint is published by the registered company Springer Nature Switzerland AG
The registered company address is: Gewerbestrasse 11, 6330 Cham, Switzerland

To my Lord Jesus Christ who guides all my works.

To my parents, Blanca and Percy, and my comprehensive wife, Patti.

To my professors, Drs. Daniel and Claudio Kirschbaum, who made possible my professional development in plastic surgery.

I like to express my gratitude to Dr. William Carter for his generous help as a surgeon and professor, who provided the best benefit to poor children in Peru.

To the Smile Train Foundation, who transformed my life making me a man of service to others.

Finally, this book is dedicated to all my patients and their parents who have taught me a lot about love for others.

Foreword 1

In the intricate realm of care for those born with cleft lip and palate, treatment of the cleft nose stands out for posing both a challenge to surgeon and a benefit to patient.

The human face, a canvas of identity and emotion, holds within its delicate structure the power to express an array of sentiments and forge connections. The nose, front and center in that canvas, is crucial for airflow function and defining in appearance. Its trilaminar structure incorporates strength, flexibility, symmetry, and three-dimensionality. Consequently, rhinoplasty occupies a revered position in plastic surgery for the technical challenge of achieving excellence. Cleft rhinoplasty embodies that technical challenge, with added dimensions: a more complex underlying anatomy, evident at birth, for which early treatment can impart early benefit, yet all of which is subject to effects of growth.

There is an urgent need to democratize excellence in cleft rhinoplasty. Cleft lip and palate are among the most common congenital anomalies, with approximately 200,000 children born with cleft lip/palate in the world each year, most of whom will have a cleft nasal deformity. The last several decades have seen the proliferation of multidisciplinary cleft care in specialized centers, achieving great outcomes. We have also witnessed dramatically improved access to basic cleft lip and palate repair in lower-resource settings, which is tremendous. Interestingly, however, as patients age from infancy to adolescence in these regions without ongoing cleft care, differences and ongoing needs emerge with respect to speech, dentition, and nose appearance and function. Patient-reported outcome tools give voice to these young people, painting a picture in which a persistent cleft nasal difference is highly stigmatizing. This is not surprising in an era where one's face—in ubiquitous digital photos, and looking back from the screen of one's mobile phone—is ever-present. Thus, there is a vast and immediate need both to effectively treat the cleft nose of millions of children and young adults and to combine cleft nasal treatment with lip repair in infants.

Fortunately, several factors are shifting the paradigm toward primary cleft rhinoplasty, which is why this book is so timely and important. First, abundant evidence shows that incorporating nasal surgery with lip repair is safe and does not impair future growth. Second, outcome studies increasingly illustrate to surgeons (and to patient families) the improved middle- and long-term outcomes achieved through primary rhinoplasty. Third, there is increasing recognition of the benefits of non-surgical nasal molding adjuncts that can be used before or after surgery to enhance the outcomes of primary rhinoplasty and availability of these adjuncts. And fourth, increased attention to the specific technical components of cleft rhinoplasty demystifies and facilitates familiarity and refinement by the surgical community.

Dr. Rossell-Perry is a uniquely qualified guide on this journey. His three-decade career, which includes both leading a large urban cleft team in Lima and regular outreach activities in rural areas of Peru, imparts deep clinical experience. Furthermore, he is a gifted clinical scientist who has both carefully studied and reported patterns of his own surgical outcomes and is well-acquainted with contemporary evidence-based care. Throughout the pages of this comprehensive guide, readers will explore the anatomical complexities and surgical techniques that define primary cleft rhinoplasty. Each chapter meticulously blends theoretical knowledge, practical insights, and visual guidance, empowering both novice and experienced surgeons to refine their skills and achieve optimal outcomes.

In a field where precision is paramount, this atlas does more than present surgical techniques; through clinical examples, it encapsulates the profound impact of primary cleft rhinoplasty on patients' lives. By restoring the physical harmony of the nose and lip, as well as the confidence and self-esteem of those affected, this procedure embodies the essence of reconstructive surgery. As you delve into the chapters that follow, may you find inspiration in the artistry of primary cleft rhinoplasty. May this atlas serve as a beacon of knowledge, guiding you toward the highest standards of patient care and surgical excellence. Together, let us continue to push the boundaries of what is possible, transforming challenges into triumphs and bringing smiles to those who need them most.

Division of Plastic, Reconstructive and Oral Surgery
Children's Hospital of Philadelphia
Philadelphia, PA, USA
July 2024

Jordan W. Swanson

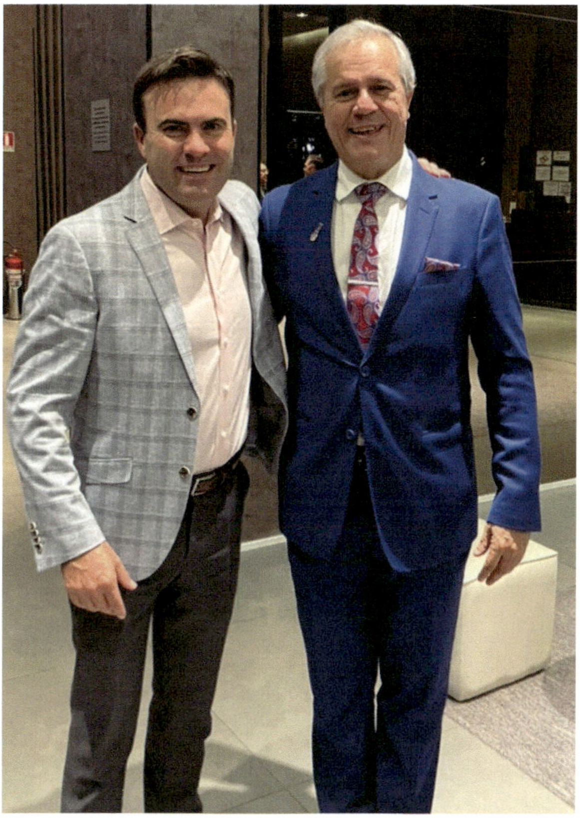

Fig. 1 Dr. Percy Rossell-Perry with Dr. Jordan Swanson during Brazilian Cleft Palate Craniofacial meeting in Campinas, São Paulo, 2024

Foreword 2

The cleft lip and palate field has been close to my heart for the past 35 years. It has been my good fortune to have been trained and later to work together with outstanding and passionate surgeons for congenital defects.

The biological revolution of the past century has seeded a flowering biotechnology revolution in the twenty-first century. The main goal for people interested in craniofacial dysmorphogenesis has always been to create lasting treatment concepts based on a better understanding of the natural history of cleft lip and palate and facial growth.

Most of the time, new book readers look for knowledge acquisition, for references to previous books, for the author's personal thoughts, for treatment protocols, and, above all, for rapid synopsis via readable images. Indeed, these ingredients are all present in the *Atlas of Primary Cleft Rhinoplasty* and are well framed by repeated landmarks in a concise and descriptive text.

A single-author book is more pleasant to read chapter after chapter than one with many co-authors from whom personal thoughts, methods, planning, and results do not emerge. Therefore, an individual's remarkable progress toward analysis and understanding fosters approaches that can produce good functional and aesthetic results.

In the wide spectrum of cleft lip and palate disorders, the function (speech, breathing, swallowing) predominates over form. But whatever the function involves, form is always present and the obsession with form will persist.

In the past decades, surgery has been able to transform malformed faces into normal ones, but newer investigations, techniques, and tools have repeatedly improved results and the speed with which they are accomplished. Very illustrative examples of surgical technique evolution are widely represented in the pages of this excellent atlas.

Cleft lip and palate surgery can usually correct disordered faces with applications of experience and great surgical skill, both of which are apparent in these chapters.

Last but not least, one can not mention enough the fundamental life changes experienced by countless children whose lip and palate abnormalities have been treated in recent decades, and also it is important to mention the support and understanding of parents and family.

Miami, FL, USA August 2024

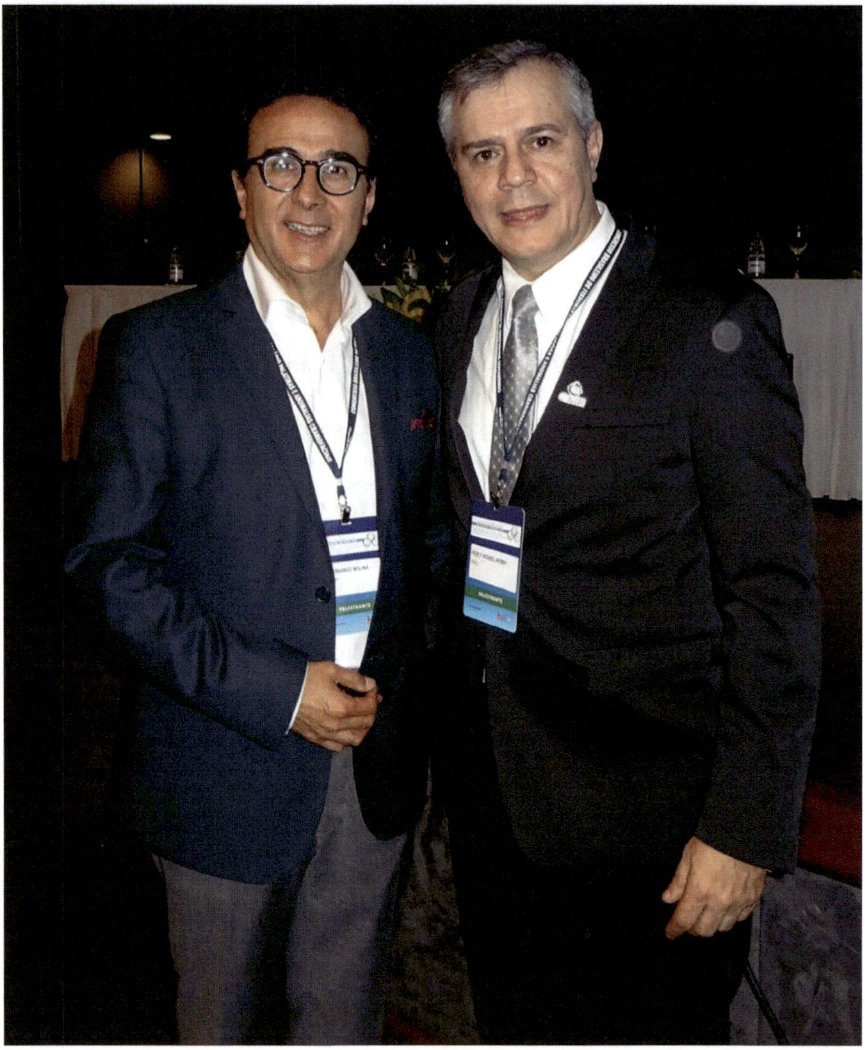

Fig. 2 Dr. Molina and Dr. Rossell-Perry during the Latin American Craniofacial Association meeting in São Paulo, Brazil, 2018

Preface

The *Atlas of Primary Cleft Rhinoplasty* is my ninth book and represents a lifetime dedicated to this field supported by close to 30 years of experience and more than 3000 operated patients.

This work is based on illustrative images of congenital nose deformity associated with the cleft lip and palate and its management is an educational tool for any resident or surgeon with interest in cleft surgery. Cleft nasal deformity is a complex challenge in plastic surgery involving the skin, cartilage, mucosa, and skeleton and the main limitation for primary cleft rhinoplasty is the repair of the soft tissues over a distorted skeleton.

Each patient requires functional and aesthetic evaluation in order to determine an individual plan for nasal reconstruction. A better understanding of the deformity has resulted in an increase in successful repair of these problems; therefore, proper strategies and interdisciplinary management must be considered to provide appropriate support for observing more consistent and satisfactory outcomes.

Surgical techniques for primary cleft lip nose repair have evolved over time. Personally, I have changed my surgical strategies during my professional practice, as cleft surgeon was more conservative during my first years. Mc Comb rhinoplasty was used initially; however, the rate of revision was greater and there was greater recurrence of nose deformity.

This is the reason why I changed the surgical strategies toward more aggressive methods with better aesthetic and functional outcomes. The rotational composite flap and the V-Y-Z rhinoplasties are good examples of this evolution. Their utility and efficacy have been evaluated and demonstrated through different scientific studies developed by the editor and published in high-impact indexed journals. High technology is also considered in the interdisciplinary management actually using 3D scan methods for pre- and postoperative treatment.

This book describes our work based on the experience of a group of experts in the management of primary cleft lip nose deformity in cleft lip and palate patients during the last 25 years.

I owe special thanks to William Carter M.D. for his lessons during my first years sharing surgical campaigns in Perú through ReSurge International (formerly Interplast).

Additionally, I am grateful for the life-changing experience I had during my visiting international scholarship at the Institute of Reconstructive Plastic Surgery of the New York University and University of California Los Angeles under the direction of Dr. Joseph Mc Carthy and Dr. Henry Kawamoto Jr., respectively.

Lima, Peru Percy Rossell-Perry

Contents

About the Author

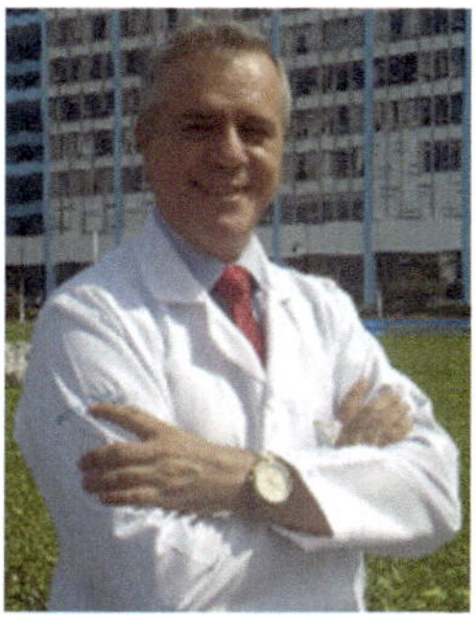

Born in Lima, Peru, he studied human medicine at San Marcos University of Lima, finishing in 1993; then, he performed a plastic surgery training at Kirschbaum Institute between 1993 and 1996 and Military Central Hospital between 1996 and 1999 supported by San Marcos University of Lima.

He was a Visitor Scholar in Craniofacial Surgery as the winner of the Plastic Surgery Education Foundation Scholarship in 2005 and visited Emory University from Atlanta in 2004, University of California Los Angeles (UCLA) in Los Angeles, and New York University in 2006 (Drs. Henry Kawamoto and Joseph Mc Carthy visited professors).

In 2011, he obtained a Master's Degree in Teaching University and a Doctorate (Ph.D.) in Human Medicine from San Marcos University of Lima in 2014. He also has a Diploma Course in Clinical Research from Harvard University, USA, in 2015.

His teaching experience began in 1987 in the Department of Human Anatomy of the School of Human Medicine at the University of San Marcos until the year 2000. Later, he taught specialty courses at the Universities of San Marcos, Cayetano Heredia, and through the Peruvian Society of Plastic Surgery. Currently, he is research professor at the Health of Science Faculty, School of Human Medicine, Peruvian University Union (UpeU), and Professor of Postgraduate Studies at the Faculty of Human Medicine, University of San Martin de Porres (USMP), Lima, Peru.

Although he is involved in many aspects of plastic surgery, his main activity is now centered on cleft lip and palate surgery.

Since 2016, Dr. Percy Rossell-Perry has been a plastic surgeon assistant at the Edgardo Rebagliati Martins National Hospital of ESSALUD, where he had performed pediatric reconstructive plastic surgery until December 2021. In addition, he was a consultant Plastic Surgeon at the Casimiro Ulloa Hospital (2004–2008), Cayetano Heredia National Hospital (2009), and other Hospitals of Lima, Peru, such as San Bartolome Hospital, Navy Hospital, and Alberto Sabogal, Edgardo Rebagliati, and Guillermo Almenara Hospitals of ESSALUD (Social Security System).

During his professional career, Dr. Percy Rossell-Perry has been awarded many times. In 2002, he was awarded with the KAELIN National Award for scientific research from ESSALUD. Later, he received the Humanitarian Award from the Interplast Foundation of the United States in 2003 and then in 2005 he won the Plastic Surgery Educational Foundation Scholarship granted by the Pierr Foundation of the United States.

In 2010, 2013, and 2019, he received the Hipólito Unanue National Award for the Best Scientific Edition for the following books: *Treatment of the Cleft Lip and Palate*, *Basic Management of Chronic Cutaneous Lesions Based on Scientific Evidence*, and *Bad Results and Complications in Cleft Lip and Palate Surgery*.

He has written many books and scientific articles. Dr. Percy Rossell-Perry is the main author of the following books: *Cleft Lip and Palate Treatment* (2009), *Unilateral Cleft Lip Surgery* (2011), *Basic Management of Chronic Cutaneous Lesions Based on Scientific Evidence* (2012), *Bilateral Cleft Lip Surgery* (2013), *Cleft Palate Surgery* (2015), *Bad Results and Complications in Cleft Lip and Palate Surgery* (2018), *Atlas of Operative Techniques in Primary Cleft Lip and Palate Repair* (2020), and *Atlas of Non-desirable Outcomes in Cleft Lip and Palate Surgery* (2022). The last textbook has been translated to the German language by Springer Ed.

He has also edited author's chapters of "Principles of Cleft Palate Repair" in *Global Cleft Care in Low-Resource Settings* (Editors: David Low and Jordan Swanson) and "Mucoperiosteal Necrosis After Palatoplasty" and "One Flap Palatoplasty" in *Surgical Atlas of Cleft Palate and Palatal Fistulae* textbook (Editor: Ghulam Fayyaz).

Since 2006 he has authored more than 50 scientific articles published in indexed journals and has received more than 700 citations.

He is on the editorial board of the *Journal of Craniofacial Surgery* and was an editorial board member of the *Plastic Reconstructive Surgery GO Journal* from 2015 to 2023, as well as a reviewer of the most important plastic surgery journals of the world (such as the *Plastic Reconstructive Surgery Journal*, *Aesthetic Plastic Surgery Journal*, *Journal of Plastic Surgery and Hand Surgery*, and *Journal of Craniofacial Surgery*).

He is a well-known international lecturer in his experience in countries such as Chile, Brazil, Mexico, Colombia, Bolivia, the United States, Egypt, and Poland and was elected as a member of the Scientific Committee of the IX and X International Cleft Lip and Palate Foundation Congress (CLEFT 2009 in Brazil) and in 2013 in the USA). Likewise, he is the chair of the Symposium "Cleft Surgery in Developing Countries" during CLEFT 2013 in the Orlando USA and member of the Task Force for the CLEFT 2022 in Edinburgh.

He is a Fellow of American College of Surgeons (FACS) and was an international member of the American Society of Plastic Surgery until 2023.

Dr. Percy Rossell-Perry was president of the Latin American Craniofacial Association (LATICFA) during the 2018–2020 period, and, actually, he is the president of the Smile Train South American Medical Advisory Council (SAMAC) and member of the Smile Train Global Research and Innovation Advisory Council (STRIAC).

Finally, recently he has been elected as a member of the Cleft Lip and Palate Chapter of the Ibero Latin American Plastic Surgery Federation (FILACP) and member of the Craniofacial Cleft Lip and Palate Chapter of the International Confederation of Plastic Surgery Societies (ICOPLAST).

Contributors

Juan Pablo Gomez Arango Department of Biomechanics, University of Manizales Colombia, Pereira, Colombia

Martha Mejia Department of Plastic Surgery, Nicklaus Children's Hospital, Miami, FL, USA

Percy Rossell-Perry Health of Science Faculty, School of Human Medicine, Peruvian University Union (UpeU), Lima, Peru

Anatomy and Physiology

1

Percy Rossell-Perry

Contents

Introduction

The nose is a complex structure that plays a significant role in facial appearance and function.

Between the sixth and ninth weeks, the upper lip and nose form from the maxillary, medial, and lateral nasal prominences at the rostral and lateral boundaries of the primitive oral cavity (Fig. 1.1).

Failure to merge between the nasal and maxillary processes on one or both sides results in cleft lip and occurs at the junction between the central and lateral segments of the upper lip.

P. Rossell-Perry (✉)
Health of Science Faculty, School of Human Medicine, Peruvian University Union (UpeU), Lima, Peru
e-mail: percy.rossell@upeu.edu.pe

P. Rossell-Perry (ed.), *Atlas of Primary Cleft Rhinoplasty*,
https://doi.org/10.1007/978-3-031-68012-0_1

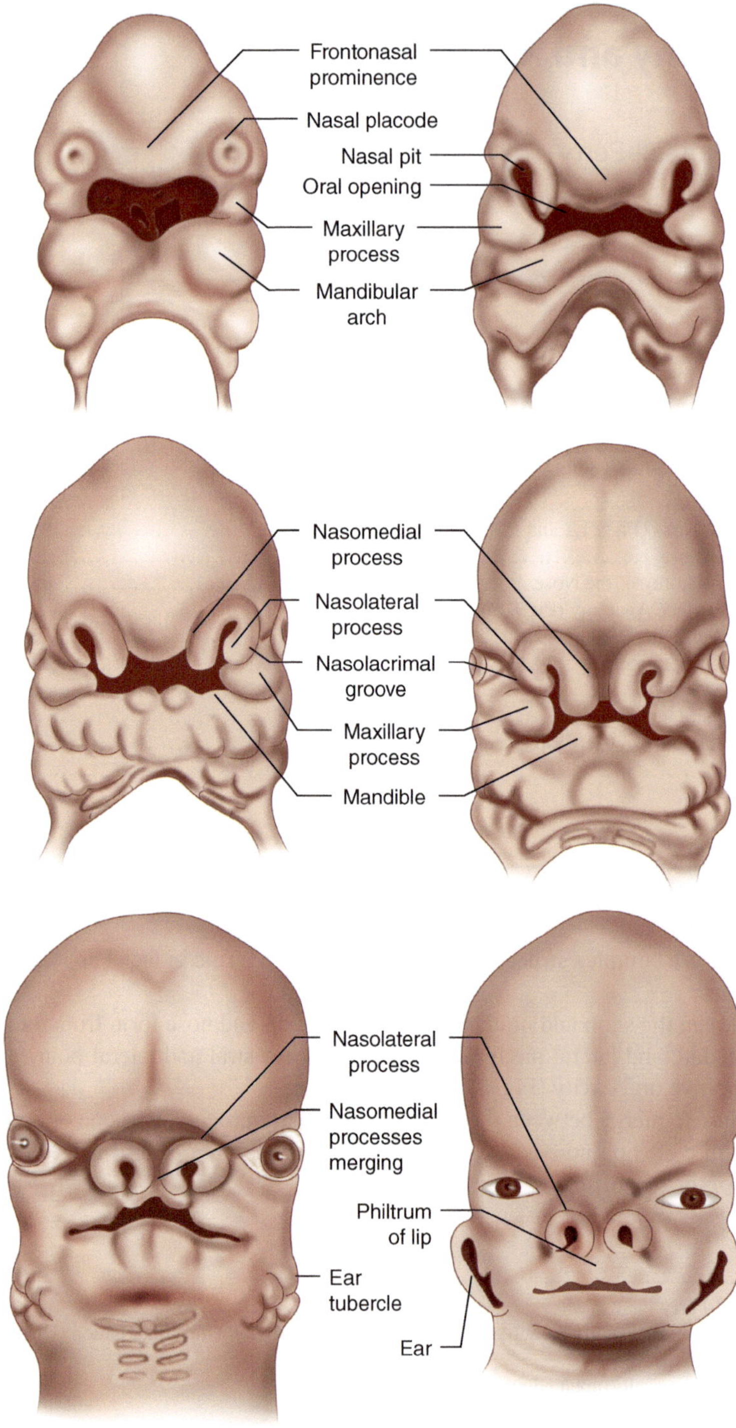

Fig. 1.1 Upper lip and nose embryology

Knowledge of the embryology, anatomy, and physiology of the nose is essential for understanding the characteristics of congenital anomalies in cleft noses.

To understand anatomical complexity, two parts are considered: external and internal.

External Nose (Figs. 1.2 and 1.3)

The external nose can be divided into three sections: upper, middle, and lower.

The external nose is entirely covered by skin with differences in location. The skin of the dorsum, columella, and sidewalls is thin and less sebaceous while the skin of the nasal tip and alae is thicker and more sebaceous and less flexible.

The skin of the upper third is thick but tapers into a thinner middle third being the dorsal skin the thinnest section. Both of them are more flexible. The lower third is thicker and has the more sebaceous skin in the nasal tip.

It is important to consider that ethnic variations in nasal skin exist. It is so Asian noses have thicker skin and more subcutaneous tissue than Caucasians.

An interesting study made by Eggerstedt et al. [1] revealed that the nasal skin and soft tissue envelope are thicker at the sellion in Latin American and Caucasian noses than in African and Asian noses. In addition, the supratip skin is thicker in African noses than in other races and the nasal tip skin was thinner in Caucasian noses.

Nasal skin thickness may influence surgical planning and postoperative outcomes.

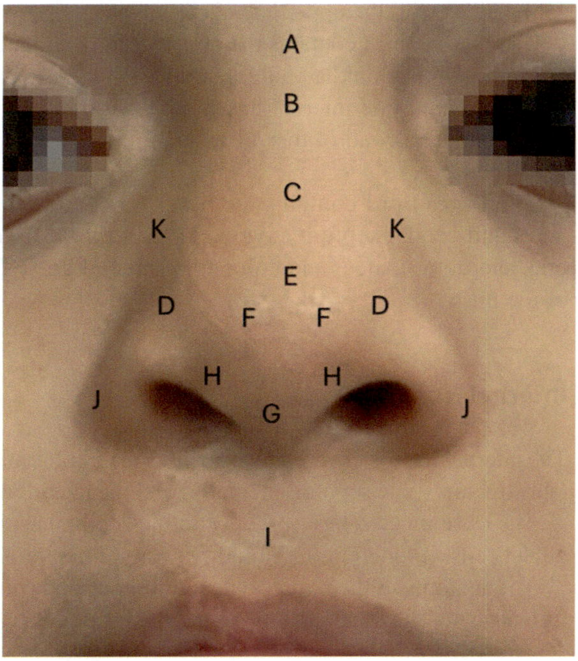

Fig. 1.2 Repaired unilateral cleft lip external nose anatomy (frontal view). A. Root. B. Bridge. C. Rinion D. Supraalar crease E. Supratip. F. Tip definition point. G. Columella. H. Soft triangle. I. Philtrum. J. Alar nasal sulcus. K. Nasofacial angle

Fig. 1.3 External nose anatomy (skeletal support)

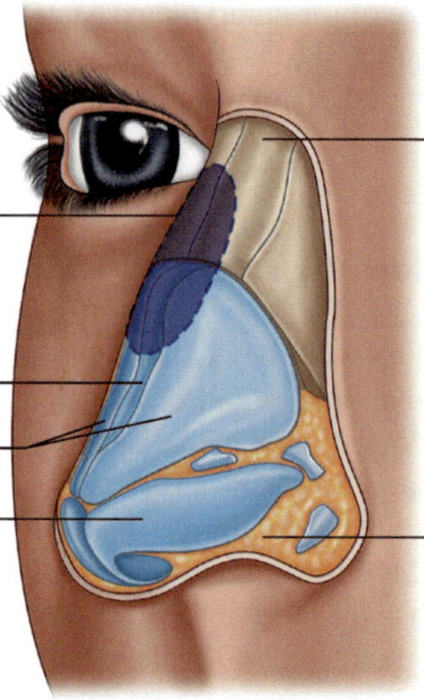

For example, any cartilaginous structure deficiency after primary nose repair may be more evident in Caucasian nose than other races because of the nature of the nasal tip skin.

Regarding the skeletal structure, the upper third of the nose is composed of the nasal bones. This rectangular structure limits with superolaterally to the lacrimal bone and inferolaterally to the nasomaxillary process of the maxilla. Its lower border overlaps with the upper lateral cartilages.

The middle third contains the upper lateral cartilages of the nose also known as the cartilaginous middle vault area. Medially, these cartilages fuse with the nasal septum creating the internal nasal valve, an important functional structure of the nose. The lateral wall of this area is composed of the lower turbinate and the pyriform aperture.

The lower third contains the nasal tip composed by the lower lateral cartilages and caudal septum covered by soft tissues to create the nasal tip (lateral crus and dome), alae, and columella (medial crus). This is the nasal valve area of the nose.

Internal Nose

The internal nose is covered by a mucous membrane and is composed of two important structures: the septum (medially) and the lateral wall (Figs. 1.4 and 1.5).

The nasal mucosa has a pseudostratified columnar ciliated epithelium and mucus goblet cells. It functions to humidify, warm, filter, protect, and eliminate debris.

The anatomy of the nasal cavity allows time and enough surface area through the turbinates for the inhaled air to be warmed and moistened.

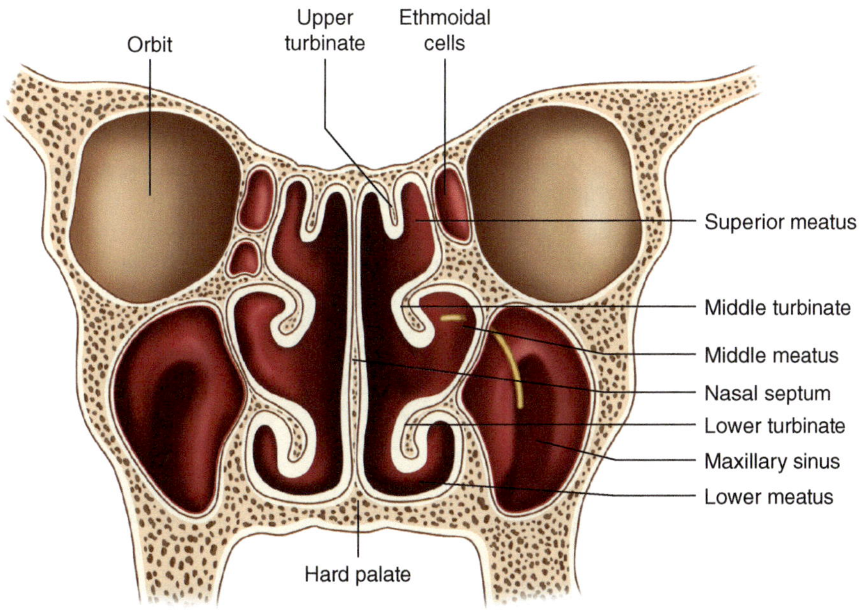

Fig. 1.4 Internal nose anatomy diagram

The nasal septum is usually located at the midline and is made of cartilage anteriorly and bone posteriorly (Figs. 1.4 and 1.5).

The anterior segment of the septum is known as the caudal septum and has a membranous portion caudal to the columella. This section is part of the nasal valve.

The posterior segment is composed mostly of the vomer, palatine bones, and the ethmoid bone (Fig. 1.5).

The nasal septum commonly deviates in individuals with unilateral cleft lip and palate resulting in variable degrees of nasal obstruction. It tends to deviate toward the cleft side with the septal base displaced off the maxillary crest (Fig. 1.6).

Early septal repositioning during primary cleft lip repair may improve aesthetic and functional nasal outcomes.

The lateral wall includes the turbinates (upper, lower, and middle) which are in communication with the meatus for nasal sinus and lacrimal drainage.

These structures are four pairs of air-filled cavities responsible for humidifying and warming inspired air (Fig. 1.4).

The meatuses are three spaces beneath each of the turbinates. The upper one drains for the sphenoid and posterior ethmoid sinuses, and the middle meatus drains for the frontal, anterior ethmoid and maxillary sinuses. Finally, the lower drain was through the nasolacrimal duct (Fig. 1.4).

The triangular shape of the nose is completed by the nasal floor which is composed by four segments: vestibular (nasal sill), primary palate (alveolus), secondary palate (hard palate), and soft palate (functional floor) (Fig. 1.7).

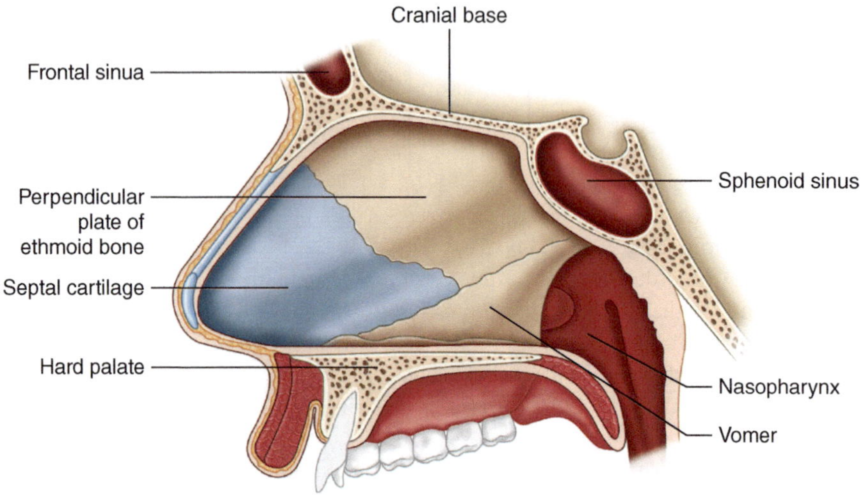

Fig. 1.5 Nasal septum diagram

Fig. 1.6 Nasal septum deviation in unilateral cleft lip patients observed during secondary cleft rhinoplasty. 1. Cleft side alar cartilage. 2. Noncleft side alar cartilage 3. Nasal septum

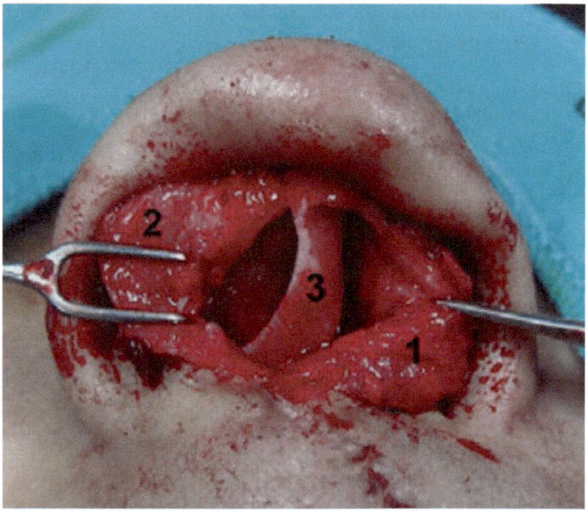

Different protocols have been developed to correct the nasal floor during cleft lip and palate repair. The Oslo protocol repairs the vestibular and vestibular nasal floor during the lip and hard palate repair while other protocols repair the primary palate segment during the mixed dentition period.

Functionally, these structures create two valves: external and internal (Fig. 1.8).

The external nasal valve is composed of the columella (medially), nasal sill (inferiorly), and nasal rim (superiorly) including the alar cartilages and nasal ala.

The internal nasal valve is limited by the septum (medially), laterally to the upper lateral cartilage and inferiorly to the head of the lower turbinate.

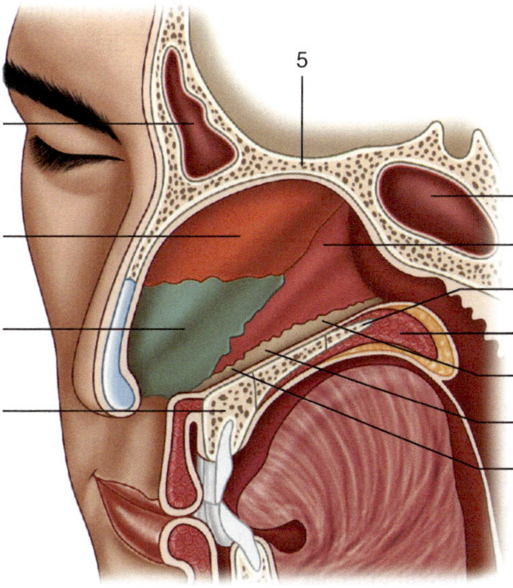

Fig. 1.7 Anatomy of the floor of the nose

Fig. 1.8 External and internal nasal valves

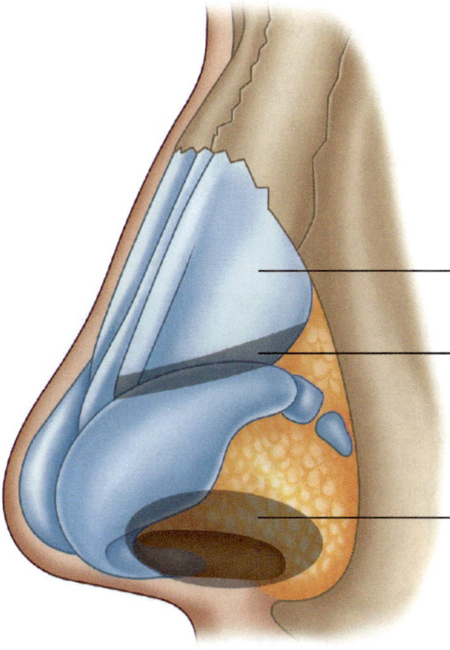

Finally, two opening structures (nares) exist, the external (anterior) structures are the nostrils, and the internal (posterior) structures are the choanae, the opening from the nasal cavity to the pharynx.

Surgical Anatomy of the Nose

The bases of nasal anatomy are presented here.

Nasal Surface Anatomy (Fig. 1.9)

The surface anatomy (or visual anatomy) includes the external features of the nose; its knowledge enables the surgeons to locate anatomical structures exteriorly, improving their clinical and surgical skills. It includes the root (superiorly), apex (inferiorly), dorsum, nostrils, and columella. A good description of the external anatomy is required using correct terminology to assist in the diagnosis and facilitate the selection of surgical options.

The following terms used for describing the surface anatomy of the nose are used:

Root: It is defined as the top of the nose and is limited to the forehead. It is above the nasal bridge and below the glabella. The depressed midpoint between them is the nasion at the point where the frontal bone meets the nasal bones.

Nasal bridge: It is also known as the nasal dorsum. This is an area that includes the nasal root and lateral borders of the nose, extending laterally to the inner canthi. It limits inferiorly to the nasal tip. The upper half of the dorsum is made of nasal bones, and the lower half of the dorsum is made of nasal cartilages. The most inferior portion of the nasal dorsum, which is limited by the nasal tip, is known as the supratip area.

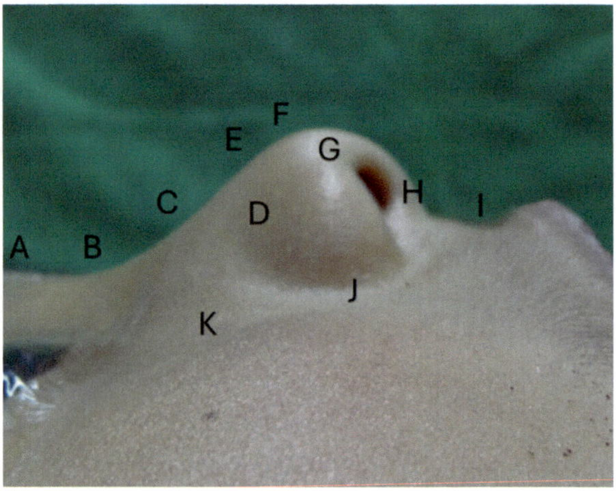

Fig. 1.9 Surface anatomy of the nose (lateral view). A. Root. B. Bridge. C. Rinion D. Supraalar crease E. Supratip. F. Tip definition point. G. Soft triangle. H. Columella. I. Philtrum. J. Alar nasal sulcus. K. Nasofacial angle

Nasal tip: This is the most prominent area of the nose and represents the medial cephalic portion (domes) of the alar cartilage.

Nasal lobule: It is an area limited by a line connecting the upper edge of the nostrils, the supratip, and the lateral alar wall. This area is subdivided into the tip, supratip, and infratip.

Ala: It is also known as the wings of the nostrils. The nasal tissue lateral to the nasal tip represents the lateral boundary of the nose and inferiorly surrounds the nostrils.

Alar lobule: It is composed of vascular fibroareolar tissue, muscle, and fat. They are the most lateral components of the nasal base. The muscular composition of the alar lobule comprises the alar portion of the nasalis, running posterior to anterior while the dilator naris anterior muscle runs cephalic to caudal.

Alar base: It represents the bottom parts of the ala and limits medially with the nasal sill [2].

Alar rim: It represents the roof of the nostrils. They surround the nostril aperture [3].

Columella: It is a bridge of tissue located between the nostril and linking the nasal tip with the upper lip. It represents the fleshy external end of the caudal septum.

Nostrils or external nares: They are a pair of openings at the end of the nose leading from the nasal cavity to the outside.

Nasal sill: The nasal sill is a protuberant soft tissue bridge, extending from columellar base to the ala of the nose and limiting inferiorly to the upper lip.

Soft triangle: It is named as "soft" triangle because of the lack of cartilage and subcutaneous tissue support. It is located between the dome and the alar lobule. It is a triangular thin skin located lateral to the tip of the nose and above the nostrils. They can be visually identified in subjects with thin skin [4].

Nasolabial angle: It denotes the angle between the columella and the upper lip. The angle between the line drawn through the midpoint of the nostril and the line drawn perpendicular to the Frankfurt line while intersecting the subnasale point is also considered.

Alar groove: It is the depression observed between the nostril and lateral nasal wall. It lies at the junction of the lower lateral crus and the alar lobule and represents a curved line that extends from the nasal tip and joins the alar facial sulcus. The groove is produced by muscular attachment between the perichondrium of the lower lateral cartilage and the vestibular mucosa as a result of bulging in the fatty layer on one side of the groove [3]. The alar groove is also known as the alar crease or alar sulcus.

Alar facial sulcus: It is also referred as alar facial groove. This depression represents a junctional area of the nasal base, the medial aspect of the cheek and the upper lip.

Nasal Aesthetic Subunits

The facial aesthetic subunit is a concept that organizes the facial skin into units that are classified by their color, texture, and thickness. There are six facial aesthetic subunits: forehead, nose, eyelids, cheeks, upper and lower lips, and scalp and ears [5]. Each one includes its respective subunits; thus, the nose has the following subunits: tip, dorsum, sidewalls, alar lobules, soft triangles, and columella (Fig. 1.10).

Tip lobule: It is located between the junction of the inferior border of the nasal dorsum superiorly and the columella inferiorly.

Nasal dorsum: This is limited by the nasal roof superiorly and the nasal tip inferiorly. Laterally it is in continuity with the nasal sidewalls.

Alar lobules: They are the sidewalls of the nasal base. It is outlined by the alar groove beginning at the nostril rim and then continues in a circular shape down to the alar crease. It is composed of subcutaneous tissue and muscles [2].

Soft triangle: Or facet, located at the apex of the nostril and limited superiorly by the medial and lateral crus of the alar cartilage and inferiorly by the nostril. It was first described by Converse and is also referred as the "Bermuda triangle of the nose" [5]. Since there is no cartilage support for the soft triangles, notching is a common complication following primary cleft rhinoplasty. The soft triangle is considered one of the most challenging nasal subunits to reconstruct, and it is extremely vulnerable [6].

Columella: It is limited by the nasal tip superiorly and nasolabial angle inferiorly.

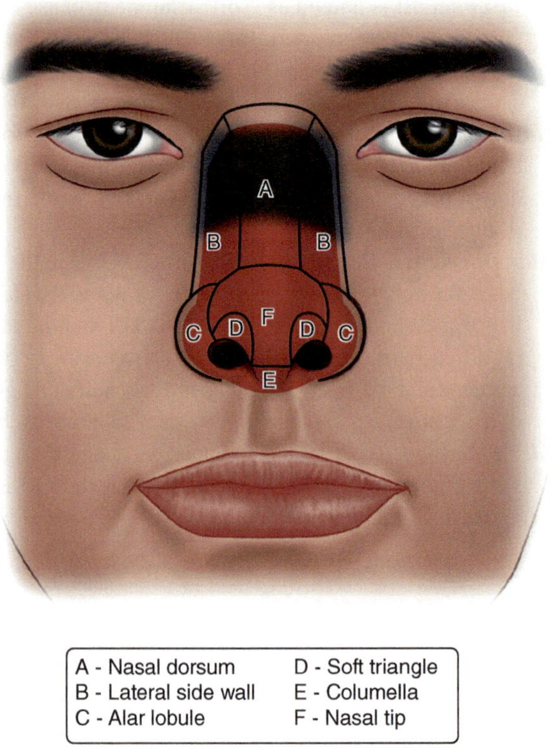

Fig. 1.10 Aesthetic nasal subunits of the nose

Nasal Components

The Nasal Tip

The nasal tip is defined as the most projecting part of the nose and located in its lower third. It is composed of the following structures:

Cartilaginous Framework (Figs. 1.11 and 1.12)

It is represented by the alar cartilages (lower lateral cartilages) and the caudal septum. Each alar cartilage has three segments: lateral crura, medial crura, and the intermediate (dome). The structural support works in combination with ligamentous structures including intercartilaginous ligaments between the upper and lower lateral cartilages, ligaments between the medial crura and the caudal septum through the membranous septum, attachments between both medial cruras, interdomal ligaments, and finally ligaments from the skin to the nasal domes [7] (Fig. 1.13).

The paired cartilages support the nasal tip as a tripod, and both medial cruras are the components of the nasal columella which together with the septum make up the support the nasal tip.

The dome (intermediate crura) provides the projection and definition to the nasal tip. There is approximately 60° of divergence between the two domes, and the point of projection of the nose is located within at the intermediate and lateral crus junction. The area between the domes is known as the supratip area or the weak triangle of Converse [8] (Fig. 1.14).

The lateral crura provides lateral support to the nasal tip, and its affection may cause aesthetic (pinched nose) and functional (airway obstruction) disorders [9].

The alar cartilage (lateral crura) is attached to the upper lateral cartilage through fibrous ligaments, and its most lateral border is attached to small sesamoid cartilages and fibrofatty tissue extending to the pyriform aperture.

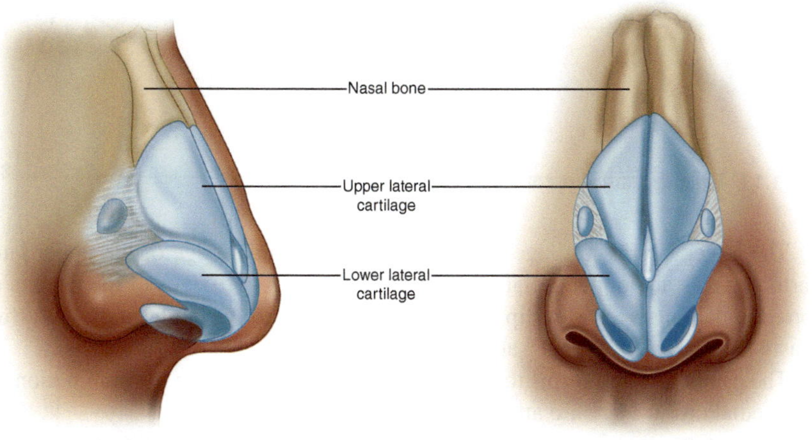

Fig. 1.11 Cartilaginous framework of the nose diagram

Fig. 1.12 Lower lateral cartilage anatomy diagram

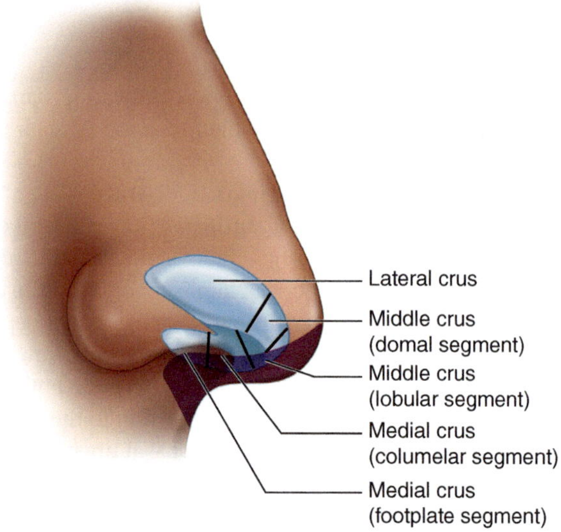

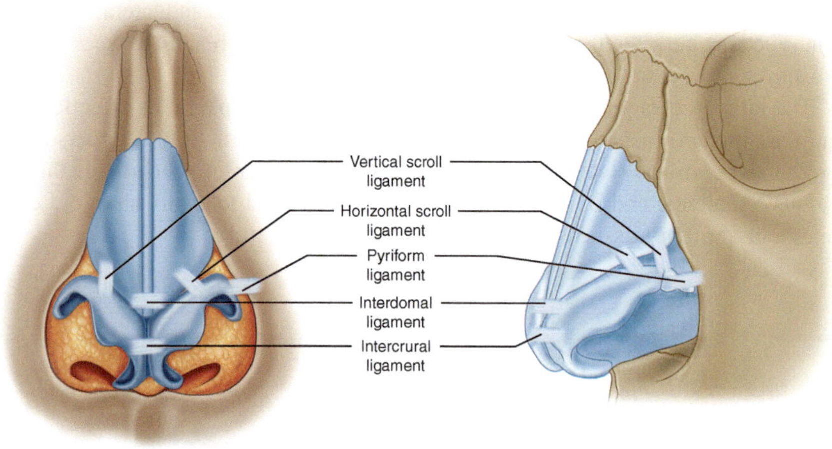

Fig. 1.13 Ligament structures of the nose diagram

The lower lateral cartilage is curving over the caudal edge of the upper lateral cartilage; this anatomical relation between the lateral cartilages of the nose is distorted in patients with cleft lip and should be corrected during primary cleft rhinoplasty (Figs. 1.15, 1.16, 1.17 and 1.18).

The caudal septum forms the central support of the nasal tip in combination with the medial crura. They are attached through ligaments.

Most of its anterior section is membranous, composed by fibrous tissue and located between the caudal end of the cartilaginous septum (anterior septal angle) and the medial crura. There is a muscular component in this area, the depressor septi

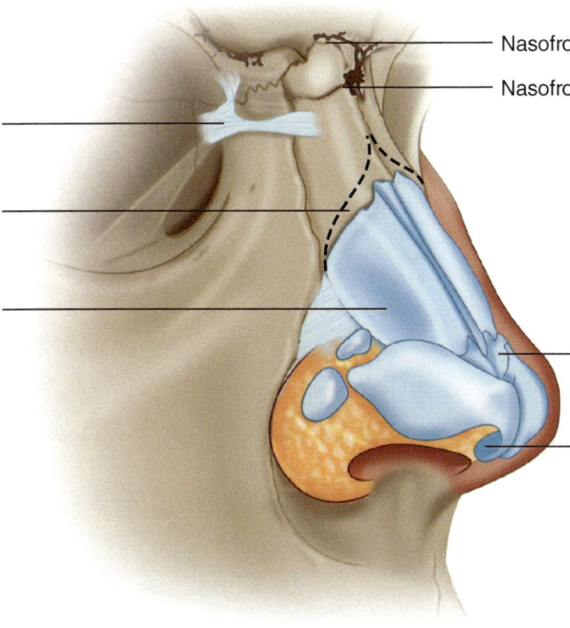

Fig. 1.14 Supratip area of the nose diagram (weak triangle of converse)

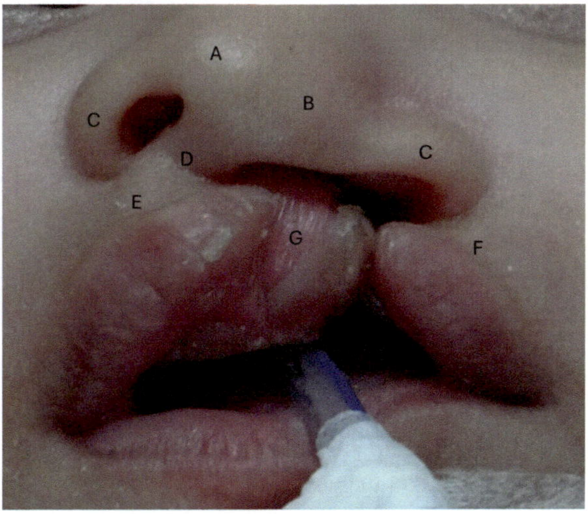

Fig. 1.15 Lower lateral cartilage displacement in unilateral cleft lip patient. A. Alar cartilage noncleft side. B. Alar cartilage cleft side. C. Alae. D. Columella E. Medial lip segment. F. Lateral lip segment. G. Premaxilla

nasi [10]. The caudal septum is also attached to the nasal spine at the posterior septal angle.

Overlaying soft tissues: The soft tissue components include skin, muscles, nerves, and vascular tissues. Depending on the thickness of the soft tissues, they may have stronger tip support than the cartilaginous structure. The thickness of the

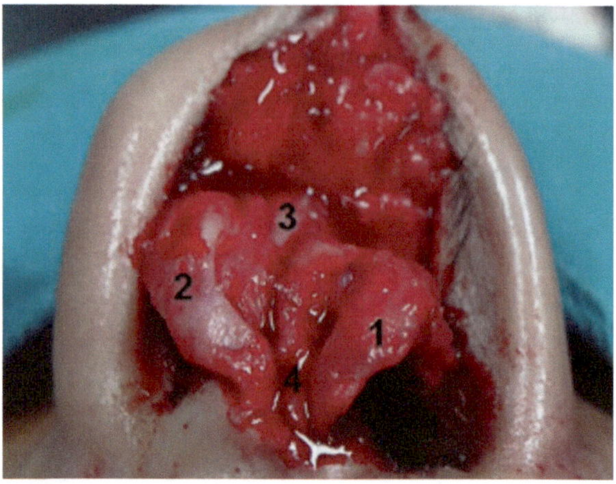

Fig. 1.16 Intraoperative view of nasal cartilages during primary unilateral cleft rhinoplasty. 1. Alar cartilage (cleft side). 2. Alar cartilage (noncleft side). 3. Dorsum. 4. Septum

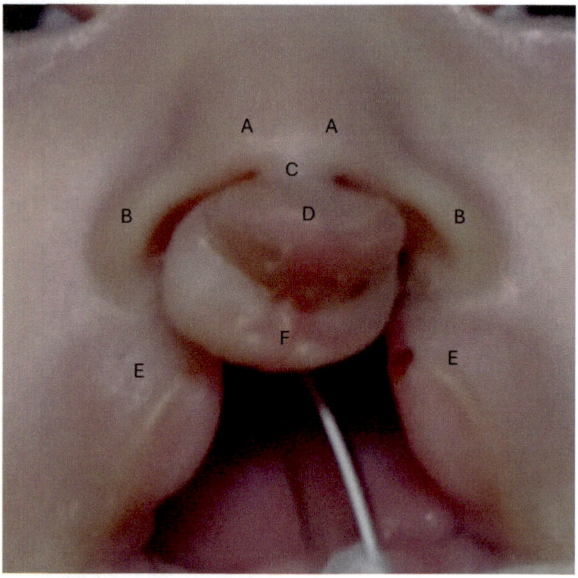

Fig. 1.17 Lower lateral cartilage displacement in bilateral cleft lip patient. A. Alar cartilages. B. Alae C. Columella. D. Prolabium E. Lateral lip segment. F. Premaxilla

nasal tip skin may also affect the outcome after primary cleft rhinoplasty and should be considered during surgical planning. The soft tissue characteristics of each subunit of the nasal tip are different, for example, the skin of the alar lobule forms a semirigid unit that maintains the graceful curve of the alar rim.

The Nasal Columella

The nasal columella is defined as the most anterior portion of the nasal septum and located between the two nostrils linking the nasal tip to the nasal base. It is a single midline structure composed of cartilage and skin and includes six components: the caudal septum, medial crura, columellar skin, membranous septum, anterior nasal spine, and depressor septi nasi muscle (Fig. 1.19).

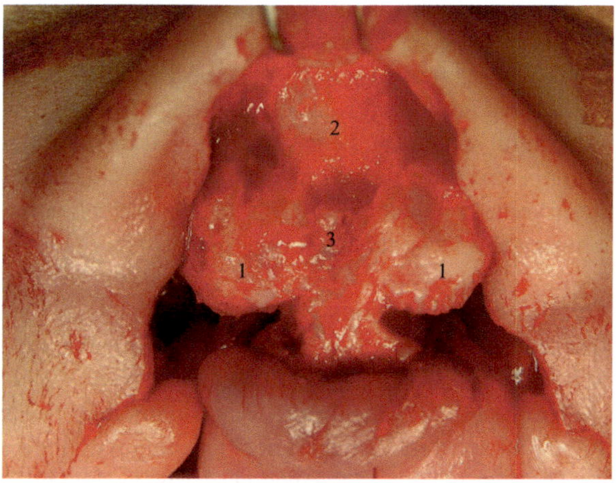

Fig. 1.18 Intraoperative view of nasal cartilages during primary bilateral cleft rhinoplasty. 1. Alar cartilages. 2. Dorsum. 3. Septum

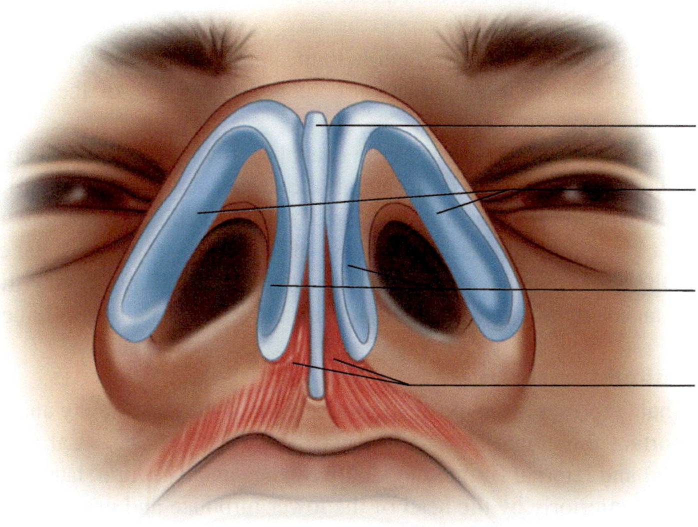

Fig. 1.19 Nasal columella structural framework diagram

This structure in combination with the caudal septum provides support and projection to the nasal tip playing a functional role in nostril patency and breathing.

The nasal columella is composed of the following main structures:

Cartilaginous Framework

It is represented by the medial crus of the alar cartilage and the caudal septum. Structural support works in combination with ligamentous structures between the medial crura and caudal septum through the membranous septum and attachments between both medial crura and caudal septum.

The medial crus is the inner portion of the alar cartilage and is situated perpendicularly to the septal nasal cartilage. The lower segment, 5 mm in length, courses laterally and often posteriorly and is called the footplate.

The caudal septum is attached through ligaments with the medial crura forming the central support of the nasal columella. Its most anterior section is membranous.

This structural support of the nasal tip frequently deviates and displaces off the nasal spine in unilateral cleft lips, and its correction is an essential component of the primary and secondary cleft rhinoplasty.

Overlaying Soft Tissues

The soft tissue components of the nasal columella include the skin, muscles, nerves, and vascular tissues.

The skin of the lateral side of the columella is fixed, thinner, less sebaceous, and tightly attached to medial crura connecting with the vestibular skin internally.

The anterior side of the medial crus is covered by mobile skin and subcutaneous tissue. There is an important muscular component in this area: the depressor septi nasi. This muscle is located between the caudal end of the cartilaginous septum and the medial crura.

It connects the incisive fossa of the maxilla to the nasal septum of the nose. This muscle draws the ala of the nose downward, reducing the size of the nostrils (Fig. 1.19).

The columella follows the direction of the caudal septum and explains its position in patient with unilateral cleft lip in whom the columella deviates toward the cleft side. Another important application is related to the bilateral cleft lips in which the columella is hidden into the nasal tip because of the malposition of the alar cartilages; in fact, the columella is not short and is only displaced. Reposition of these structures using an adequate surgical technique may allow us to repair the columella.

The Nasal Vestibule

The nasal vestibule represents the most anterior section of the nasal cavity and represents an important functional area. It is located between the two nasal valves: external (nostrils) and internal (limited medially by the caudal septum, laterally by the limen nasi and inferiorly by the head of the lower turbinate and nasal sill) [11] (Fig. 1.20).

The nasal vestibule is the narrowest portion of the nasal cavities, and any alteration that reduces the lumen (such as scar contractures) is bound to have a great impact on airflow. It is a specialized respiratory organ limited laterally by the ala, medially by the caudal septum and columella, and superiorly by the limen nasi (or limen vestibuli), and its inferior limitation is the nostril.

The area of the internal nasal valve should be preserved during primary cleft rhinoplasty in order to prevent functional disorders.

The limen nasi is an important structure of the nasal vestibule and represents the junction between the upper and lower lateral cartilages (scroll region). It is the place where the intercartilaginous incision is made to access the nasal dorsum and also performed during the rotational composite flap and VYZ techniques of primary cleft

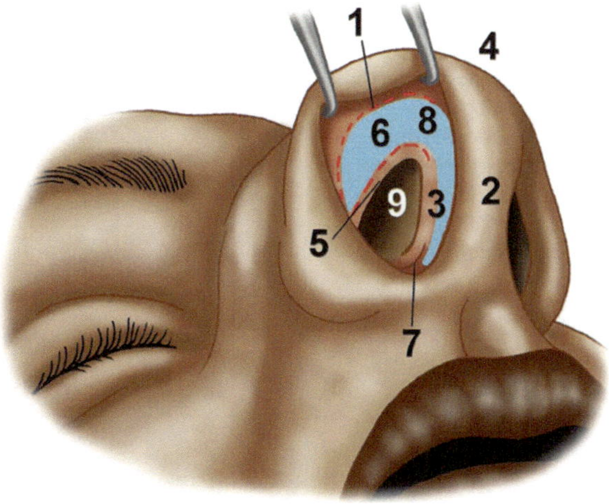

Fig. 1.20 The vestibule of the nose diagram. 1. Alar margin. 2. Nasal columella. 3. Caudal septum. 4. Nasal tip. 5. Intercartilaginous border. 6. Alar cartilage (sky blue area). 7. Nostril sill. 8. Internal nasal valve angle. 9. Nostril

rhinoplasty. This structure separates the vestibule from the nasal cavity and represents the change from the vestibular skin to the respiratory epithelium of the nasal cavity.

This area between the upper lateral and lower lateral cartilages is a cul-de-sac, known as the infundibulum or diverticulum. It has a distortion in cleft lip patients and requires reposition of the lower cartilage over the upper cartilage (mucocutaneous junction). The nasal vestibule is enclosed by the nasal cartilages and lined by skin (hair-bearing, sebaceous, and sweat glands) until reaching the marginal line (caudal border of the lower lateral cartilage). This is a keratinized stratified squamous epithelium.

Above the marginal line until the limen nasi, the lower lateral cartilage is covered by a transitional epithelium which is a thinning of the stratified epithelium. The difference between these two linings is easily identified because they have different colors.

Below the marginal border (caudal border of lower lateral cartilage), the color is the same as the color of the skin of the face and above the marginal border until the limen nasi the area is reddish because of the transition of the epithelium (Fig. 1.21).

This anatomical reference is very important to locate the place of marginal incision used for the nasal approach during rhinoplasty and the surgical techniques used for primary cleft rhinoplasty used by the author.

Due to functional nature, the nasal vestibule area is severely affected by scar contractures and synechia which can cause breathing disorders.

Recurrence of the nasal deformity after primary cleft rhinoplasty may be explained by scar contracture of the nasal vestibule lining and support the success of the surgical techniques based on vestibular lengthening, such as Potter.

The author developed a vestibular lengthening method using a combination of V-Y advancement flap (Potter) with a lateral Z plasty (Berkeley) in a similar form as the presurgical orthopedic (NAM) that temporarily expands the nasal vestibule and named it as "the surgical nasoalveolar molding" [12–14].

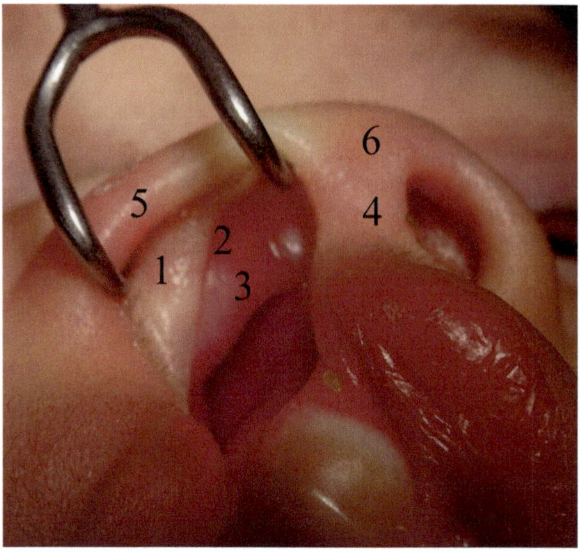

Fig. 1.21 Characteristics of the nasal vestibule, marginal, and intercartilaginous borders. 1. Nasal vestibule 2. Marginal border 3. Area below the marginal border that covers the alar cartilage. 4. Columella. 5. Alae. 6. Nasal tip

The development of scars in this functional area may increase the risk of scar contractures; therefore, postoperative use of nasal conformers is mandatory for at least 6 months.

The Nasal Septum

This bony and cartilaginous structure is covered by nasal mucosa located in the midline separating the right and left nostrils, extending from the nares to the choanae.

It provides support to the columella, nasal tip, vault, and mucosa influencing nasal airflow.

Bony-Cartilaginous Framework (Fig. 1.22)

The framework of the nasal septum is composed of four parts: septal cartilage, perpendicular plate of the ethmoid bone, vomer, and maxillary crest. Minor contributions are made by palatine, nasal, and frontal bones [15].

The septal cartilage ("quadrangular cartilage") is a hyaline type and articulated with bones and cartilaginous structures of the nose, posteriorly with the perpendicular plate of the ethmoid bone (posterosuperiorly) and the vomer (posteroinferiorly).

Its inferior margin joins the nasal crest and the anterior nasal spine of the maxilla. The maxillary crest has a maxilla component (anteriorly) and a palatal component (posteriorly). The anterosuperior border of the septal cartilage is articulated with the two triangular upper lateral cartilages. This articulation forms an angle between 10° and 15° which represents anteriorly the angle of the internal nasal valve, an important functional structure of the nose [16].

The anterior portion of the caudal septum articulates with the nasal columella through the membranous septum.

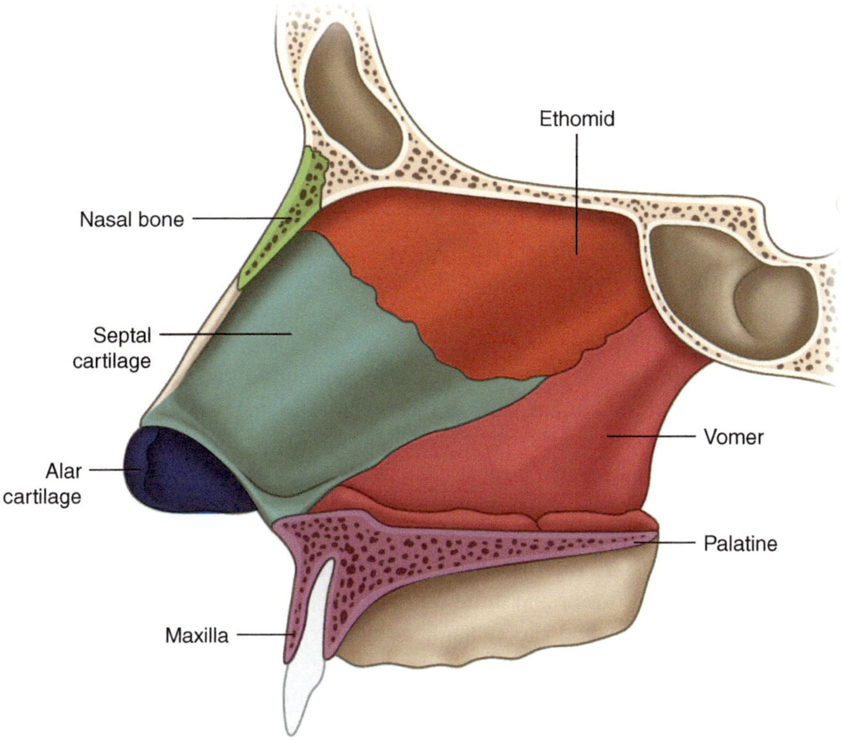

Fig. 1.22 The nasal septum bony cartilaginous framework diagram

The area between the nasal bone, septal cartilage, bony septum, and upper lateral cartilages which is firmly connected by fibrous tissue is the keystone area, a critical zone for maintaining the stability of the nasal dorsum.

The vomer is an unpaired bone located in the midline and articulated with the septal cartilage, maxilla, palatine, ethmoid, and sphenoid bones. It has an important relation with the premaxilla. This bone is also known as incisive or intermaxillary bone (Goethe's bone because of his description in 1784) and represents the primary palate [17].

The junction between the vomer and premaxilla (vomero-premaxillary suture) is an important facial growth site, and the surgical procedures involving this area were found to inhibit of maxillary growth. This area should be preserved, especially during premaxilla setback procedures [17].

Overlying Mucosa

The nasal septum is covered with a mucosal layer that warms air passing through the nasal cavity.

Nasal septum deviation is a common disorder observed in unilateral cleft lip and palate and affects the nasal physiology reducing the airflow and causing congestion and difficulty breathing in these patients. This structure often shows convexity toward the cleft side, and the direction of the deviation is toward the noncleft side. The nasal columella follows the deviation of the caudal septum portion.

Surgical correction of its caudal portion is performed during the primary cleft rhinoplasty.

Internal Lateral Wall

The lateral wall of the nasal cavity is composed of curved shelves of bone known as the turbinates. They are a fingerlike and project into the nasal cavity creating pathways for the air to flow called meatus. There are three pairs of turbinates and four pairs of meatuses (Figs. 1.4 and 1.23).

The function of the turbinate is to increase the surface area of nasal mucosa and the contact with the inspired air which is heated and humidified.

They also disrupt the laminar flow of the air, making it slow and turbulent.

The three turbinates are superior, middle, and inferior.

The inferior turbinate is the largest and has immune functions because it is the first to come in contact with the outside air. Additionally, it is enlarged in unilateral cleft lip patients [18].

The four meatuses are inferior (between the inferior turbinate and nasal floor), middle (between the inferior and middle turbinates), superior (between the middle and superior turbinate), and the sphenoethmoidal recess (located superiorly and posteriorly to the upper turbinate).

The lateral wall also contains the following openings which drain a variety of structures as follows: sphenoid sinus, ethmoidal air cells, maxillary sinus, frontal sinus, and nasolacrimal duct.

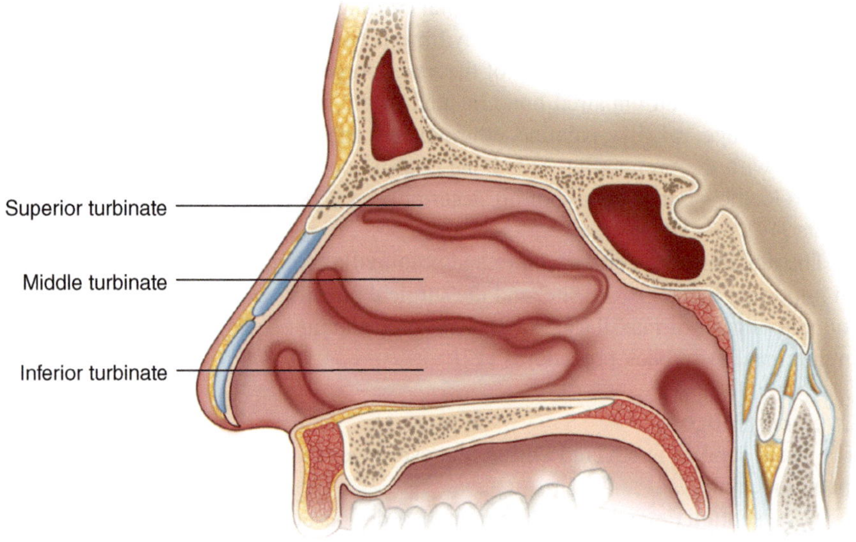

Fig. 1.23 Internal lateral wall of the nose diagram

Bony Framework (Fig. 1.4)

The bone structure of the lateral wall of the nasal cavity consists of the frontal process of the maxilla, lacrimal region, the ethmoid bone, perpendicular section of the palatine bone, and medial pterygoid plate of the sphenoid.

The ethmoid bone is located at the midline of the anterior cranial fossa and forms also the roof of the nasal cavity and the medial wall of the orbits.

The cribriform plate forms the roof of the nasal cavity and contains small perforations allowing olfactory nerve fibers to cross.

Laterally, two small cuboidal bone structures are located between the orbits and the nasal cavity. These are the ethmoidal labyrinths which include the ethmoidal sinus and cells. The sphenopalatine foramen (a structure between sphenoid and palatine bones) is located at the level of the superior meatus. This foramen communicates the nasal cavity and the pterygopalatine fossa. The sphenopalatine artery, nasopalatine, and superior nasal nerves passed through this region.

Overlying Mucosa

The nasal mucosa covering the lateral wall and turbinates contains many blood vessels. This mucosa has respiratory epithelium, which consists of pseudostratified ciliated columnar cells with goblet cells. The inferior turbinate is exclusively covered with a pseudostratified ciliated and not ciliated columnar epithelium with more goblet cells on its lateral side.

This structure may shrink or swell in response to the quality of the inspired air.

Septal deviation can be associated with turbinate hyperplasia leading to nasal obstruction in patients with unilateral cleft lip and palate [18, 19].

The Nasal Floor

The nasal cavity is limited by the following structures (Figs. 1.24 and 1.25):

- Roof: It is the olfactory area formed by nasal, frontal, sphenoid, and ethmoid bones covered by respiratory mucosa.
- Medial wall: It is represented by the nasal septum. It is formed by perpendicular plate of ethmoid, vomer, and septal cartilage.
- Lateral wall: This is formed by the maxilla, ethmoid, and the palatine bones. It includes the turbinates and meatuses.
- Floor: The skeletal framework is formed by the maxilla and palatine bones.

Four sections can be clearly identified in the nasal floor.

Anterior (vestibular): This section corresponds to the vestibular nasal floor (nasal sill).

Primary palate (premaxilla): This is the most anterior portion of the palate and includes the premaxilla bone which bears the incisor teeth. Close to the junction with the palatine process of the maxilla is the incisive foramen which transmits branches of the sphenopalatine artery and the nasopalatine nerve.

Secondary palate (hard palate): The hard palate includes the anterior two-thirds of the palate, and it is composed by the palatine processes of the maxilla and the horizontal plates of the palatine bones.

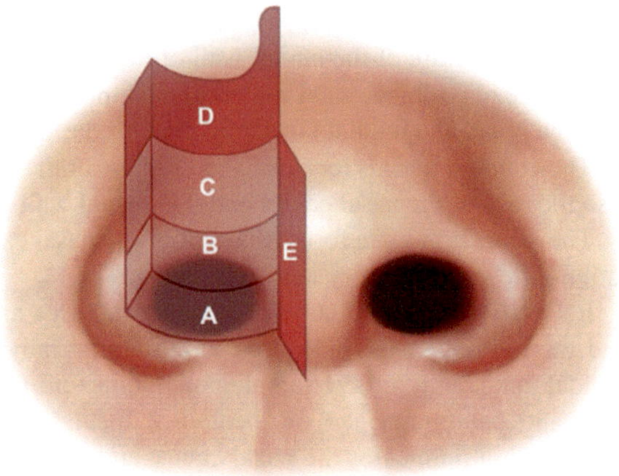

Fig. 1.24 Nasal floor segment diagram. A. Nostril sill. B. Primary palate. C. Secondary palate. D. Soft palate. E. Nasal septum

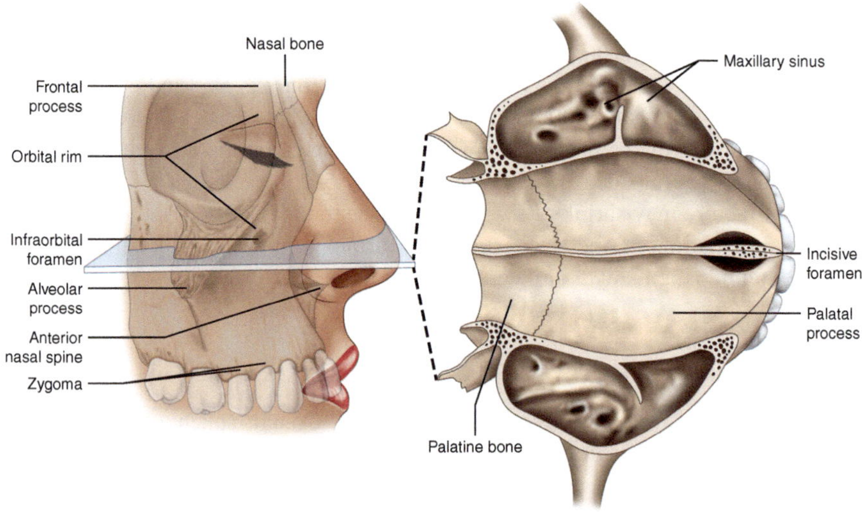

Fig. 1.25 Anatomical diagram of the nasal floor skeletal framework

Soft palate: It represents the posterior third of the palate, and this is the functional part of the nasal floor and appears during velopharyngeal closure.

The nasal floor is absent in the complete cleft lip and palate (Veau III and IV types), and it is repaired depending on the surgical protocol used (Table 1.1) (Figs. 1.26 and 1.27).

The author's protocol is based on cleft lip repair at 3–6 months of age and the whole palate repair at 9–12 months of age. Later the primary palate section is repaired during alveolar bone grafting during the mixed dentition period [20].

Two-stage hard palate delayed closure (Gothenburg protocol) involves closing the soft palate section first and then the hard palate. Primary palate section is closed

Table 1.1 Nasal floor closure regarding the cleft palate repair protocol

Nasal floor	One stage	Delayed hard palate Gothenburg	Delayed soft closure Oslo	LIMA protocol[a]
Segment I	3–6 months	3–6 months	3–6 months	3–6 months
Segment II	7–9 years	7–9 years	3–6 months	5 years
Segment III	9–12 months	3 years	3–6 months	9–12 years
Segment IV	9–12 months	6 months	9–12 months	9–12 years

[a]The Lima protocol for cleft palate repair considers delayed hard palate closure for severe bilateral cleft lip and palate

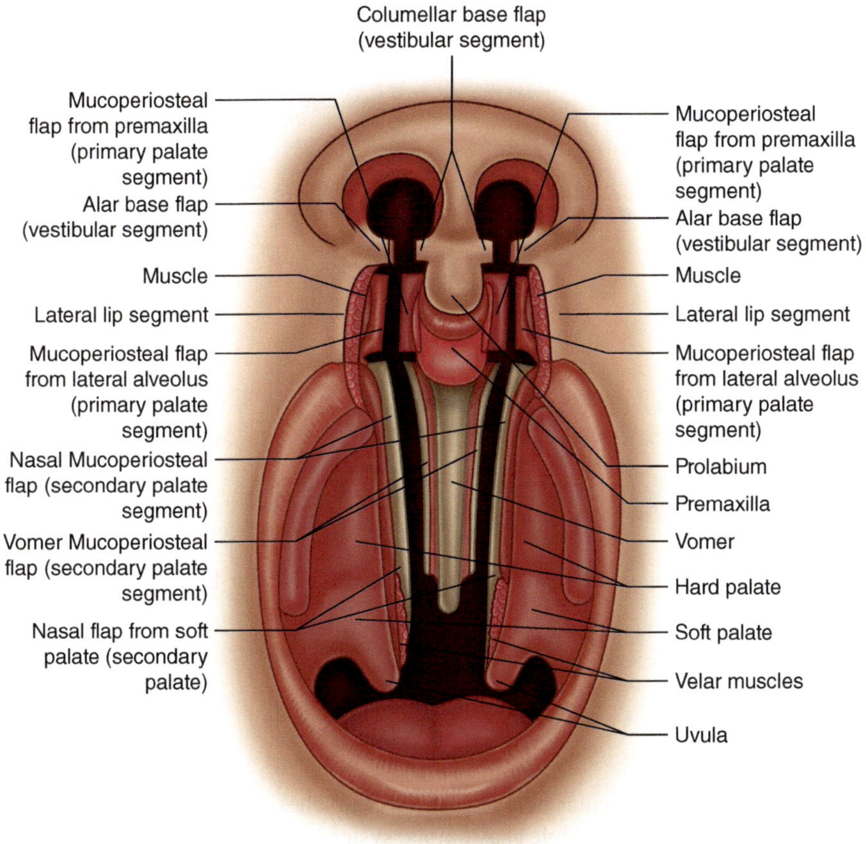

Fig. 1.26 Bilateral cleft lip and palate nasal floor repair

during alveolar bone grafting [21]. A variant, the Milan protocol, performs the lip and nose repair at the same time as the soft palate.

The two-stage soft palate delayed closure (Oslo protocol) close first the primary and hard palate using the vomer flap and the soft palate later. The cleft lip is repaired previously at 3 months of age during hard palate closure [22].

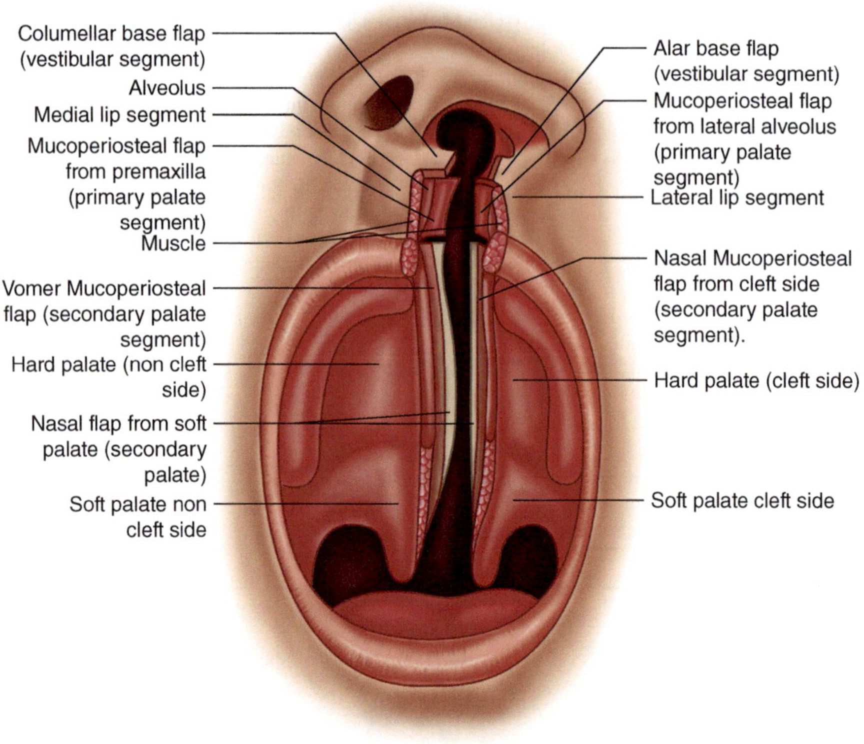

Fig. 1.27 Unilateral cleft lip and palate nasal floor repair

These are the main protocols; however, many of them have been published actually.

Nasal Systems

Vascular System

The nose has a rich vascular network, and its branches originate from the carotid arteries and conform to multiple anastomotic systems. The internal carotid branches are the anterior and posterior ethmoidal arteries, and the external carotid branches are sphenopalatine, greater palatine artery, superior labial artery, and lateral nasal artery (from the facial artery). The main contributor to this vascular network is the facial artery through the lateral nasal artery.

Saban et al. [23] described several arterial arcades around nasal tip following the upper and lower border of the alar cartilage of the nose.

The arcade located around the lower border of the alar cartilage (marginal arcade) connects both marginal arteries, and the arcade located around the upper border of the alar cartilage (upper and lower lateral cartilage junction) connects both lateral nasal arteries (Fig. 1.28). Both arcades are connected to branches of the superior labial artery, another branch of the facial artery.

The main external arteries of the nose are as follows (Figs. 1.29, 1.30 and 1.31):

Dorsal nasal artery (external nasal artery): This is the terminal branch of the ophthalmic artery (branch of the internal carotid artery) receiving branches from the supratrochlear artery. Two terminal branches: one lateral anastomoses with the angular artery and the other medial travel along the dorsum of the nose and form anastomoses with its contralateral fellow [24].

Lateral nasal artery: It supplies most of the blood supply to the nasal tip. It is a branch of the facial artery (external carotid branch) and ascends along the side of the nose. These arteries provide the vascular arcades (upper and lower) around the nasal tip and branches for the ala and dorsum (anastomoses with the dorsal nasal artery) and the anastomoses with the contralateral fellow. It has other anastomoses with branches of the infraorbital artery.

Columellar artery: Vascular supply of this important segment of the nose is composed by anastomoses between vascular arcades of the lateral nasal artery and branches from the superior labial arteries.

The main internal arteries of the nasal cavity are the following [25] (Figs. 1.32 and 1.33):

Ethmoid arteries (anterior and posterior): From the ophthalmic artery, they supply the roof of the nasal cavity.

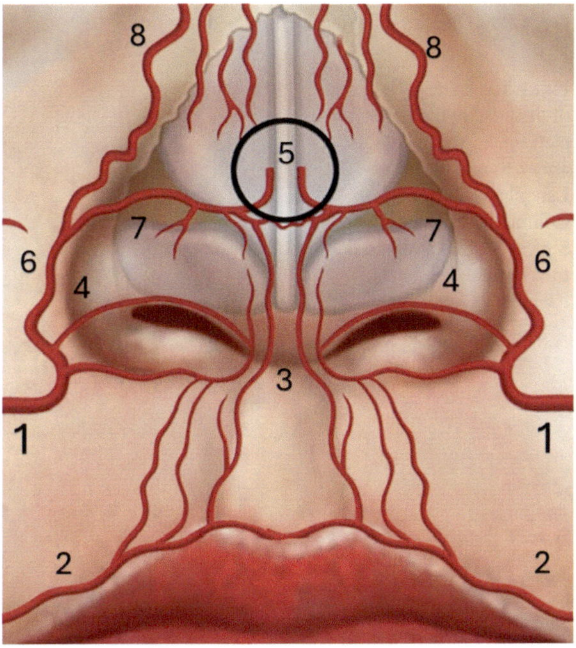

Fig. 1.28 External arteries of the nose: nasal arcades. 1. Facial artery. 2. Upper labial artery. 3. Columellar arteries. 4. Marginal arcade. 5. Arcade anastomosis. 6. Lateral nasal artery. 7. Intercartilaginous arcade. 8. Angular artery

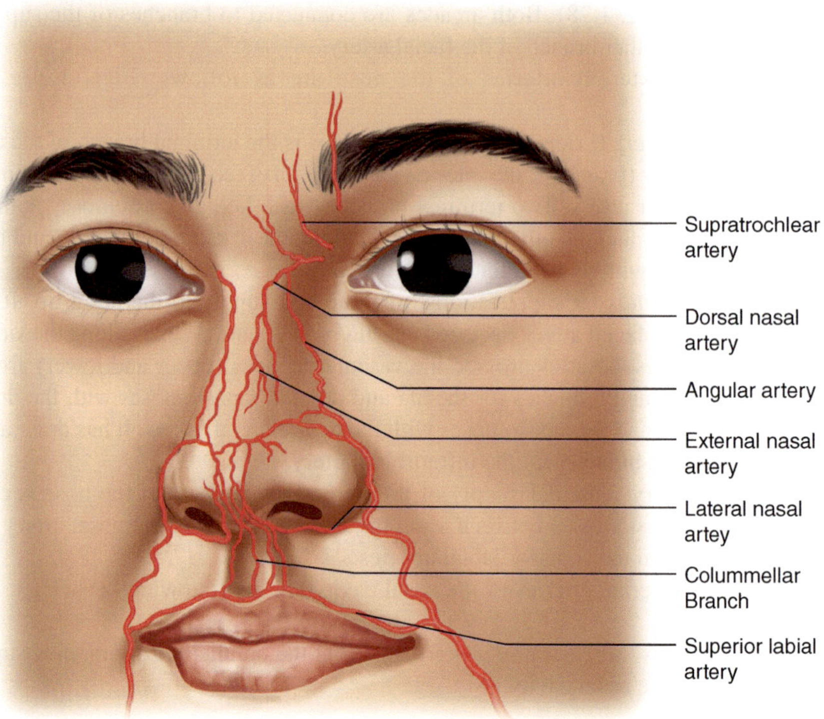

Fig. 1.29 Diagram of external arteries of the nose

Fig. 1.30 External arteries of the nose in the unilateral cleft lip. 1. Medial nasal artery. 2. Angular artery. 3. Lateral nasal artery. 4. Columellar branches. 5. Superior labial artery. 6. Inferior labial artery. 7. Facial artery

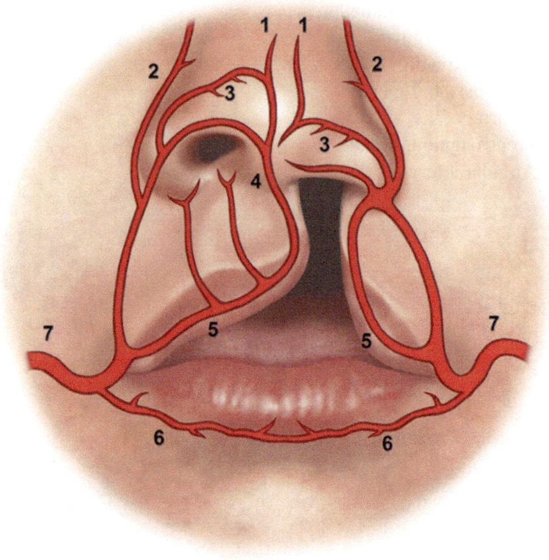

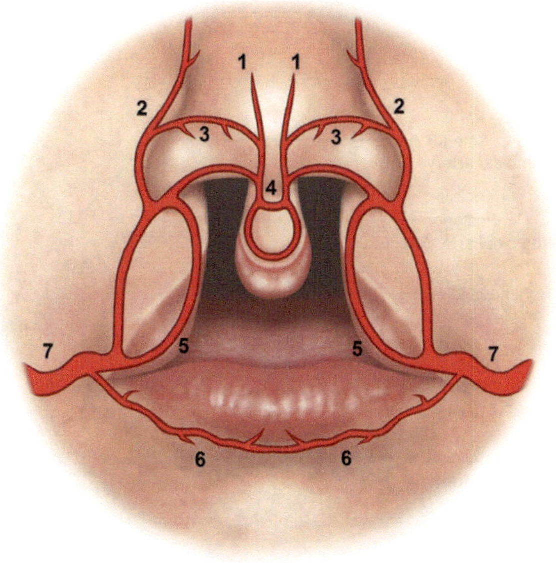

Fig. 1.31 External arteries of the nose in the bilateral cleft lip. 1. Medial nasal artery. 2. Angular artery. 3. Lateral nasal artery. 4. Columellar branches. 5. Superior labial artery. 6. Inferior labial artery. 7. Facial artery

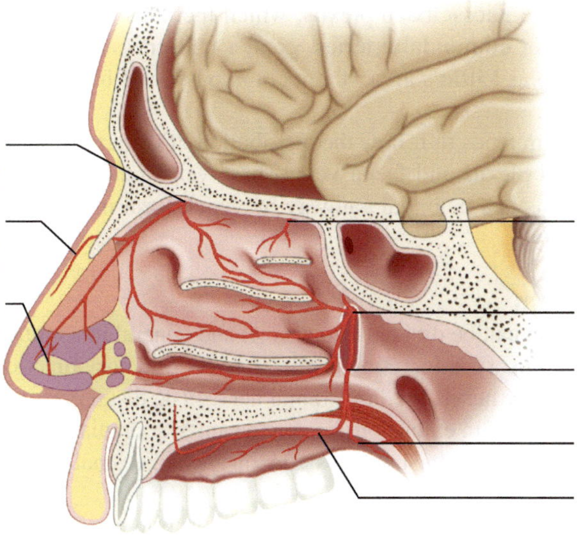

Fig. 1.32 Diagram of the main internal arteries of the lateral wall nasal cavity

Sphenopalatine: This artery originates from the maxillary artery (a branch of the external carotid artery) and provides two major branches: the lateral and medial. The lateral branch ramifies over the lateral wall (turbinates) and the medial branch ramifies to the nasal septum.

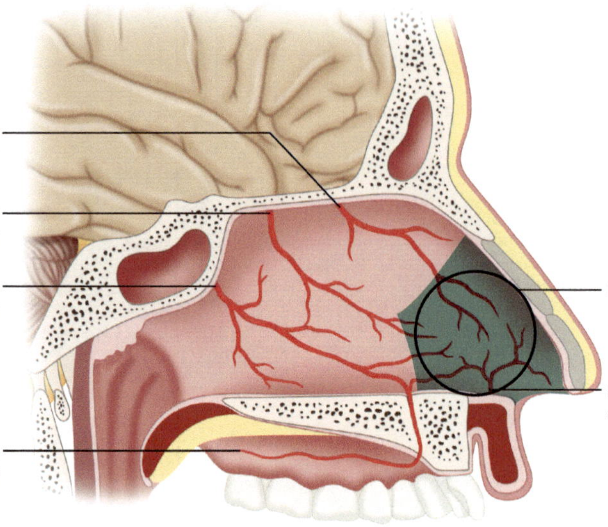

Fig. 1.33 Diagram of the main internal arteries of the internal wall nasal cavity

The internal arteries conform an important vascular plexus supplying the nasal septum: the Kiesselbach plexus, which includes the sphenopalatine, anterior and posterior ethmoidal arteries, greater palatine, and superior labial arteries. Known also as Little's area, it is a common site of bleeding in young adults [26] (Fig. 1.33).

Venous system tends to follow the distribution of the arterial system. They drain to the pterygoid plexus and facial vein. These veins join the dural sinuses which explains why this is a potential pathway by which local infection may spread into the cranial cavity.

Nervous System

Nasal innervation can be divided into special and general innervation [27].

The special sensory innervation is related to the olfactory function and is carried out by the olfactory nerve, the first cranial nerve. The distal portion of these nerves (olfactory bulbs, a brain extension) lies on the anterior cranial base which is located above the nasal cavity. Its branches run through the small holes of the cribriform plate.

The general sensory innervation provides sensation as touch, temperature, and pain. Innervation of the nasal cavity is delivered by the nasopalatine nerve (from the maxillary nerve) and the nasociliary nerve (from the ophthalmic nerve).

The innervation of the nasal external skin is supplied by the trigeminal nerve (Fig. 1.34), and the nasal muscles are innervated by the buccal branch of facial nerve, the seventh cranial nerve.

The nasociliary nerve is a branch of the ophthalmic nerve (one of the three divisions of the trigeminal nerve) that provides sensory innervation to the upper face

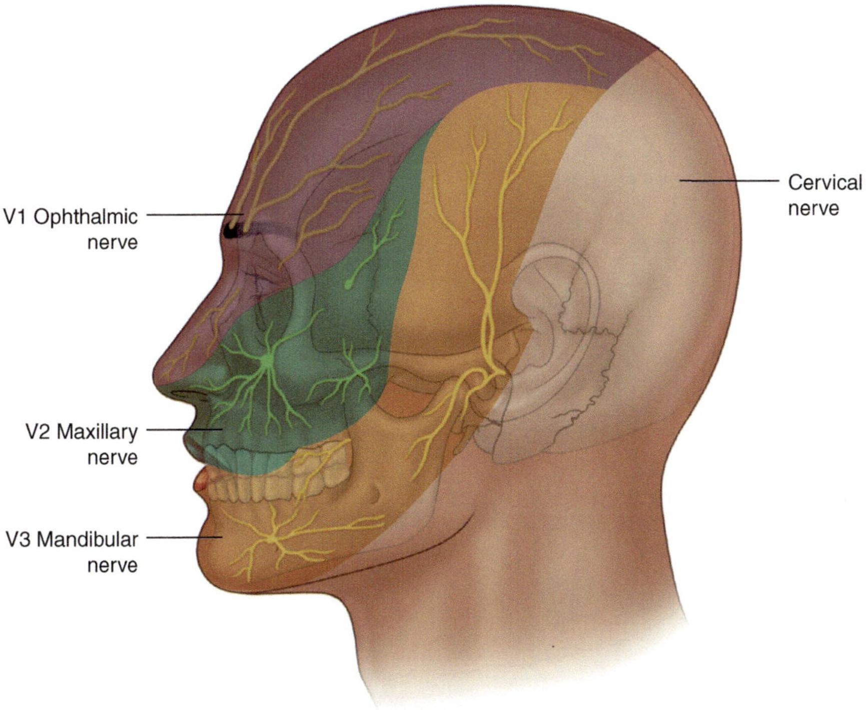

Fig. 1.34 Facial distribution of the trigeminal nerve facial distribution

and scalp, more specifically cutaneous and mucosal innervation to the apex and ala of the nose and anterior nasal cavity.

Its terminal branches are the infratrochlear and external nasal nerves. It also provides the ciliary and anterior and posterior ethmoidal nerves (Fig. 1.35).

The external nasal nerve exits between the lower border of the nasal bone and the upper lateral cartilage; it is the place where the local anesthetic block is performed.

Branches of the maxillary division of the trigeminal nerve (internal branches of the infraorbital nerve) innervate the ala of the nose as well as the caudal septum and nasal vestibule. The anesthetic block of this nerve is an important resource for post-operative pain management based on multimodal protocol.

The nasal septum general sensory innervation and nasal lateral walls are innervated by the nasopalatine nerve (a branch of the second division of the trigeminal nerve) and the nasociliary nerve (a branch of the ophthalmic division of the trigeminal nerve).

The paranasal sinuses are innervated by the anterior and posterior ethmoidal nerves and branches of the ophthalmic (nasociliary nerve) and maxillary nerve division of the trigeminal nerve [28] (Fig. 1.36a, b).

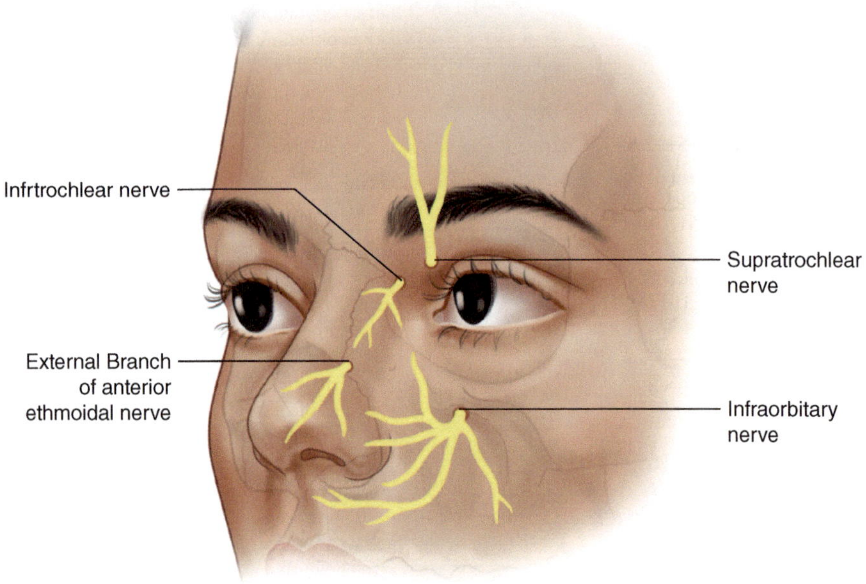

Fig. 1.35 External nasal branches of the trigeminal nerve

Finally, the motor innervation for the nasal muscles is provided by branches of the seventh cranial nerve, specifically the buccal branch with the exception of the procerus which is innervated by the temporal branch of this nerve.

Musculoaponeurotic System

Nasal Superficial Musculo Aponeurotic System (SMAS)

The SMAS is an organized fibrous network composed of collagen and elastin fibers that extend across the face separating the deep and superficial adipose tissue. It was initially described by Mitz and Peyronie in 1976 [29].

This system has a specific morphology according to the region and plays an important role in facial expression by connecting facial muscles to the skin.

The nasal SMAS is an extension of the facial SMAS and consists of a unique layer divided at the level of the internal nasal valve into deep and superficial layers. Both layers conform to the ligaments of the nasal tip.

The deep layer of the nasal SMAS inserts laterally into the internal nasal valve and medially passes anterior to the caudal septum and posterior to the interdomal ligament. Another nasal ligament is the midline ligament of the nose described by Pitanguy [30]. This structure influences the equilibrium of the dorsum-tip relationship, and it originates from the nasalis muscle fascia and finishes at the caudal edge of the septum (Fig. 1.37).

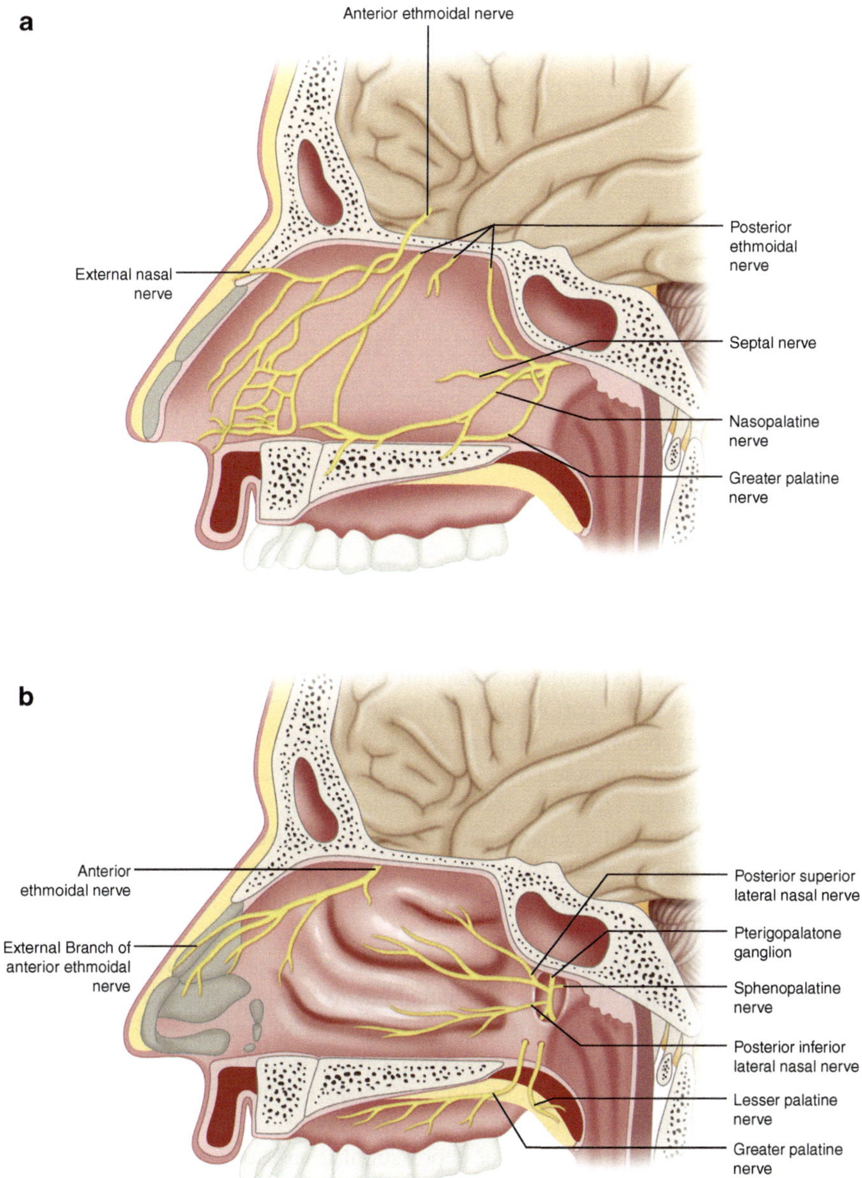

Fig. 1.36 Internal nasal nerves. (**a**) Medial wall (septum). (**b**) Lateral wall

Nasal Muscles (Figs. 1.38, 1.39 and 1.40)

A number of muscles inserted into the external nose and contributes to the facial expression and nasal function. All of them are innervated by the facial nerve (seventh cranial nerve). They are procerus, nasalis, myrtiformis, depressor septi nasalis, and levator labii superioris alaeque nasalis muscle [31].

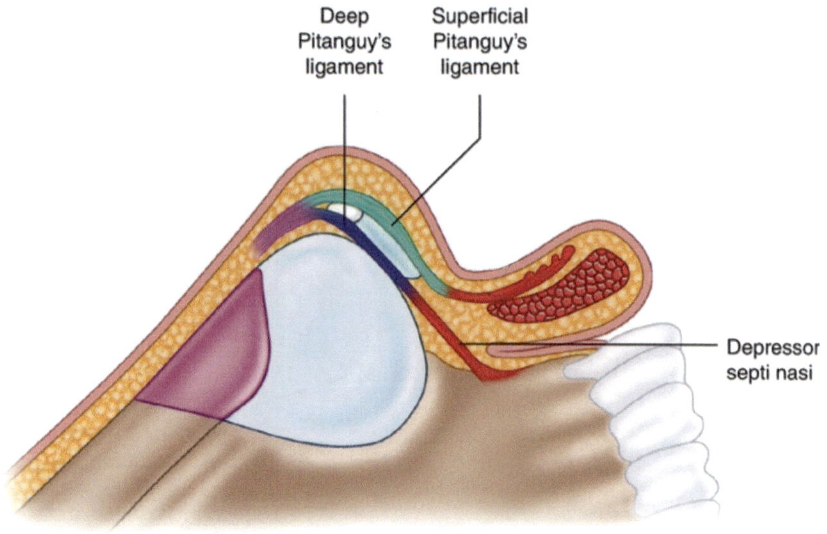

Fig. 1.37 The nasal SMAS (superficial musculo aponeurotic system) and Pitanguy's ligament

Procerus muscle: It is a small pyramidal muscle located covering the lower part of nasal bone and upper part of upper lateral cartilage. This muscle pulls the skin between the eyebrows downward assisting in flaring the nostrils.

Nasalis muscle: This muscle covers the nasal dorsum and has two components: transverse and alar. The transverse part is also known as compressor naris and the alar component as dilator naris. The dilator naris muscle acts to widen and narrow the nostril, preventing the collapse of the nostril during inhalation.

The compressor naris muscle has two major and minor components (not always present).

The compressor naris wrinkles the nasal skin and compresses the nasal aperture.

Myrtiformis muscle: This is a muscle that begins from the myrtiform fossa at the anterior surface of the maxilla. It was first described by Sappey in 1876. Its fibers end up with attachments to the fibroadipose tissue under the base of the lower lateral cartilage. This muscle works by narrowing the nostrils while acting with the depressor septi nasi via the fibers inserted into the septal base.

Depressor septi nasalis muscle or depressor alae nasi muscle connects the incisive fossa of the maxilla to the nasal septum. This muscle extends the airway pulling the nasal tip and narrowing the labiocolumellar angle. Its section is practiced during cosmetic rhinoplasty. In patients with unilateral cleft lip, the function of the normal side is increased bringing dislocation and malformation of the base of the columella and caudal septum [32].

Levator labii superioris alaeque nasalis muscle: This is a muscle composed of two parts and acts to widen the nostril and elevate the nostril and upper lip producing a snarling facial expression. This is why this muscle is known as the "Elvis Presley muscle."

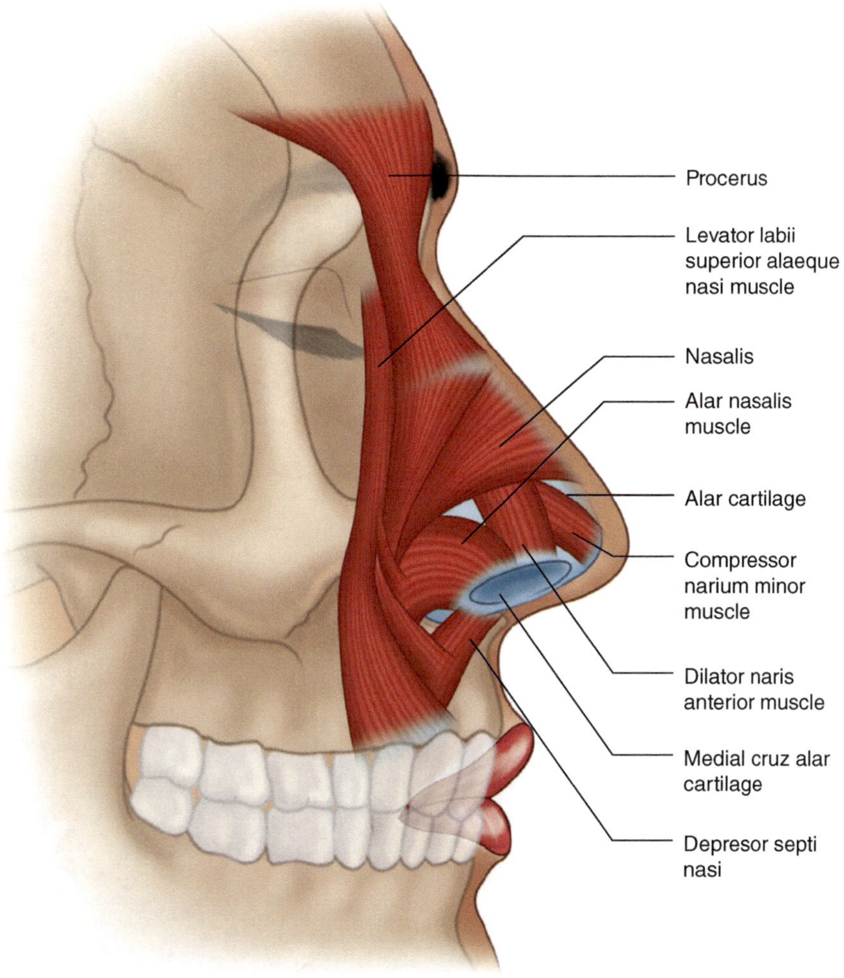

Fig. 1.38 Nasal muscles

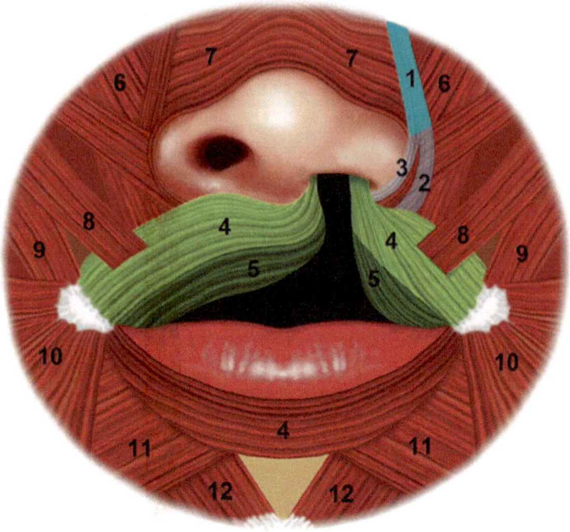

Fig. 1.39 Unilateral cleft lip labial nasal muscles. 1. Levator labii superioris alaeque nasi muscle. 2. Labial division of this muscle. 3. Nasal division of this muscle. 4. Orbicularis oris muscle (marginal portion). 5. Orbicularis oris muscle (peripheral portion). 6. Levator labii superioris. 7. Nasalis. 8. Zygomaticus minor. 9. Zygomaticus major. 10. Depressor anguli oris. 11. Depressor labii inferioris. 12. Mentalis

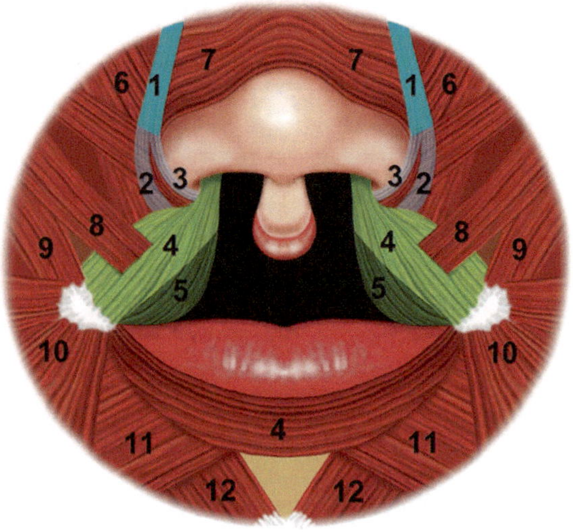

Fig. 1.40 Bilateral cleft lip labial nasal muscles. 1. Levator labii superioris alaeque nasi muscle. 2. Labial division of this muscle. 3. Nasal division of this muscle. 4. Orbicularis oris muscle (marginal portion). 5. Orbicularis oris muscle (peripheral portion). 6. Levator labii superioris. 7. Nasalis. 8. Zygomaticus minor. 9. Zygomaticus major. 10. Depressor anguli oris. 11. Depressor labii inferioris. 12. Mentalis

Nasal Physiology

The nose is part of the respiratory system and has three main functions: olfaction, breathing, and immunity. These can be described as follows:

(a) Sense of smell.
(b) Conforms the most anterior part of the airway.
(c) The inhaled air is warmed and moisturized through the nasal cavities.
(d) Through the turbinates and ciliated epithelium, the nose acts as a filter to remove foreign agents.
(e) The nose plays an essential role in speech and phonetics.

Functionally, the nose has three regions: vestibule, respiratory, and olfactory regions (Fig. 1.41)

Respiratory region, covered by pseudostratified columnar ciliated epithelium and mucus goblet cells. It functions to humidify, warm, filter, protect, and eliminate debris. The anatomy of the nasal cavity allows time and enough surface area through the turbinates for the inhaled air to be warmed and moistened.

Olfactory region: This is located at the top of the nasal cavity and lined by olfactory mucosa.

Nasal vestibule is the anterior external opening of the nasal cavity and limited by the internal and external nasal valves. Its circumference is lined with hair bearing skin; the vibrissae have a job filtering larger airborne particles increasing the resistance of the external nasal valve. The most important regional sections of potential airflow restriction are the external and internal nasal valves. They represent the narrowest cross sections of the nasal airway.

External Nasal Valve This area is limited superolaterally by the caudal border of the upper lateral cartilage, anterolaterally by the alar rim, medially by the caudal septum and the columella, inferiorly by the nasal sill, and posteriorly with the internal nasal valve opening. The primary structural support of the external nasal valve is the upper lateral cartilage.

Mink was the first to identify the nasal valve in 1903.

This is the dynamic section of the nose, composed of skin and cartilages; it is subject to the action of the nasal muscles changing its anatomy by compression or dilatation of the nasal vestibule [33, 34] (Fig. 1.42).

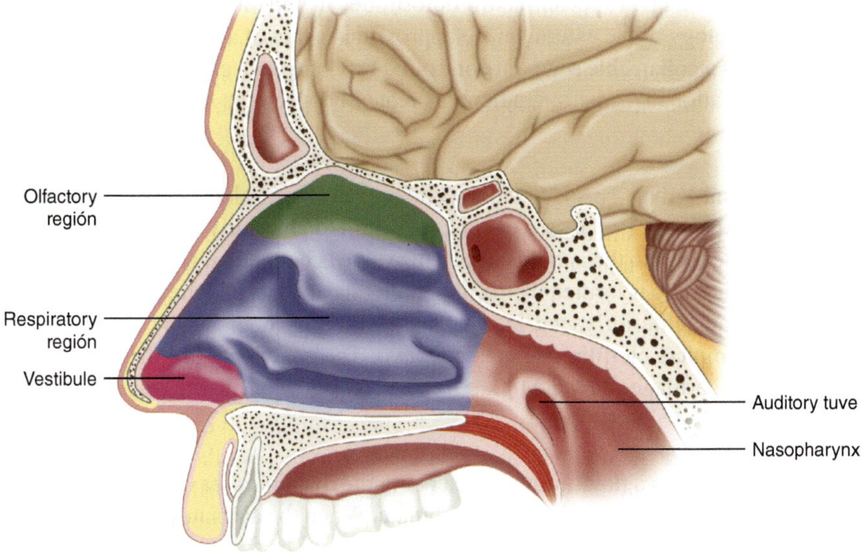

Fig. 1.41 Functional regions of the nose

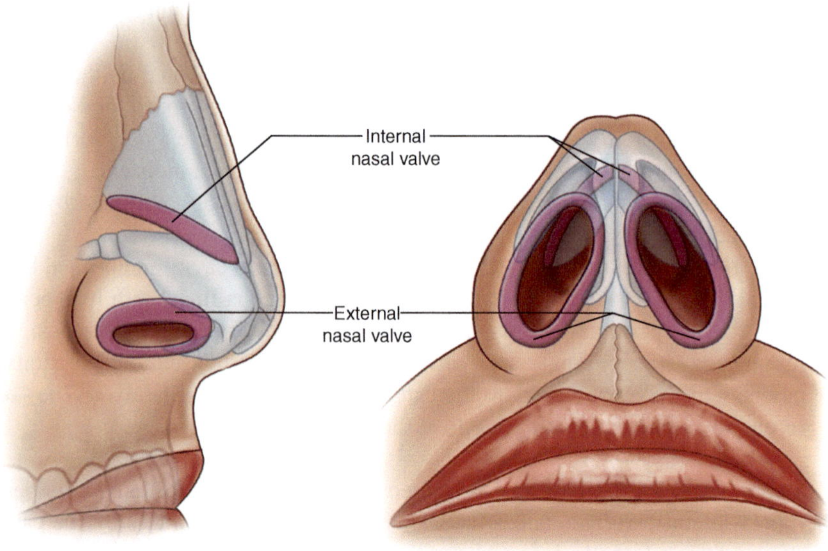

Fig. 1.42 Internal and external nasal valves of the nose

A critical area of the external nasal valve is the soft triangle; this name comes from the lack of cartilage support as it is formed only of skin and soft tissue (Fig. 1.43).

This is the area between the dome and the nostril rim and has functional and aesthetic considerations during primary rhinoplasty because this is often neglected in this surgery. Overcorrection techniques or techniques such as Mulliken technique resect the soft triangle to repair nostril deformities in patients with cleft lip.

The physiology of the external nose approximates that of a Starling resistor. This rigid tube has a collapsible segment controlled by changes in external pressure [35]. During inspiration, a pressure gradient is created between the nasopharynx and the atmosphere.

Internal Nasal Valve This is the narrowest area of the nasal vestibule where inspiratory and expiratory turbulence occurs; it is limited anteriorly to the ostium internum and posteriorly to the isthmus nasi. This valve is bounded medially by the nasal septum and laterally is limited by the upper lateral cartilage and the anterior head of lower turbinate. Inferiorly, the internal nasal valve is bounded by the nasal sill (absent in complete cleft lip and palate forms). The angle between the septum and upper lateral cartilage (called Mink's nasal valve) is 10–15° in Caucasian people [36, 37] (Figs. 1.44 and 1.45).

This valve acts as a flow-limiting area being the dynamic area of the upper lateral cartilage and the mucosa of the lower turbinate. When the air is inspired, it is forced through this area increasing its speed and pressure. The transverse portion of the nasalis muscle provides stabilization of the nasal valve preventing its collapse.

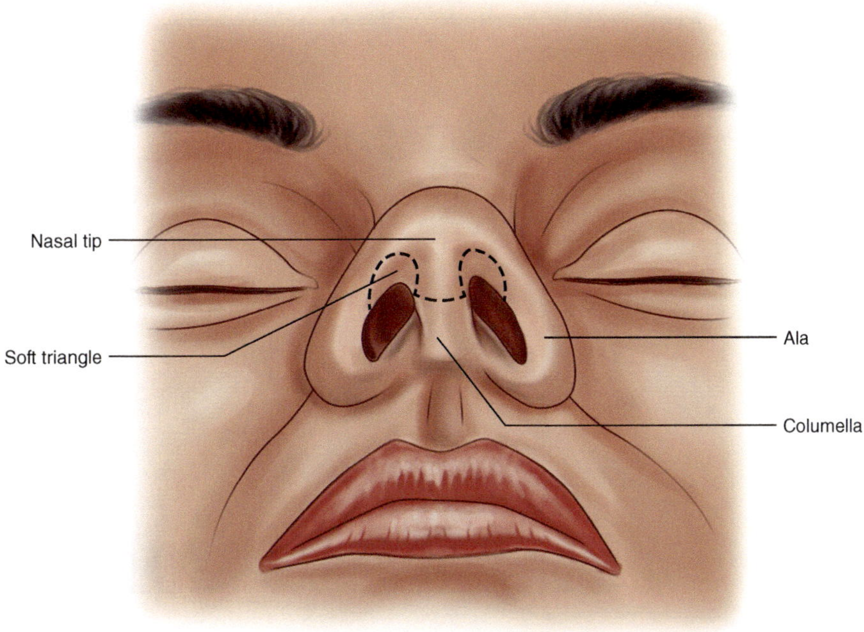

Fig. 1.43 The soft triangle of the nose

Fig. 1.44 Mink's nasal valve

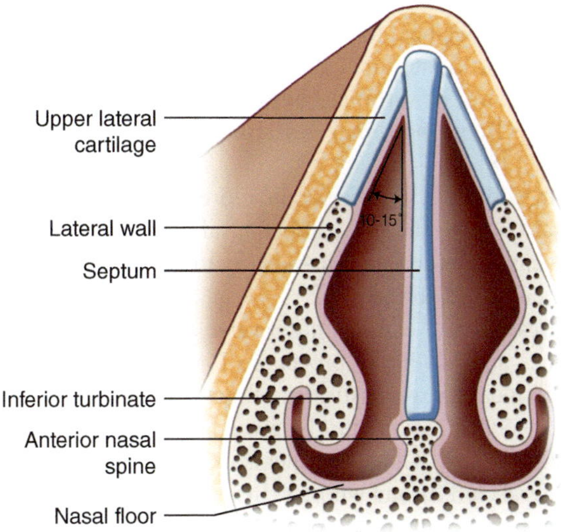

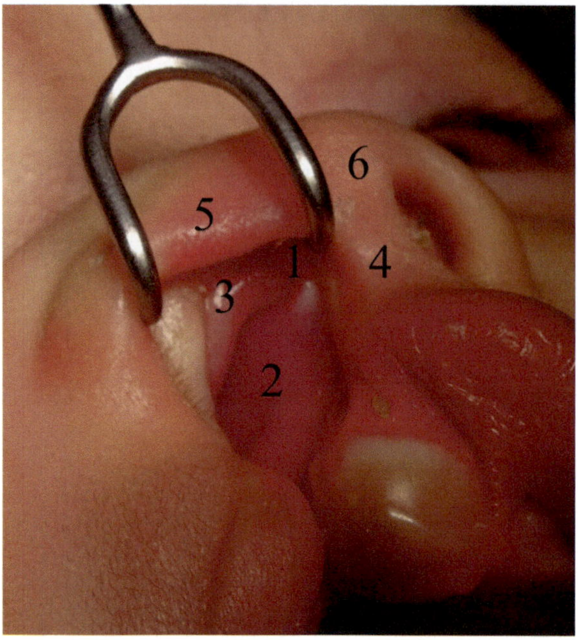

Fig. 1.45 Mink's nasal valve anatomy in a patient with unilateral cleft lip and palate. Internal nasal valve angle. 2. Nasal septum. 3. Intercartilaginous border. 4. Columella. 5. Alae. 6. Nasal tip

A reduction in this area will lead to nondesirable effects on the inspiratory and expiratory currents. Scar contracture of the nasal vestibule or synechiae produced by cleft rhinoplasty may cause this problem (Fig. 1.46).

The nasal airway is physiologically related to the resistance. The most important structure is the internal nasal valve which represents almost 50% of the total airway resistance; therefore small changes in the size of the internal nasal valve (related to anatomical disturbances like septal deviation, valve collapse, scar contracture, or turbinate hypertrophy) can have major effects on airflow resistance. Often, the septal deviation into the cleft side occurs at the internal nasal valve [38].

In addition, any scar contracture generated by primary interventions over the nasal vestibule area may affect nasal valve function; therefore the use of postoperative nasal conformers is mandatory to prevent these serious complications which are difficult to be corrected.

Resection of external nasal valve soft tissues (practiced via overcorrection techniques and Mulliken' procedure for bilateral cleft lip nose repair) may affect its anatomical characteristics and functionality.

Special attention must be given to the use of the Mulliken technique for bilateral cleft lip repair. This technique is used for primary cleft rhinoplasty in patients with bilateral cleft lip and whose skin is removed from the soft triangle and intercartilaginous border (limen nasi). In addition the author recommends skin excision from lateral vestibule wall to correct vestibular webs. Primary soft tissue resection is not recommended since there is no excess of skin and any resection creates a disbalance creating aesthetic and functional problems.

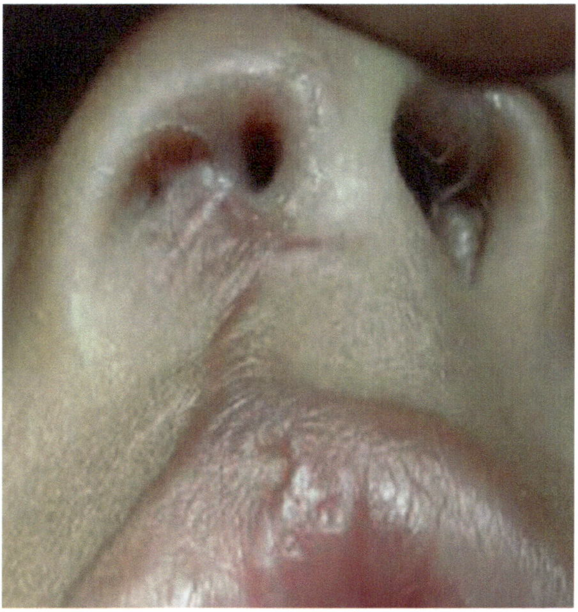

Fig. 1.46 Scar contracture of the nasal vestibule

In addition, it produces a more difficult scenario and is produced for any secondary correction if it is needed.

More studies are necessary in order to guarantee the safety of these procedures.

Based on the author's philosophy, the primary correction for nasal deformity in patients with cleft lip and palate should preserve soft tissues, elongate the nasal vestibule, prevent the development of scar contractures (using postoperative nasal conformers), and consider the caudal septum reposition in severe forms.

Based on the author's experience during the last 30 years as a cleft surgeon, this protocol guarantees good aesthetic and functional outcomes and prevents common complications associated with this surgery.

Applied Anatomy to Cleft Lip Nose

The nasal deformity associated with the cleft lip is thought to result from a combination of tissue hypoplasia and anatomic malposition.

Maxillary hypoplasia and displacement of lower lateral cartilages in association with septal deviation (in unilateral) are the main characteristics of the nasal deformity.

These congenital malformations explain the aesthetic and functional disturbances observed in cleft lip and palate patients.

The following are the anatomical changes observed in patients with unilateral and bilateral cleft lip.

Unilateral cleft lip (Figs. 1.16 and 1.47):

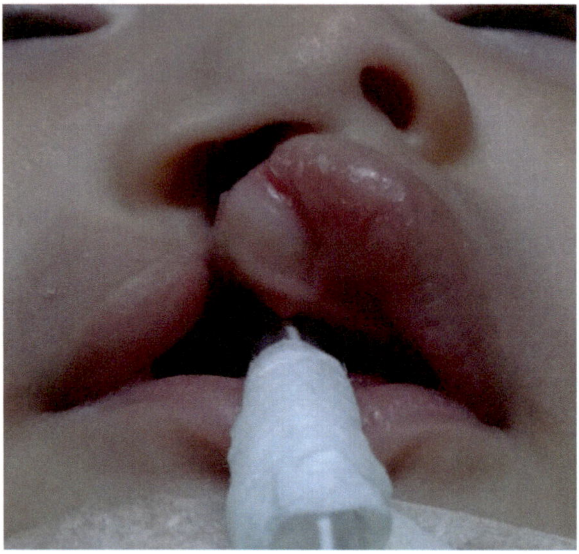

Fig. 1.47 Unilateral cleft lip nasal deformity

(a) Nasal septum deviation to the noncleft side.
(b) Deficient maxilla on the cleft side.
(c) Nasal tip asymmetry.
(d) Nostril is wider and retrodisplaced on the cleft side.
(e) The ala at the cleft side is inferiorly and laterally positioned.
(f) Columellar deviation. It is not "short" at the cleft side and is only malpositioned.
(g) Cleft side dome is retrodisplaced and alar cartilage underprojected.
(h) Cleft side alar cartilage displaced caudally and laterally.
(i) Angle between lateral and medial crura is increased.
(j) Weak attachment of the lower lateral cartilage to the upper lateral cartilage contributing to weakened sidewall and nasal obstruction during inspiration.
(k) Nasal sill absence (in complete forms).
(l) Alar cartilages are similar in shape and thickness; it is only malpositioned at the cleft side in unilateral forms.

Bilateral cleft lip (Figs. 1.18 and 1.48):

(a) "Short columella" in appearance: in fat it is not short and is only laterally displaced.
(b) Wide nostrils and deflected inferiorly.
(c) Broad and depressed nasal tip.
(d) Depressed and overhanging columella.
(e) Nasal septum deviation is uncommon, only in asymmetric forms of bilateral cleft lip.
(f) Caudal septum is displaced inferiorly and posteriorly.
(g) Nasal tip symmetry but underprojected.
(h) Alar cartilages are displaced caudally and laterally.
(i) Protrusive premaxilla. Severity of the malformed anatomy of the nose is associated with the severity of the skeletal malformation.

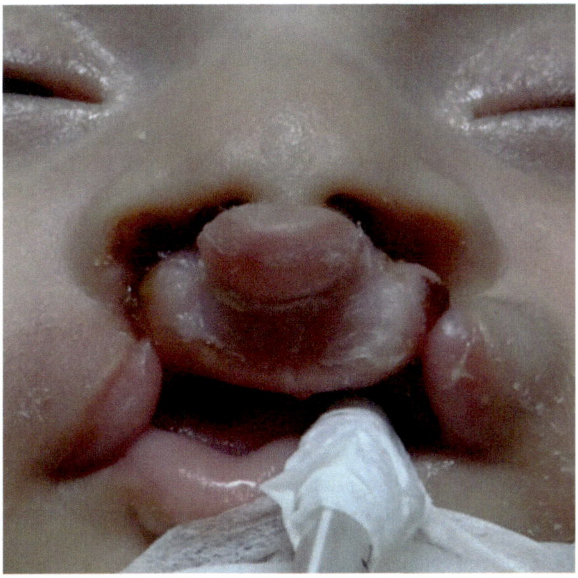

Fig. 1.48 Bilateral cleft lip nasal deformity

(j) Absence of nasal sill (in complete forms).
(k) Internal nasal valve is compromised by weakened support of the upper lateral cartilages.
(l) Bilateral maxillary hypoplasia.

References

1. Eggerstedt M, Rhee J, Buranosky M, Batra PS, Tajudeen BA, et al. Nasal skin and soft tissue thickness variation among differing races and ethnicities: an objective radiographic analysis. Facial Plast Surg Aesthet Med. 2020;22(3):188–94.
2. Daniel R, Glasz T, Molnar G, Palhazi P, Saban Y, Journel B. The lower nasal base: an anatomical study. Aesthet Surg J. 2013;33(2):222–32.
3. Ali-Salaam P, Kashgarian M, Davila J, Persing J. Anatomy of the caucasian alar groove. Plast Reconstr Surg J. 2002;110(1):261–6.
4. Bayram A, Kilavuz A, Serin G. The importance of soft triangle in rhinoplasty. J Craniofac Surg. 2016;27(6):e536–7.
5. Bochnia F. Usefulness of the subunit principle in nasal reconstruction. An Bras Dermatol. 2017;92(Suppl 1):159–62.
6. Cohn J, Shokri T, Othman B, Sokoya M. Surgical techniques to improve the soft tissue triangle in rhinoplasty: a systematic review. Facial Plast Surg. 2020;36:120–8.
7. Daniel RK. The nasal tip: anatomy and aesthetics. Plast Reconstr Surg. 1992;89(2):216–24.
8. Daniel RK. Anatomy and aesthetics of the nasal tip. Plast Reconstr Surg. 1992;89:216.
9. Busca GP, Amasio ME, Staffieri A. La chirurgia della punta nasale [The surgery of the tip of the nose]. Acta Otorhinolaryngol Ital. 2002;22(3 Suppl 70):7–29.
10. Rohrich RJ, Huynh B, Muzaffar AR, Adams WP Jr, Robinson JB Jr. Importance of the depressor septi nasi muscle in rhinoplasty: anatomic study and clinical application. Plast Reconstr Surg. 2000;105(1):376–83.
11. Cottle M. The structure and function of the nasal vestibule. AMA Arch Otolaryngol. 1955;62(2):173–81.

12. Rossell-Perry P. Primary unilateral cleft lip nasal deformity repair using VYZ plasty: an anthropometric study. Indian J Plast Surg. 2017;50(02):180–6.
13. Potter J. Some nasal tip deformities due to alar cartilage abnormalities. Plast Reconstr Surg. 1954;13(5):359–66.
14. Berkeley W. The cleft lip nose. Plast Reconstr Surg. 1959;23:567.
15. Beeson WH. The nasal septum. Otolaryngol Clin N Am. 1987;20(4):743–67.
16. Cem Miman M, Deliktaş H, Özturan O, Toplu Y, Akarçay M. Internal nasal valve: revisited with objective facts. Otolaryngol Head Neck Surg. 2006;134(1):41–7.
17. Trevizan M, Consolaro A. Premaxilla: an independent bone that can base therapeutics for middle third growth. Dental Press J Orthod. 2017;22(2):21–6.
18. Dentino KM, Sierra-Vasquez D, Padwa BL. Inferior turbinate asymmetry is a feature of the unilateral complete cleft lip and palate nasal deformity. J Oral Maxillofac Surg. 2016;74(4):797–803.
19. Sun J. Comparison of inferior turbinate hypertrophy in pediatric patients with cleft lip and palate. Master's Thesis University of Pittsburgh, 2023.
20. Rossell-Perry P, Luque-Tipula M. The Lima surgical protocol for cleft palate repair. J Craniofac Surg. 2020;31(6):1533–8.
21. Friede H, Lilja J, Lohmander A. Long-term, longitudinal follow-up of individuals with UCLP after the Gothenburg primary early veloplasty and delayed hard palate closure protocol: maxillofacial growth outcome. Cleft Palate Craniofac J. 2012;49(6):649–56.
22. Semb G, Rønning E, Åbyholm F. Twenty-year follow-up of 50 consecutive patients born with unilateral complete cleft lip and palate treated by the Oslo Cleft Team, Norway. Semin Orthod. 2011;17(3):207–24.
23. Saban Y, Chiara Andretto A, Bouaziz D, et al. Nasal arterial vasculature. Medical and surgical applications. Arch Facial Plast Surg. 2012;14:429–36.
24. Pilsl U, Anderhuber F. The external nose: the nasal arteries and their course in relation to the nasolabial fold and groove. Plast Reconstr Surg. 2016;138(5):830e–5e.
25. MacArthur FJ, McGarry GW. The arterial supply of the nasal cavity. Eur Arch Otorrinolaringol. 2017;274:809–15.
26. Ritter FN. The vasculature of the nose. Ann Otol Rhinol Laryngol. 1970;79(3):468–74.
27. Uddman R, Sundler F. Innervation of the upper airways. Clin Chest Med. 1986;7(2):201–9.
28. Ogle O, Weinstock R, Friedman E. Surgical anatomy of the nasal cavity and paranasal sinuses. Oral Maxillofac Surg Clin. 2012;24(2):155–66.
29. Mitz V, Peyronie M. The superficial musculo-aponeurotic system (SMAS) in the parotid and cheek area. Plast Reconstr Surg. 1976;58(1):80–8.
30. Pitanguy I. Surgical importance of a dermocartilaginous ligament in bulbous noses. Plast Reconstr Surg. 1965;36(2):247–53.
31. Patel RG. Nasal anatomy and function. Facial Plast Surg. 2017;33(01):003–8.
32. Rohrich RJ, Huynh B, Muzaffar AR, et al. Importance of the depressor septi nasi muscle in rhinoplasty: an anatomic study and clinical application. Plast Reconstr Surg. 2000;105:376–83.
33. Aksoy F, Veyseller B, Yıldırım YS, Acar H, Demirhan H, Özturan O. Role of nasal muscles in nasal valve collapse. Otolaryngol Head Neck Surg. 2010;142(3):365–9.
34. Bruintjes TD, Van Olphen AF, Hillen B, Huizing EH. A functional anatomic study of the relationship of the nasal cartilages and muscles to the nasal valve area. Laryngoscope. 1998;108(7):1025–32.
35. Kienstra MA, Gassner HG, Sherris DA, Kern EB. Effects of the nasal muscles on the nasal airway. Am J Rhinol. 2005;19(4):375–81.
36. Fattahi T. Internal nasal valve: significance in nasal air flow. J Oral Maxillofac Surg. 2008;66(9):1921–6.
37. Murthy VA, Reddy RR, Pragadeeswaran K. Internal nasal valve and its significance. Indian J Otol Head Neck Surg. 2013;65:400–1.
38. Fischer H, Gubisch W. Nasal valves-importance and surgical procedures. Facial Plast Surg. 2006;22(04):266–80.

History of the Primary Cleft Rhinoplasty

2

Percy Rossell-Perry

Contents

Introduction

For a long time, there was a concern regarding the impact of primary nasal repair in patients with cleft lip and palate. Surgeons have considered the potential effect of the growth of the nose and other nondesirable side effects, and their recommendation was to delay the surgery until adulthood. Gustav Aufricht in 1955 mentioned: "Please do not touch the nasal tip until the child is at least a teenager" [1]. This surgeon (Joseph's student and assistance) stated that a high rate of relapse is observed after primary cleft rhinoplasty during long-term follow-up (Figs. 2.1 and 2.2).

Controversy exists regarding the use of primary rhinoplasty, because some authors approved the conventional idea that early repair during primary rhinoplasty interferes with nasal growth [2–4]; however, sufficient scientific evidence that exists support its safety and utility [5–8]. A recent systematic review concluded that primary cleft rhinoplasty during cleft lip repair results in good outcomes with limited

P. Rossell-Perry (✉)
Health of Science Faculty, School of Human Medicine, Peruvian University Union (UpeU), Lima, Peru
e-mail: percy.rossell@upeu.edu.pe

P. Rossell-Perry (ed.), *Atlas of Primary Cleft Rhinoplasty*,
https://doi.org/10.1007/978-3-031-68012-0_2

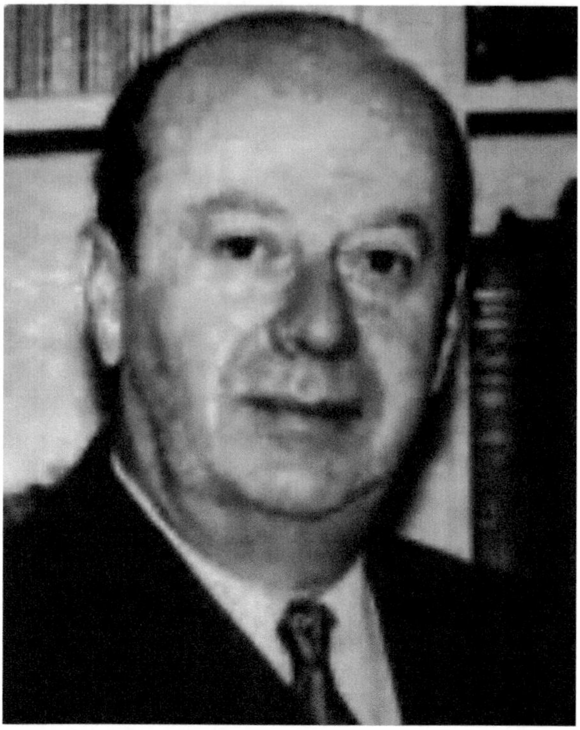

Fig. 2.1 Gustav Aufricht (1894–1980)

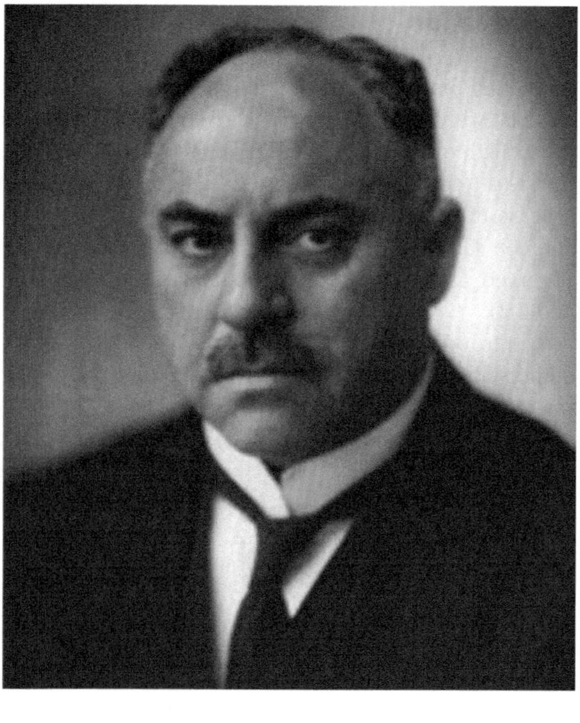

Fig. 2.2 Jacques Joseph (1865–1934)

or no effect on nasal growth [9]. Personally, based on my experience and published studies, I have confirmed the low rate of relapse and nondesirable effects after long-term follow-up [10–13].

The psychological impact of the sequelae in patients with cleft lip and palate during their childhood and adolescence has been increasingly considered, and many surgical methods have been proposed in order to improve the quality of life of these patients. However, primary nasal repair becomes important for cleft surgeons and considered actually in any cleft protocol as a standard of care. Blair and Brown first described a cleft rhinoplasty technique in 1931 and later Harold McComb's contributions regarding the abnormal gross anatomy and better understanding of the cleft nose deformity; different techniques have been published in this field [14, 15].

Most of the techniques described for nose deformity repair in cleft lip patients were used initially for secondary deformities and later used for primary correction; Blair and Brown, Gillies and Kilner, and Potter's are good examples of these methods.

The techniques used for bilateral cleft rhinoplasty have lagged behind those used for unilateral cleft lip because of the complexity of bilateral cleft nasal deformity. The first strategies developed to address bilateral cleft nose deformity were the Cronin and Millard's methods. Both methods were initially used for secondary correction [16, 17]. Cronin used bipedicled composite flaps from the nostril sills to elongate the nasal columella, and Millard promoted the "forked flap" method which consists of a two-stage procedure. Tissue from the prolabium is banked during lip closure and transposed to the columella in early childhood (therefore, Millard did not address the nasal deformity primarily).

Later during the 1990s, there were two important advances in bilateral cleft rhinoplasty: the evolution to primary single-stage nasolabial closure (the Trott and Mulliken methods) and the use of presurgical orthopedics [18, 19].

During the early 1990s, the use of an innovative technology named as Naso Alveolar Molding (NAM) was introduced by Grayson [20] as a columella lengthening method for bilateral cleft lips and has been used to improve congenital anatomy and facilitate the primary nasal repair; however, there is a lack of scientific support to validate its efficacy. This chapter presents a review of the history of cleft lip nasal repair to the reader.

The Unilateral Cleft Lip Nasal Deformity

Reports describing the development of primary cleft rhinoplasties have been published since the 1920s. In 1925, Blair and Brown introduced a surgical technique for cleft nose repair based on the rotation of the alar lobule complex as a pioneer in attempting primary nasal correction at the time of the lip closure. However, this method was mostly used for secondary deformities [1] (Figs. 2.3, 2.4 and 2.5).

Most likely, the first attempt at primary nasal repair was the correction of the nasal floor performed by Veau (1931), but the outcomes were consistently bad [1]. Vilroy Blair's and Barrett Brown's concepts were modified over the next 40 years

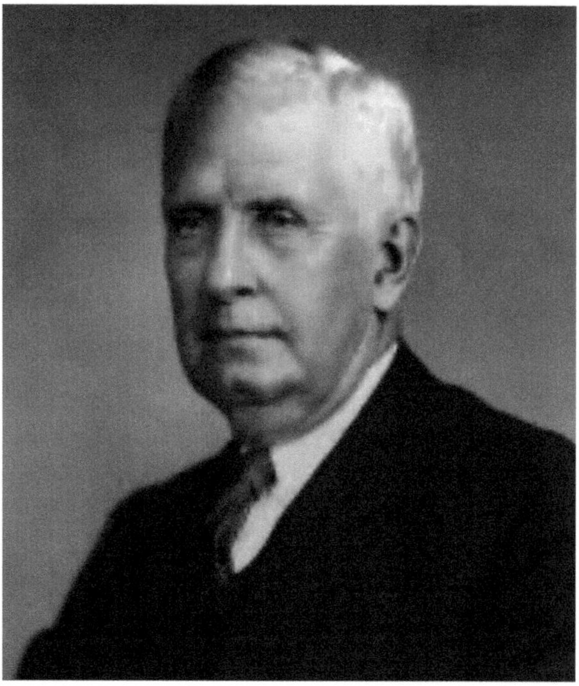

Fig. 2.3 Vilray Blair (1871–1955)

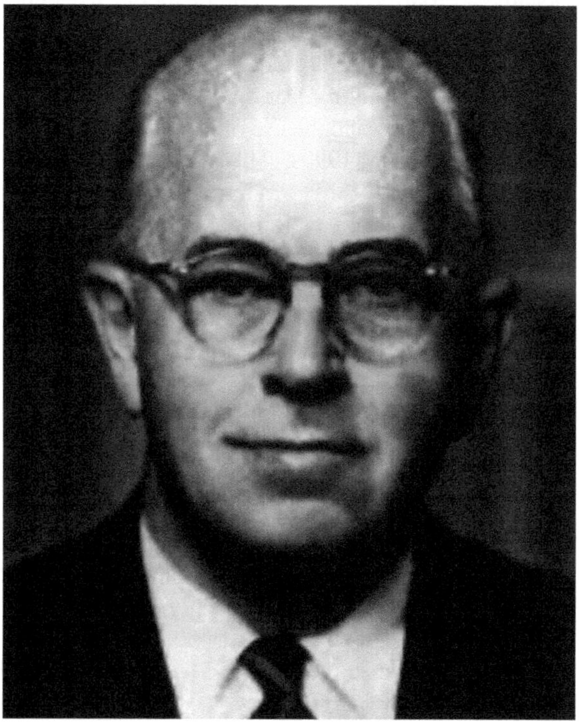

Fig. 2.4 James Barrett Brown (1899–1971)

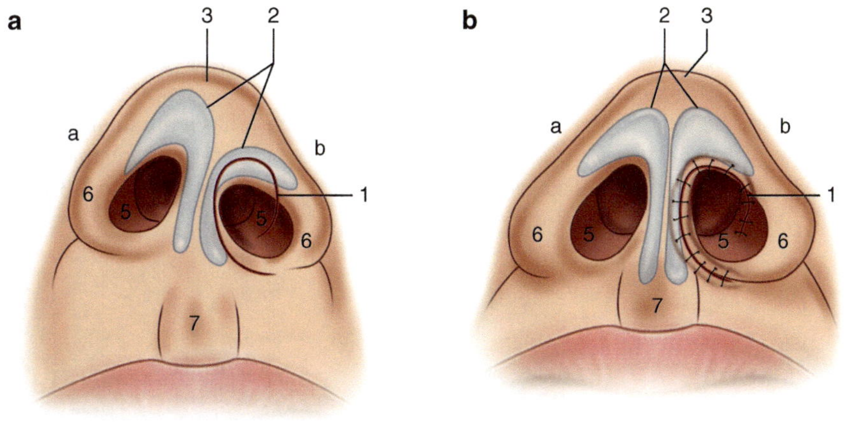

Fig. 2.5 Blair and Brown's cleft rhinoplasty. Initially used as a treatment for secondary deformities. (**a**) Preoperative view. (**b**) Postoperative view. a: Noncleft side. b: Cleft side. 1. Black line: Surgical marking following alar base and margin of the nostril. 2. Dotted line: Position of the alar cartilages on both sides. 3. Nasal tip. 4. Columella. 5. Nostrils. 6. Alar bases. 7. Nasal philtrum

by different authors. Gillies and Kilner performed one of these modifications in 1932, and their method was known as the "alar shift" operation, which consists of the use of a composite chondrocutaneous hemicolumellar flap [21] (Figs. 2.6, 2.7 and 2.8). Later, their technique of medial to lateral composite chondrocutaneous flap displacement was modified by Potter in 1954 [22] who performed lateral to medial advancement in a V-Y form, which is actually one of the more popular repairs (Fig. 2.9). A modification of the Potter's concept (combined with skin excision from the affected alar rim) was published by Victor Spina in 1968 and used in secondary and primary correction of the unilateral cleft lip nose. This method is likely one of the first published descriptions of primary unilateral cleft rhinoplasty [23]. Columellar lengthening (an important step in addressing the nasal deformity) was probably initially described by Millard Jr. in 1955 using the C flap during the rotational advancement lip repair (Millard type II variation of the technique) [1] (Figs. 2.10 and 2.11).

Later, Berkeley in 1959 proposed the primary correction of the nasal tip based on the open tip approach with a heminasal rotation and treating the shortness of the lateral wall of the nasal vestibule using a Z plasty [24] (Figs. 2.12 and 2.13).

It is important to mention that most of the methods proposed during those years were described for the treatment of secondary nose corrections in patients with unilateral cleft lip and later used for primary repair. This situation was due to the rejection of primary nose treatments because of concerns about the growth of the nose during that time and the observed poor outcomes that we mentioned before. During those years, there was a lack of studies describing the abnormal gross anatomy in patients with cleft lip nasal deformity. It was not known until the Harold McComb's studies were published in 1975 [15] (Figs. 2.14 and 2.15).

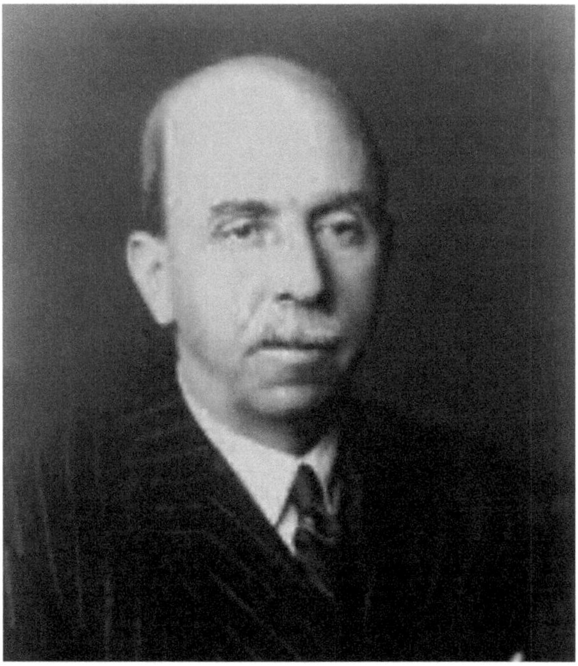

Fig. 2.6 Sir Harold Delf Gillies (1882–1960)

Based on his findings, he proposed a surgical technique that was probably the most popular during those years. The method consists of the use of an elevating mattress suture introduced using straight needles after nasal dissection from within the vestibule through the alar cartilage and skin into the nasion area. Finally, these sutures are tied using bolsters and the affected alar cartilage is elevated (Fig. 2.15). These sutures are removed on the fifth postoperative day. The main limitation of this method is the high rate of relapse.

Another technique used initially for secondary correction of the cleft nose and later for primary repair was the reverse U-shaped incision described by Tajima in 1977 [25]. The method involves placing a semilunar incision (reverse U) placed on the dorsum of the nostril and creating a composite flap that is moved upward and medially using stitches to correct the nose. This method is still used actually for primary cleft rhinoplasty in combination with overcorrection of the affected nostril [26] (Fig. 2.16).

Some authors combine the reverse U incision with marginal skin incision producing an overcorrection of the nostril [27].

Later in 1986, Kenneth Salyer published a more conservative technique based on extended nasal soft tissue dissection for reshaping and repositioning them using temporary stent transcutaneous sutures [28] (Figs. 2.17 and 2.18).

During recent decades, few innovations have been reported, and most of the published techniques are modifications of the conventional methods. One example is the Potter's and Berkeley's combination published by the editor of this book and named as V-Y-Z [10]. This is another method widely used initially in secondary

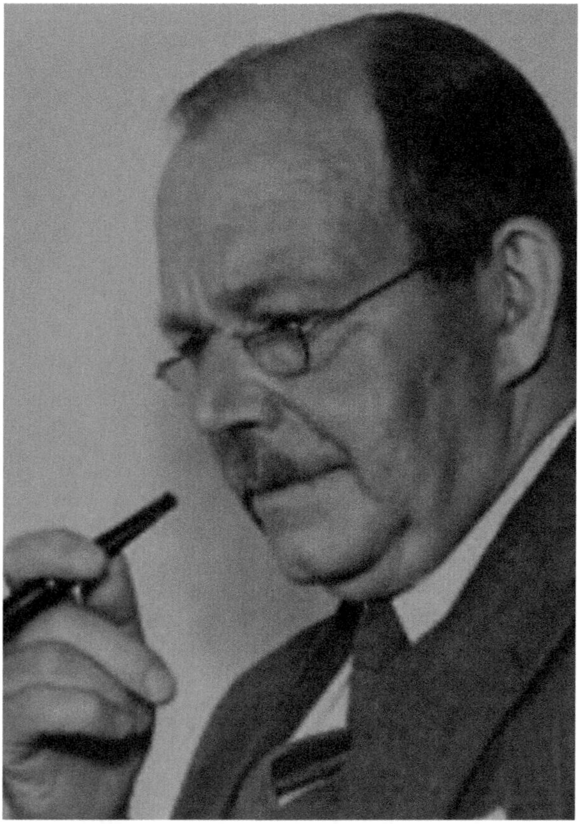

Fig. 2.7 Thomas Pomfret Kilner (1890–1964)

cleft rhinoplasty and later proposed for primary cases with success. Another contribution of the author, recently published in 2020, is the rotational composite flap technique used to correct minor deformities associated with incomplete cleft lip nasal deformity. The method combines a marginal and a small intercartilaginous incision to elevate a composite flap including vestibular skin and alar cartilage for repositioning. The flap is medially displaced in a rotational form [29].

Finally, Raymond Tse, a plastic surgeon from Ontario Canada, published an innovative method for avoiding the nasal tip dissection based on primary septoplasty in 2019, a more conservative method; however, more scientific evidence is required to validate this method [30]. His published study does not include long-term postoperative images, and statistical analysis was performed comparing with controls.

We may conclude that there are different efficient methods for primary nose correction, and their utility should be analyzed based on different variables such as postoperative complications, long-term outcomes, and facial growth disturbance.

In summary, actually it is important to clarify that the primary repair of the nose during cleft lip repair in unilateral clefts is the gold standard, and there is a consensus regarding its utility and safety.

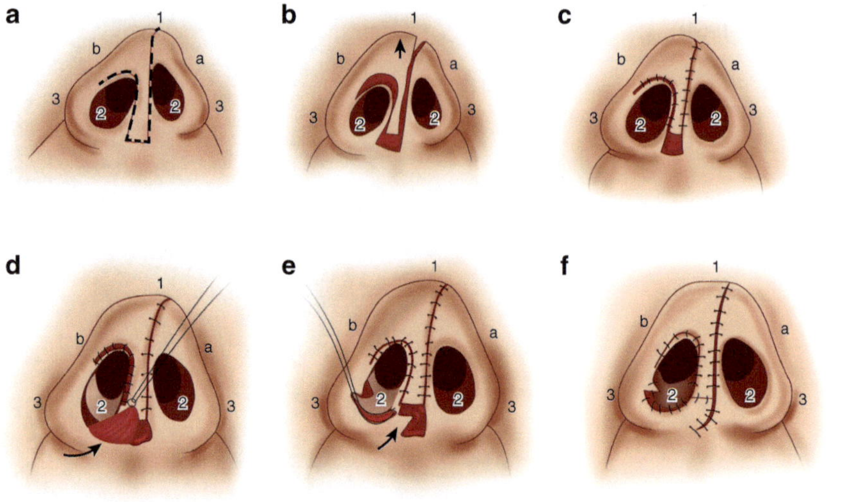

Fig. 2.8 The "alar shift" Gillies and Kilner's modification of Blair and Brown's cleft rhinoplasty. Initially, used as a treatment for secondary deformities. (**a**) Preoperative view. Dotted line: Surgical marking. (**b**) Intraoperative view. Surgical incision following marking. (**c**) Intraoperative view: Cleft side alar cartilage reposition. (**d**) Intraoperative view. Muscular repair. (**e**) Intraoperative view. A vestibular incision was made to release the nasal sill through small lateral z plasty. (**f**) Postoperative view. a: Noncleft side. b: Cleft side. 1. Nasal tip. 2. Nostrils. 3. Alar bases

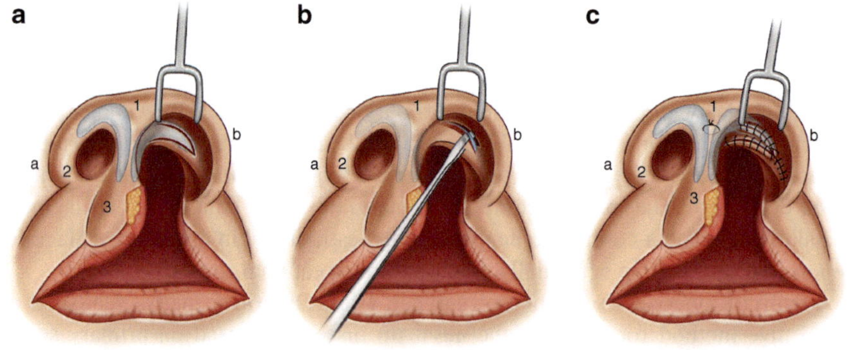

Fig. 2.9 The "V-Y" advancement flap cleft rhinoplasty described by John Potter rhinoplasty was initially used as a treatment for secondary deformities. (**a**) Preoperative view. Black line: V vestibular composite flap marking following marginal border and intercartilaginous border. (**b**) Intraoperative view: V composite flap (vestibular skin and cartilage) elevation. (**c**) Postoperative view. V to Y advancement and cleft side alar cartilage reposition. a: Noncleft side. b: Cleft side. 1. Nasal tip. 2. Alar bases. 3. Nasal philtrum

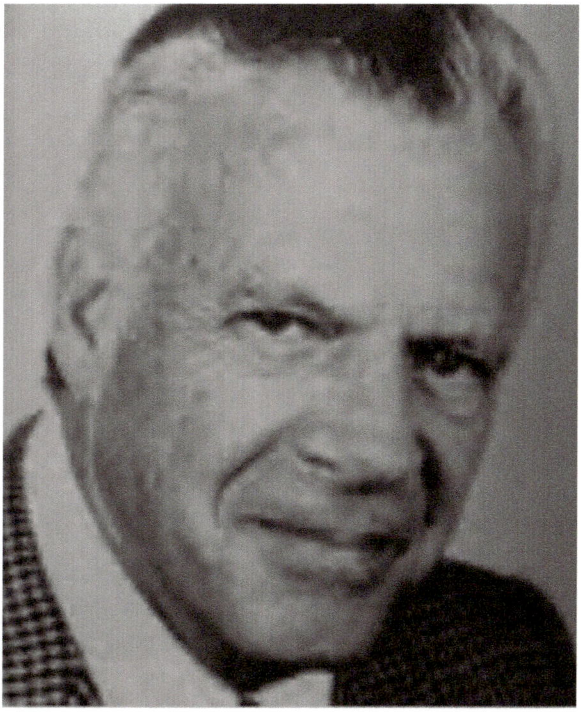

Fig. 2.10 David Ralph Millard Jr. (1919–2011)

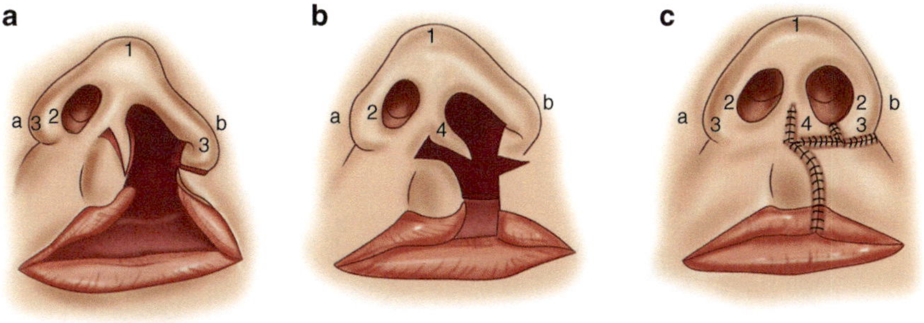

Fig. 2.11 The columellar lengthening, Millard's concept for primary unilateral cleft rhinoplasty during the rotation advancement method for cleft lip repair (Millard's II type cheiloplasty). (**a**) Preoperative view. Black line: Cleft lip markings. (**b**) Intraoperative view: Surgical incisions and flap transposition. (**c**) Postoperative view. a: Non cleft side. b: Cleft side. 1. Nasal tip. 2. Nostrils. 3. Alar bases. 4. C flap

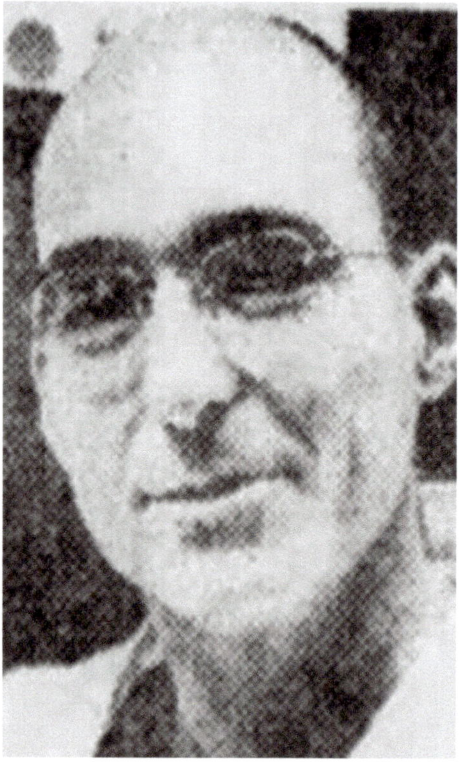

Fig. 2.12 Berkeley

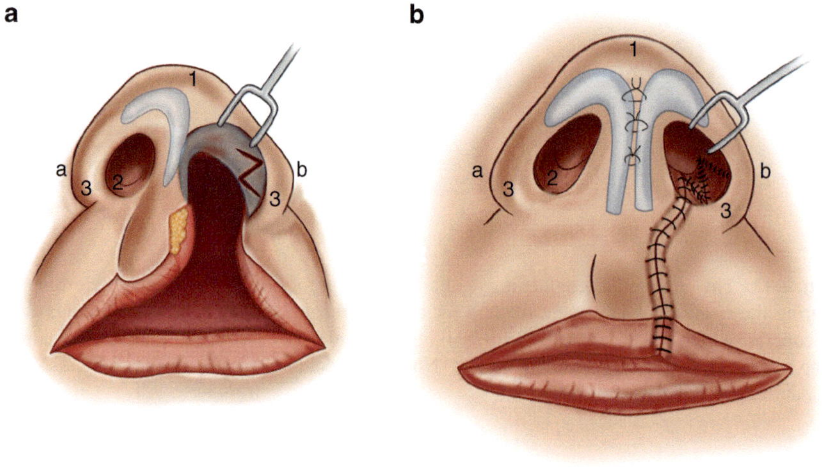

Fig. 2.13 The vestibular lengthening using lateral Z plasty. (**a**) Preoperative view. Black line: Lateral Z plasty design. (**b**) Postoperative view: Z plasty transposition and alar cartilage reposition using interdomal transcutaneous sutures. a: Noncleft side. b: Cleft side. 1. Nasal tip. 2. Nostrils. 3. Alar bases

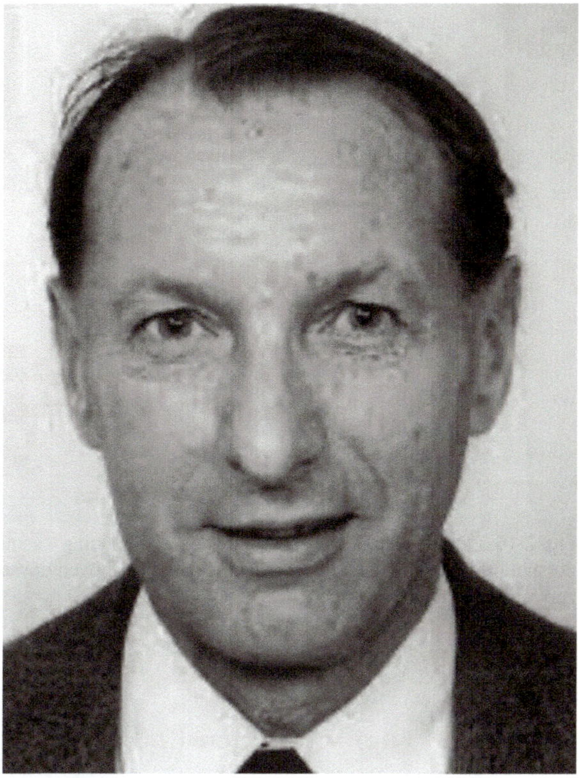

Fig. 2.14 Harold Keith McComb (1924–2012)

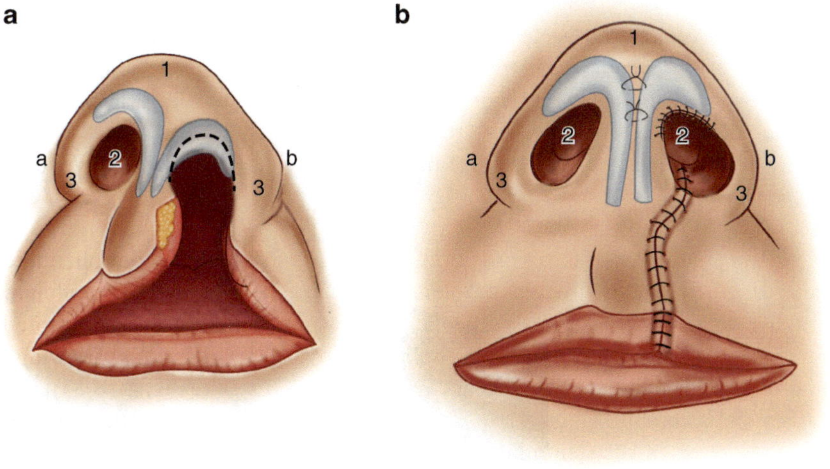

Fig. 2.15 The Mc Comb method is based on transcutaneous stitches. (**a**) Preoperative view. Shadow area: Zone of surgical dissection releasing the soft tissues from the skeleton. (**b**) Postoperative view. Cleft side alar cartilage reposition using transcutaneous stitches. a: Noncleft side. b: Cleft side. Arrow: Direction of the transcutaneous stitches. 1. Vertical transcutaneous stitch. 2. Lateral transcutaneous stitch

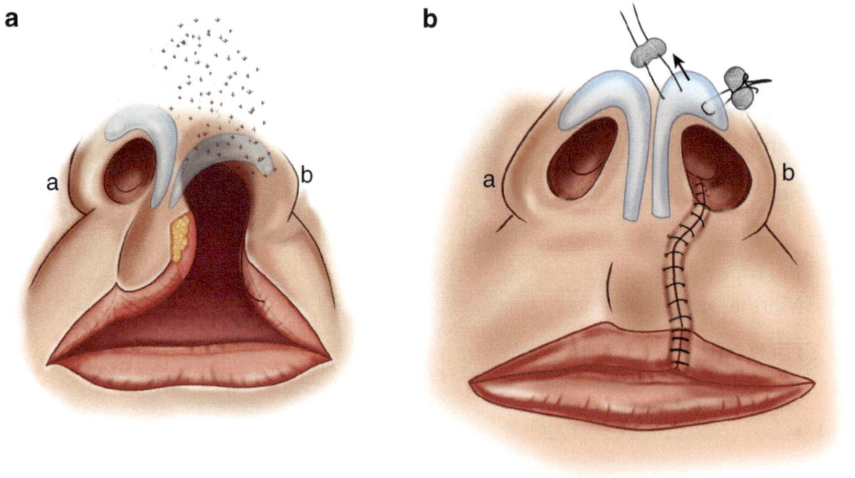

Fig. 2.16 The reverse U-shaped incision involves placing a semilunar incision (reverse U) on the dorsum of the nostril and creating a composite flap moved upward and medially using stitches to correct the nose

Fig. 2.17 Kenneth Salyer (1936–2020)

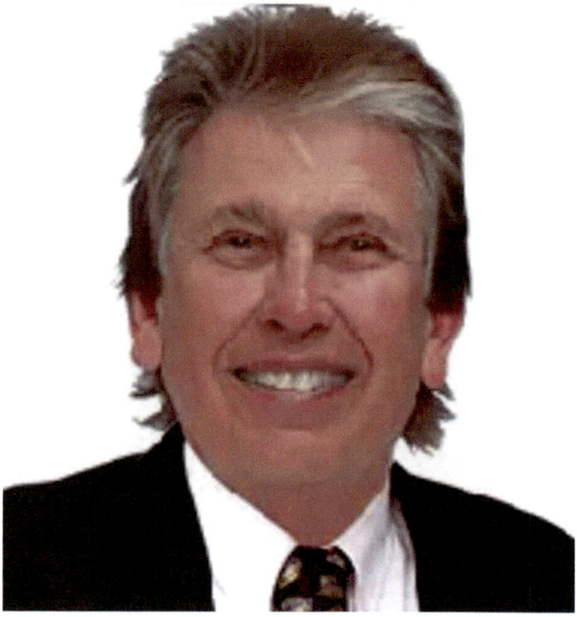

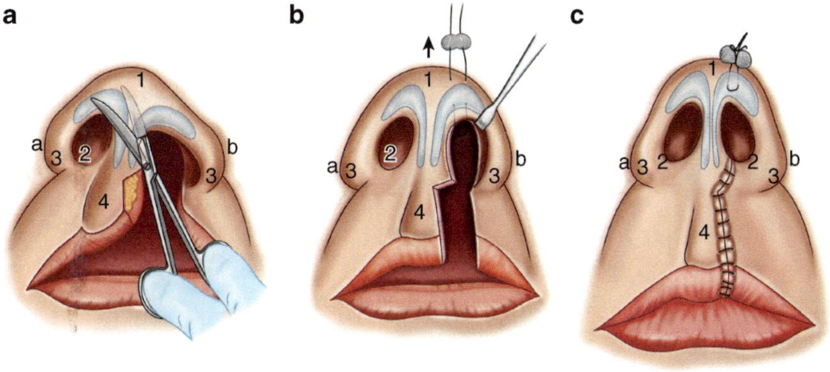

Fig. 2.18 Salyer's primary cleft rhinoplasty. (**a**) Preoperative view. After lip surgical incisions, nose dissection is performed through the medial incision. The alar cartilage on the left side is completely released. (**b**) Intraoperative view: Cleft side alar cartilage is repositioned using a vertical transcutaneous stitch. (**c**) Postoperative view. Final lip and nose closure a: Noncleft side. b: Cleft side. 1. Nasal tip. 2. Nostrils. 3. Alar bases. 4. Nasal philtrum

The Bilateral Cleft Lip Nasal Deformity

With respect to the primary bilateral cleft lip nasal deformity, primary attention was given to delayed closure of nasal deformities for secondary repair via staged columellar lengthening methods.

Initially, tissue excision during cleft rhinoplasty was introduced by Joseph [1] who performed skin resection over the marginal incision-placed cephalad to the alar rim in 1931. This method was actualized later by Mulliken [31]. Ralph Millard Jr. proposed a staged method for columellar lengthening using lip tissues and was known as "banked fork flap" technique. This procedure uses tissue from the prolabium for columellar lengthening as a secondary procedure. In fact, Millard's bilateral cleft rhinoplasty does not include primary nose repair [1] (Fig. 2.19).

Previously, Cronin described a method for bilateral cleft lip nose repair using nasal tissue as bilateral nasal floor advancement flaps in a V-Y form [1] (Figs. 2.20 and 2.21). After first descriptions by Cronin in 1958 using V-Y flaps from the nostril sills and Millard in 1967 with the "forked flap" two-stage method, there were not any important contributions until the 1990s.

During this decade, important contributions have been made to address bilateral cleft nose deformity. McComb described initially a primary forked flap method for nasal repair that delays the cleft lip repair. However, later this author associated the primary rhinoplasty with bilateral lip adhesion, highlighting the importance of the synchronous correction of the lip and nose. Finally, he described a bilateral cleft rhinoplasty using an external incision and opening the nasal tip for alar cartilage reposition. This author (based on his anatomical studies) postulated that the shortened columella is the consequence of lateral cartilage malposition being spread too laterally and flattening the columellar height instead of shortening of this nasal component [32].

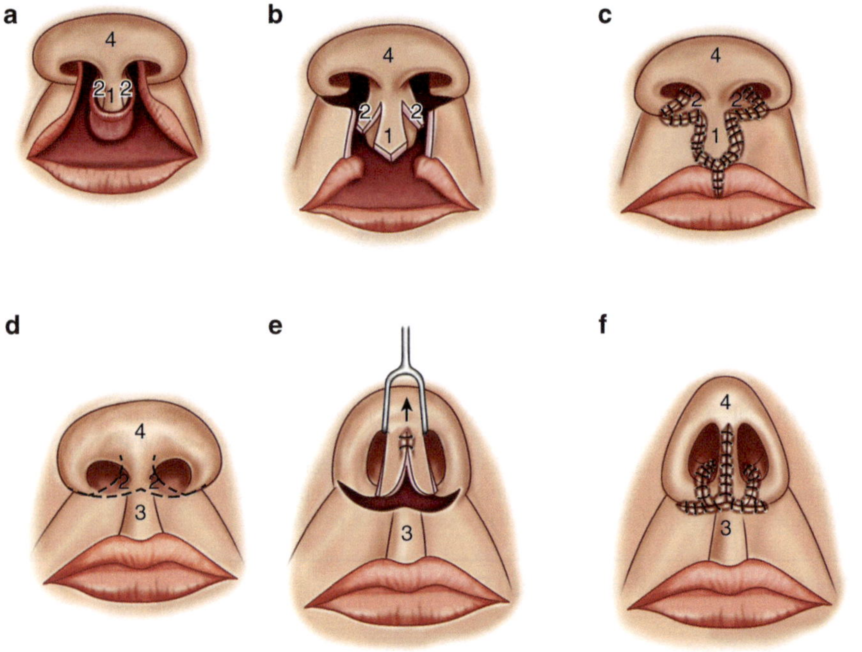

Fig. 2.19 Millard's "banked fork flap" method for primary cleft rhinoplasty in patients with bilateral cleft lip and palate. (**a**) Preoperative marking for bilateral cleft lip repair. (**b**) Bilateral cleft lip surgical incisions and dissection. (**c**) Postoperative view of bilateral cleft lip repair. (**d**) Second stage. Dotted line: intranasal and banked fork flap incisions. (**e**) Intraoperative view: Surgical dissection and forked flaps elevation. (**f**) Postoperative view after columellar and nasal tip repair. 1. Prolabium. 2. Forked flaps. 3. Nasal philtrum. 4. Nasal tip

Fig. 2.20 Thomas Cronin (1906–1993)

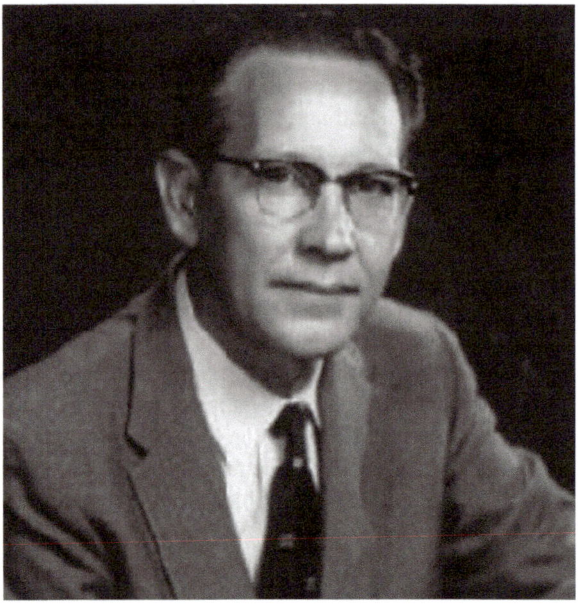

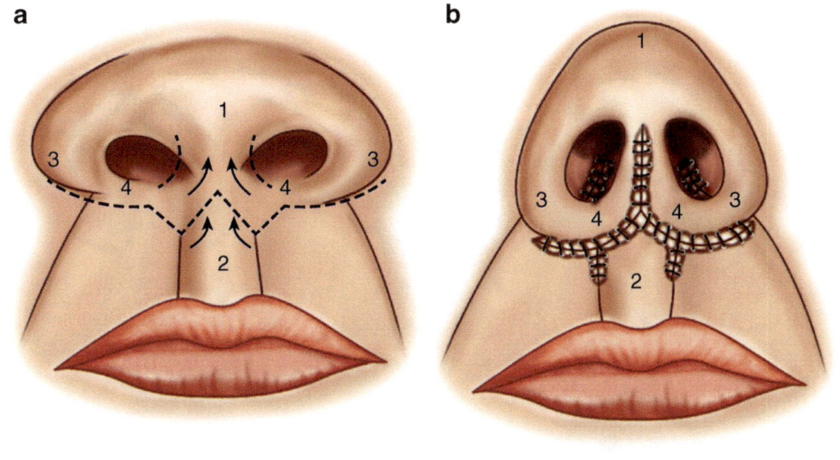

Fig. 2.21 Cronin's bilateral cleft rhinoplasty using the V-Y method. (**a**) Preoperative view. Dotted line: Marking the creation of bilateral bipedicle flaps. External perialar incisions combined with a membranous septum internal incision. Arrows: Direction of rotation toward the nasal tip. (**b**) Postoperative view: Nose repaired after V-Y advancement of nasal sill bilateral flaps showing columellar lengthening and nasal tip projection. 1. Nasal tip. 2. Nasal philtrum. 3. Alar bases. 4. Nasal sill

During recent years, bilateral deformity treatment has evolved from double- to single-stage methods. In 1991, Trott and Mohan developed a single-stage nasolabial repair method based on open rhinoplasty for alar cartilage reposition during lip repair [33] (Fig. 2.22). The same year Bardach proposed an open rhinoplasty to correct the nose deformity at later age as a secondary procedure [34]. Later during this decade, Mulliken based on his concept that "the columella is in the nose" (a single-stage nasolabial repair) performed a synchronous lip and nasal deformity repair. The method elevates the alar cartilages and repositioned them through marginal incisions. This technique was an innovative concept different from previous columellar lengthening methods. It is important to mention that the Mulliken's procedure uses tissue excision from the soft triangle and nasal vestibule to produce a "columellar lengthening" (Figs. 2.23 and 2.24). The use of soft triangle excision has been combined with a Tajima reverse-U incision for nasal repair including overcorrection of the nasal deformity, but the functional impact of this procedure remains unknown (Fig. 2.25).

During recent decades, the primary repair of the bilateral nasal deformity has been associated with the use of presurgical orthopedics, improving the management of the premaxilla, a key point in the success of bilateral nasal repair.

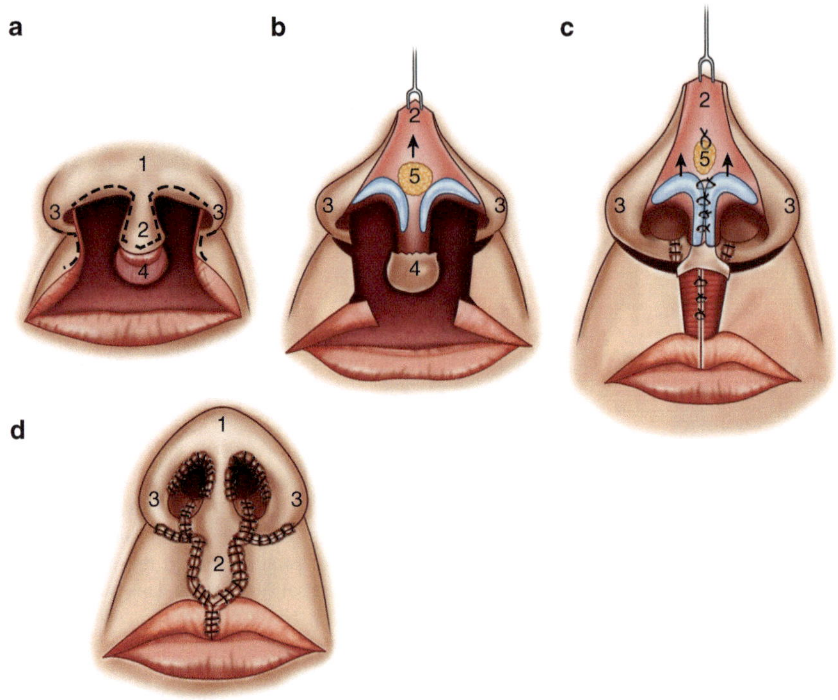

Fig. 2.22 Trott and Mohan's bilateral single-stage cheilorhinoplasty using an open approach. (**a**) Preoperative view. Dotted line: Markings. (**b**) Intraoperative view: Lip and nose dissection. The prolabial columellar flap was elevated to expose the alar cartilages and nasal skeleton. (**c**) Reposition and suturing of the alar cartilage and suturing of fibro fatty subcutaneous tissue to the nasal tip over the alar domes. (**d**) Postoperative view. 1. Nasal tip. 2. Prolabium. 3. Alar bases. 4. Premaxilla. 5. Fibro fatty tissue

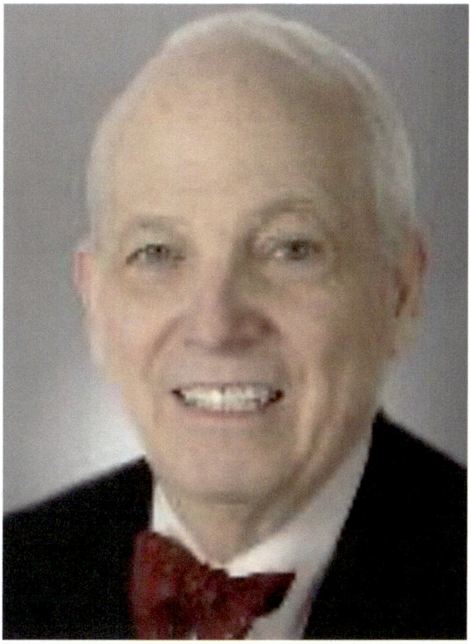

Fig. 2.23 John Mulliken

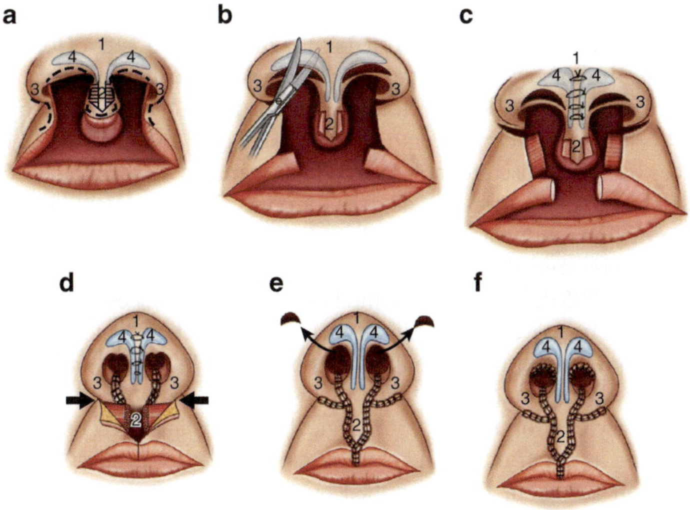

Fig. 2.24 Mulliken's synchronous bilateral cleft lip and nose technique. (**a**) Preoperative view. Dotted line: Markings. (**b**) Intraoperative view: Nose dissection through the bilateral marginal incisions. (**c**) Intraoperative view: Alar cartilage is repositioned through the bilateral marginal incisions and fibro fatty tissue resection. D: Intraoperative view: Alar base shortening. E: Intraoperative view: Skin resection over the marginal incisions and nasal vestibule. F: Postoperative view. 1. Nasal tip. 2. Prolabium. 3. Alar bases. 4. Alar cartilage

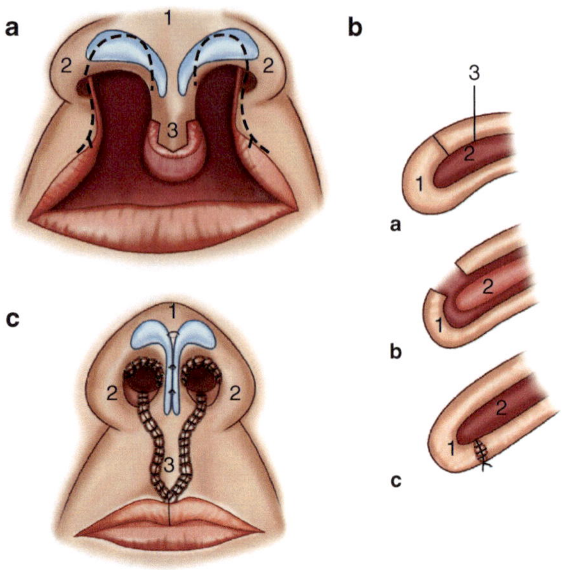

Fig. 2.25 The bilateral reverse U-shaped incision Tajima cleft rhinoplasty. (**a**) Preoperative view. Dotted line: U reverse and lip surgical marking. (**b**) Treatment of the skin at the level of the U reverse incision. (1: Skin. 2: Cartilage. 3: Dissection line.) 1. Nasal tip. 2. Alar bases. 3. Prolabium

Use of Presurgical Orthopedics

The ability of presurgical orthopedics to improve the quality of the lip and nose after primary cleft lip repair has been reported in the literature. In 1689, Hoffmann used facial binding to narrow the cleft preventing postsurgical dehiscence, and later Desault used a similar method to retract the premaxilla in bilateral cleft lip and palate patients [1]. Since the eighteenth century, bandages and mechanical compression devices have been used to mold the maxillary arch in these patients. Van Camp and Bardeleben used compression devices for presurgical treatment [1].

The use of lip taping was initially described by Hullihen in 1844 stressing the importance of presurgical preparation of clefts using an adhesive tape binding [2]. Later Brown in 1905 described the method as follows: "produces a narrowing effect by stretching the lip muscles and skin on each side" reducing the need for soft tissue to establish continuity of the orbicularis oris muscle [1]. The use of lip taping was well described and reported in the literature by Pool in 1994 as presurgical management for primary cleft lip repair [35]. Surgical methods are also considered in this group, working as a soft tissue and skeletal preparation for primary repair. This is the surgical lip adhesion, first described by Gustav Simon in 1864, and is used mostly for complete bilateral cleft lips by attaching flaps from the lateral lip segments to the prolabium to reshape the lip and alveolus prior to the primary repair. In 1954, starting in the modern school, Mc Neil combined a frame with elastic bandages for protruding maxillary component management and then used an active plate series to mold the alveolar segments into the desired position [36]. In 1966, Griswold reported the use of an elastic band system to apply compression for protruding premaxilla correction from birth until 6–12 weeks of age in bilateral cleft lip

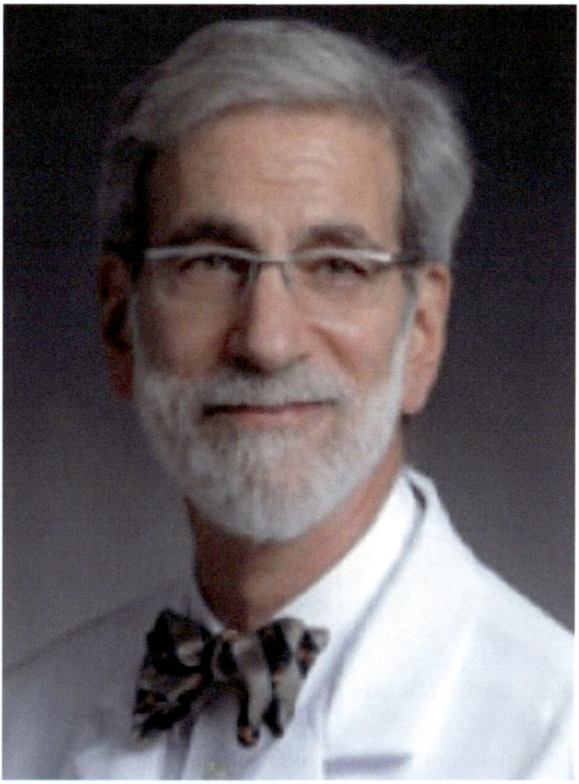

Fig. 2.26 Barry Grayson

and palate patients [37]. However, none of these previous methods address the nose deformity. Based on the Matsuo's neonatal ear molding concept, which proposes that the ear cartilage can be permanently shaped because of the effect of circulating maternal estrogen in the child [38], an innovative method was initially described by Grayson [39] (Fig. 2.26). This author proposed presurgical columellar elongation using an orthopedic device and primary retrograde nasal repair in a single-stage bilateral cleft lip and nose reconstruction. The method was described as Naso Alveolar Molding (NAM), and it is currently used worldwide as an alternative method (Fig. 2.27).

The utility of this orthopedic device is well accepted as a nonsurgical method for premaxilla management in bilateral cleft lip and palate patients. Premaxilla reposition and maxillary alignment are essential in order to provide an adequate scenario for nasal repair. Different presurgical methods (surgical and nonsurgical) have been described for this purpose without major differences in their effects. However, its use as a nasal shaper is under discussion because the temporal effect of the nasal molding has been observed and the requirement for primary rhinoplasty is necessary for long-term outcomes. The efficacy of presurgical orthopedics for nasal repair remains a strong debate actually because of the lack of scientific support to demonstrate it. A recent modification of the taping method was described as

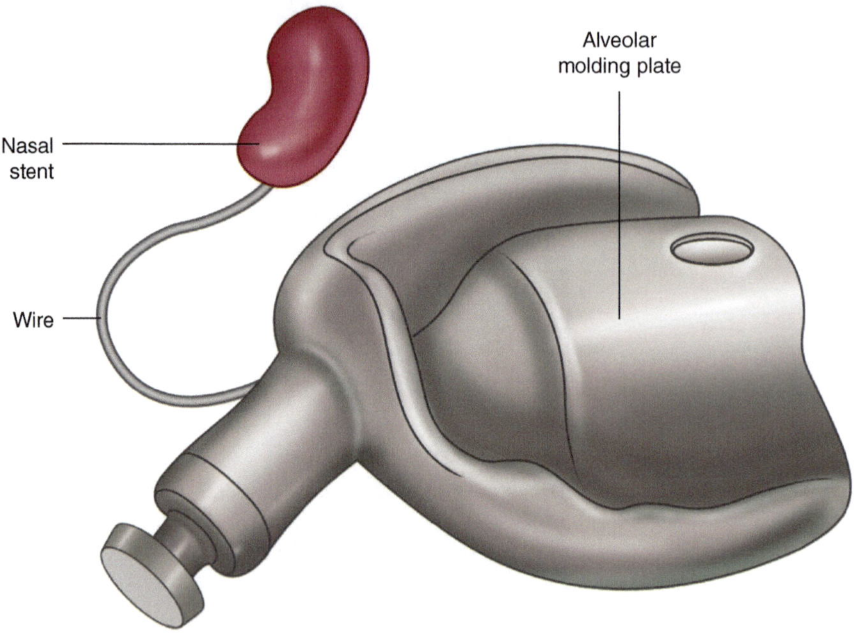

Fig. 2.27 The Naso Alveolar Molding (NAM) device

Dynacleft and used in combination with nasal elevators to mold the nasal cartilage [40].

It is a self-adhesive tape that helps to align skeletal and soft tissues in patients with cleft lip and palate. Dynacleft nasal elevators are plastic hooks that lift and support nasal tissues from a tether strip. A gentle adhesive placed against the child's forehead pulls it. The hook repositions the nasal structures; however, there is a lack of scientific evidence supporting this method.

Postoperative Nasal Conformers

Different strategies have been developed to improve or maintain nasal outcomes after primary cleft rhinoplasty. There is a tendency for the nose deformities to relapse, and several authors have developed different devices to maintain operative outcomes and prevent scar contractures inside the nose guaranteeing a long-term outcomes [2–4] (Fig. 2.28). Nasal devices have been created using different materials (acrylic and silicone) for that purpose. Even when they are used to prevent nose relapse, these devices are mostly useful for scar contracture prevention based on a recent study published by us [41]. There is a lack of scientific evidence supporting its effect to maintain or improve aesthetic nasal outcomes.

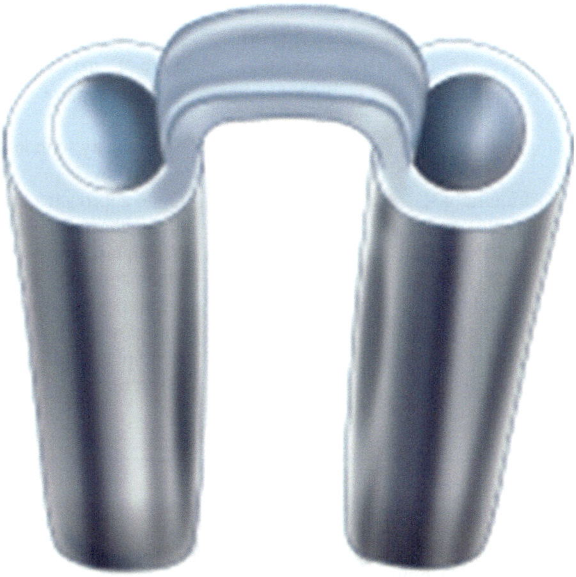

Fig. 2.28 Postoperative nasal conformers

Its utility is also related to the type of primary cleft rhinoplasty technique; therefore its use is mandatory for more aggressive techniques including vestibular incisions. For example, its use is essential after using the V-Y-Z technique; the extended incisions and vestibular scars may cause severe complications, such as scar contractures and synechia. The use of nonconventional devices such as wire hooks is commonly used to correct surgical technique deficiencies; however, there is a lack of scientific evidence to support these devices, and they may cause injuries and nondesirable outcomes.

Recent Advances

There are not relevant innovations regarding surgical techniques; therefore most of the published methods during the last years are modifications of previous descriptions (Table 2.1).

Recent advances in cleft nose deformity management are mostly in the field of molding plates and/or nasal stents. Three-dimensional technology has been used to design these orthopedic devices more efficiently.

This technology provides a more precise, accurate, and time-efficient management of the cleft lip nose deformity; however, more studies are required to validate its efficacy. Most of these studies are descriptive, short term, and limited to unilateral forms; therefore, it is difficult to validate its efficacy and actually is a common debate in cleft meetings.

Table 2.1 Recent advances in primary cleft rhinoplasty [9]

Author	Age of repair	Type of repair	Approach
Salyer [7]	Not described	Only tip repair	Through lip repair
Gosla-Reddy [42]	<1 year	Septoplasty without tip dissection	Vestibular
Yoshimura [43]	2 weeks	Open approach + rim incision	Marginal
Lonic [26]	3 months	Open approach + rim incision	Marginal
Rossell-Perry [10]	3–6 months	Septoplasty + tip dissection	Vestibular
Lu et al. [44]	3 months	Open approach + rim incision	Marginal
Pinto et al. [45]	8 months	Septoplasty + tip dissection	Alar base extension
Bschorer et al. [46]	4–6 weeks	Tip only repair	Through lip repair
Tse et al. [30]	Not described	Septoplasty without tip dissection	Through lip repair

References

1. Millard DR. A rhinoplasty tetralogy: corrective, secondary, congenital, reconstructive. Little Brown & Company; 1996.
2. Huffman W, Lierle D. Studies on the pathologic anatomy of the unilateral harelip nose. Plast Reconstr Surg. 1949;4:225–34.
3. Kane A, Pilgram T, Moshiri M, Marsh J. Long-term outcome of cleft lip nasal reconstruction in childhood. Plast Reconstr Surg. 2000;105:1600–8.
4. Karp E, Scott A, Martin K, Zavala H, Chinnadurai S, Roby B. Developing an eye tracking protocol to determine children's visual perception of secondary cleft lip deformity. Cleft Palate Craniofac J. 2020;57:321–6.
5. Haddock NMR, Cutting M, C. Long-term effect of primary cleft rhinoplasty on secondary cleft rhinoplasty in patients with unilateral cleft lip–cleft palate. Plast Reconstr Surg. 2012;129(3):740–8.
6. Broadbent T, Woolf R. Cleft lip nasal deformity. Ann Plast Surg. 1984;12:216–34.
7. Salyer K, Genecov E, Genecov D. Unilateral cleft lip-nose repair: a 33-year experience. J Craniofac Surg. 2003;14:549–58.
8. Salyer K. Early and late treatment of unilateral cleft nasal deformity. Cleft Palate Craniofac J. 1992;29:556–69.
9. Zelko I, Zielinski E, Santiago C, Alkureishi LW, Purnell CA. Primary cleft rhinoplasty: a systematic review of results, growth restriction, and avoiding secondary Rhinoplasty. Plast Reconstr Surg. 2023;151(3):452e–62e.
10. Rossell-Perry P. Primary unilateral cleft lip nasal deformity repair using VYZ plasty: an anthropometric study. Indian J Plast Surg. 2017;50(02):180–6.
11. Rossell-Perry P. The surgical nasoalveolar molding: a rational treatment for unilateral cleft lip nose deformity and literature review. Plast Reconstr Surg Glob Open. 2020;8(8):e3044.
12. Rossell-Perry P, Olivencia-Flores C, Delgado-Jimenez MP, Ormeño-Aquino R. Surgical nasoalveolar molding: a rational treatment for bilateral cleft lip nose and systematic review. Plast Reconstr Surg Glob Open. 2020;8(9):e3082.
13. Rossell-Perry P, Gavino-Gutierrez A. Mixed dentition period follow-up of primary unilateral cleft nose deformity repair. Plast Reconstr Surg Glob Open. 2023;11(10):e5313.
14. Blair V. Nasal deformity associated with congenital cleft of the lip. JAMA. 1925;84:185–7.
15. Mc Comb H. Treatment of the unilateral cleft lip. Plast Reconstr Surg. 1975;55(5):596–601.

16. Cronin TD. Lengthening the columella by the use of skin from nasal floor and alae. Plast Reconstr Surg. 1958;21(6):417–26.
17. Millard R Jr. Closure of bilateral cleft lip and elongation of columella by two operations in infancy. Plas Recons Surg. 1971;47(4):324–31.
18. Trott JA, Mohan NA. A preliminary report on one stage open tip rhinoplasty at the time of lip repair in bilateral cleft lip and palate: the Alor Setar experience. Br J Plast Surg. 1993;46(3):215–22.
19. Mulliken J. Primary repair of bilateral cleft lip and nasal deformity. Plast Reconstr Surg. 2001;108(1):181–94.
20. Grayson B, Cutting C, Wood R. Preoperative columella lengthening in bilateral cleft lip and palate. Plast Reconstr Surg. 1993;92:1422–3.
21. Gillies H, Kilner T. Hare lip operation for the correction of secondary deformities. Lancet. 1932;2:1369–75.
22. Potter J. Some nasal tip deformities due to alar cartilage abnormalities. Plast Reconstr Surg. 1954;13(5):359–66.
23. Spina V. Repair of unilateral cleft lip nose. Cleft Palate J. 1968;5(4):356–63.
24. Berkeley W. The cleft lip nose. Plast Reconstr Surg. 1959;23:567.
25. Tajima S, Maruyama M. Reverse U incision for secondary repair of cleft lip nose. Plast Reconstr Surg. 1977;60(2):256–61.
26. Lonic D, Morris D, Lo L. Primary overcorrection of the unilateral nasal deformity. Ann Plast Surg. 2016;77(Suppl 1):S25.
27. Lonic D, Morris D, Lo L. Primary overcorrection of the unilateral nasal deformity: quantifying the results. Ann Plast Surg. 2016;Suppl 1:S25–9.
28. Salyer K, Genecov E, Genecov D. Unilateral cleft lip-nose repair–long-term outcome. Clin Plast Surg. 2004;31(2):191–208.
29. Rossell-Perry P. Rotational composite flap technique for primary incomplete cleft nose deformity. Plast Reconstr Surg Glob Open. 2020;8(6):e2870.
30. Tse R, Mercan E, Fisher D, Hopper R, et al. Unilateral cleft lip nasal deformity: foundation based approach to primary rhinoplasty. Plast Reconstr Surg. 2019;144(5):1138–49.
31. Mulliken J. Primary repair of bilateral cleft lip and nasal deformity. Plast Reconstr Surg J. 2001;108(1):181–94.
32. McComb H. Primary repair of the bilateral cleft lip nose: a 10-year review. Plast Reconstr Surg. 1986;77:701–16.
33. Trott JA, Mohan N. A preliminary report on one stage open tip rhinoplasty at the time of lip repair in bilateral cleft lip and palate: the Alor Setar experience. Br J Plast Surg. 1993;46(3):215–22.
34. Bardach J. Correction of the secondary bilateral nasal deformity: Bardachs technique. In: Bardach J, Salyer K, editors. Surgical techniques in cleft lip and palate. St. Louis: Mosby; 1991. p. 13.
35. Pool R, Farnworth T. Preoperative lip taping in the cleft lip. Ann Plast Surg. 1994;32(3):234.
36. McNeil C. Orthodontic procedures in the treatment of congenital cleft palate. Dent Rec (Glasgow). 1950;70:126–32.
37. Griswold M, Sage W. Extraoral traction in the cleft lip. Plast Reconstr Surg. 1966;37(5):416–21.
38. Matsuo K, Hirose T. Nonsurgical correction of cleft lip nasal deformity in the early neonate. Ann Acad Med Singap. 1988;17(3):358–65.
39. Grayson B, Brecht L, Santiago P, Wood R, Kwon S. Presurgical columellar elongation and primary retrograde nasal reconstruction in one-stage bilateral cleft lip and nose repair. Plast Reconstr Surg. 1998;101(3):630–9.
40. Vinson L. The effect of DynaCleft® on cleft width in unilateral cleft lip and palate patients. J Clin Pediatr Dent. 2017;41(6):442–5.

41. Rossell-Perry P, Romero-Narvaez C, Gavino-Gutierrez A, Figallo-Hudtwalcker O. Postoperative nasal conformers in cleft rhinoplasty: are they efficacious? J Craniofac Surg. 2023;28:10–97.
42. Gosla-Reddy S, Nagy K, Mommaerts MY, Reddy RR, Bronkhorst EM, Prasad R, Kuijpers-Jagtman AM, Bergé SJ. Primary septoplasty in the repair of unilateral complete cleft lip and palate. Plast Reconstr Surg. 2011;127(2):761–67.
43. Yoshimura, Yohko, et al. Secondary correction of bilateral cleft lip deformity with simultaneous Abbe flap and nasal repair. J Maxillofac Surg. 1998;26(1):17–21.
44. Lu TC, Yao CF, Lin S, Chang CS, Chen PK. Primary septal cartilage graft for the unilateral cleft rhinoplasty. Plast Reconstr Surg. 2017;139(5):1177–86.
45. Pinto V, Piccin O, Burgio L, Summo V, Antoniazzi E, Morselli PG. Effect of early correction of nasal septal deformity in unilateral cleft lip and palate on inferior turbinate hypertrophy and nasal patency. Int J Pediatr Otorhinolaryngol. 2018;108:190–5.
46. Bschorer F, Schneider D, Schön G, Heiland M, Bschorer R. The microsurgical approach in primary cleft rhinoplasty-an anthropometric analysis. J Oral Maxillofac Surg. 2018;76(10):2183–91.

Classification

3

Percy Rossell-Perry

Contents

Introduction

The author's philosophy for cleft lip nose management is based on individualized treatment of the congenital deformity since there is a need for an adequate classification and descriptive diagram that will allow for the selection of the surgical strategy. Conventional descriptions are limited to illustrate the affected anatomical level but not the severity of the deformity which is the most important criterion for individualized treatment. Veau's classification (1928) describes cleft palate classifica-

P. Rossell-Perry (✉)
Health of Science Faculty, School of Human Medicine, Peruvian University Union (UpeU), Lima, Peru
e-mail: percy.rossell@upeu.edu.pe

P. Rossell-Perry (ed.), *Atlas of Primary Cleft Rhinoplasty*,
https://doi.org/10.1007/978-3-031-68012-0_3

tion only according to the affected levels (I–IV) from the isolated to the bilateral forms; however, it is still used and considered in most of the studies related to the cleft palate surgery [1] (Figs. 3.1 and 3.2).

Similarly, Spina described the position of the cleft in relation to the incisive foramen and classified the clefts into four groups (I–IV) [2]. None of these classifications considered a description of the nose deformity; most likely, the first widely accepted method was the Kernahan and Stark's classification, which was published in 1958; they used a striped Y form method to identify the affected segment, but this method has the same limitation as previous method and does not include the severity of the deformity [3] (Fig. 3.3).

The clock diagram, a novel system developed by the author of this chapter, better illustrates the nature of the cleft deformity and its degree of severity. Based on this classification of severity, four basic components are used to describe the cleft deformity: the nose, lip, primary palate, and secondary palate [4] (Figs. 3.4, 3.5, 3.6, 3.7, and 3.8).

Three degrees of severity are assigned for each component and represented in this diagram by a four-point code to be used as an interdisciplinary form of communication. Recently, Fisher et al. [5] published an objective method for grading the cleft lip severity including the nose deformity using the columellar angle for that purpose.

We used a combination of conventional and innovative classifications for nose deformity description to provide a more individualized treatment.

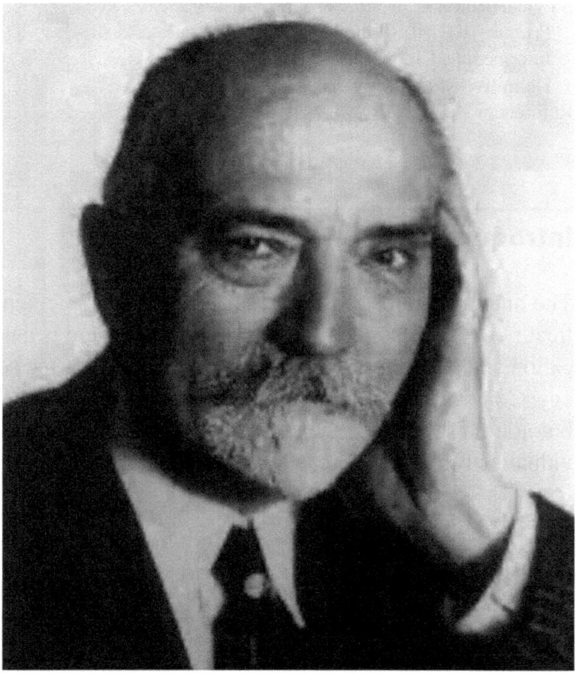

Fig. 3.1 Victor Veau (1871–1949)

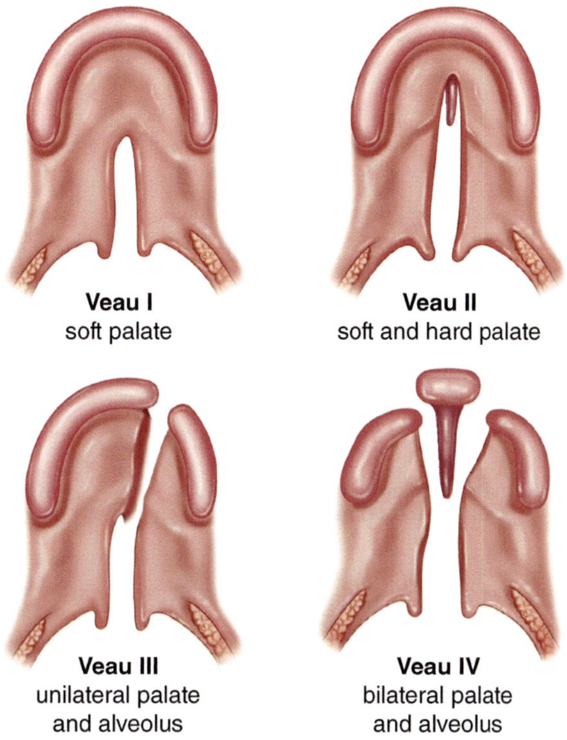

Fig. 3.2 Veau's classification for cleft palate

The complete or incomplete nature of the cleft lip is associated with differences in nose anatomy which requires different forms of treatment. Additionally, the unilateral or bilateral form of the cleft lip present a characteristic distortion of the nose.

Both criteria are essential for establishing a surgical protocol for the cleft lip nose deformity management; however, this conventional description is not enough for evaluating the severity of the distortion, and additional description is required.

The classification of severity and the clock diagram described by the author provide additional information regarding the degree of severity for each component of the cleft; however I accept that it is still limited in describing the complex nature of nose deformity associated with the cleft lip. Soft tissue and skeletal components should be considered to establish an adequate individualized surgical plan.

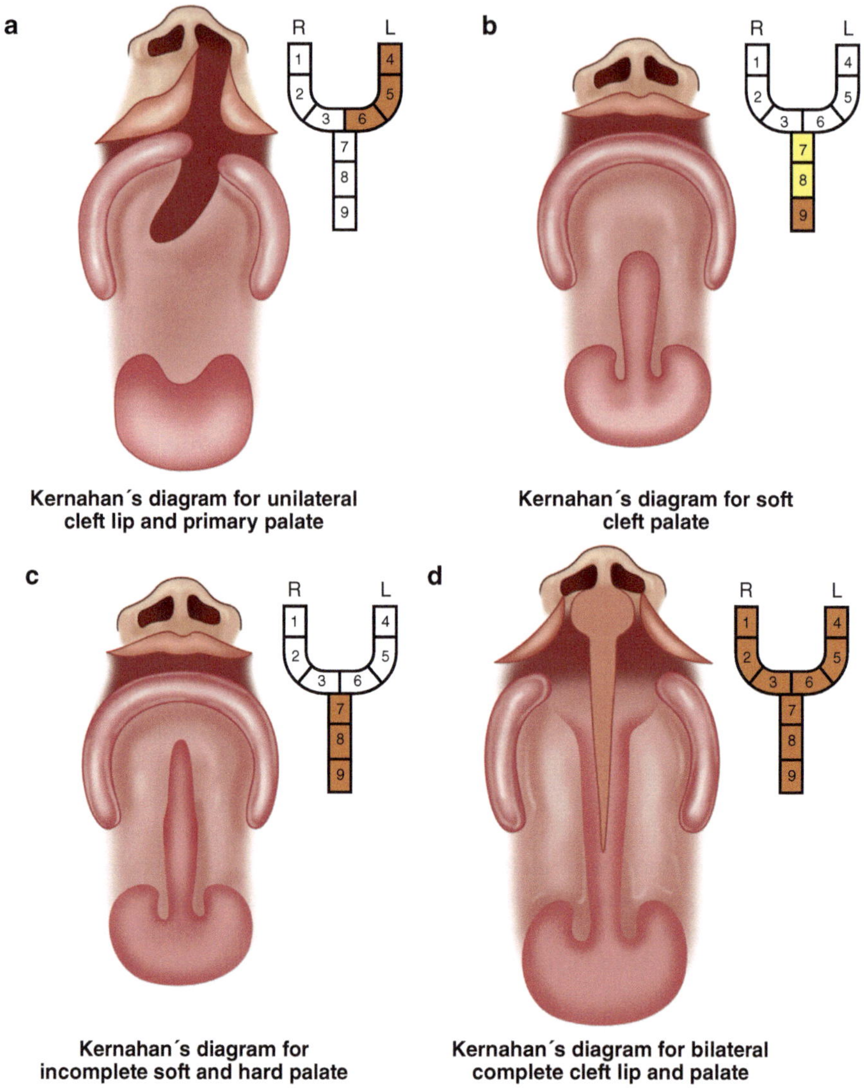

Fig. 3.3 Kernahan and Stark striped Y-shaped cleft lip and palate diagram. (**a**) Kernahan's diagram for unilateral cleft lip and primary palate. (**b**) Kernahan's diagram for soft cleft palate. (**c**) Kernahan's diagram for incomplete soft and hard palate. (**d**) Kernahan's diagram for bilateral complete cleft lip and palate

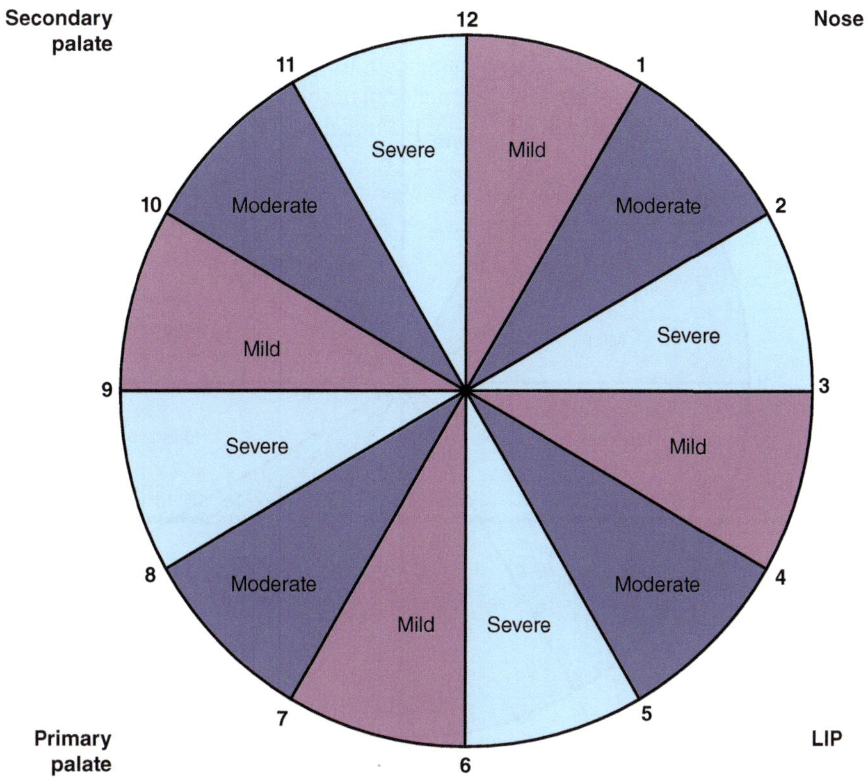

Fig. 3.4 Clock diagram of the Lima Outreach Surgical center clock diagram

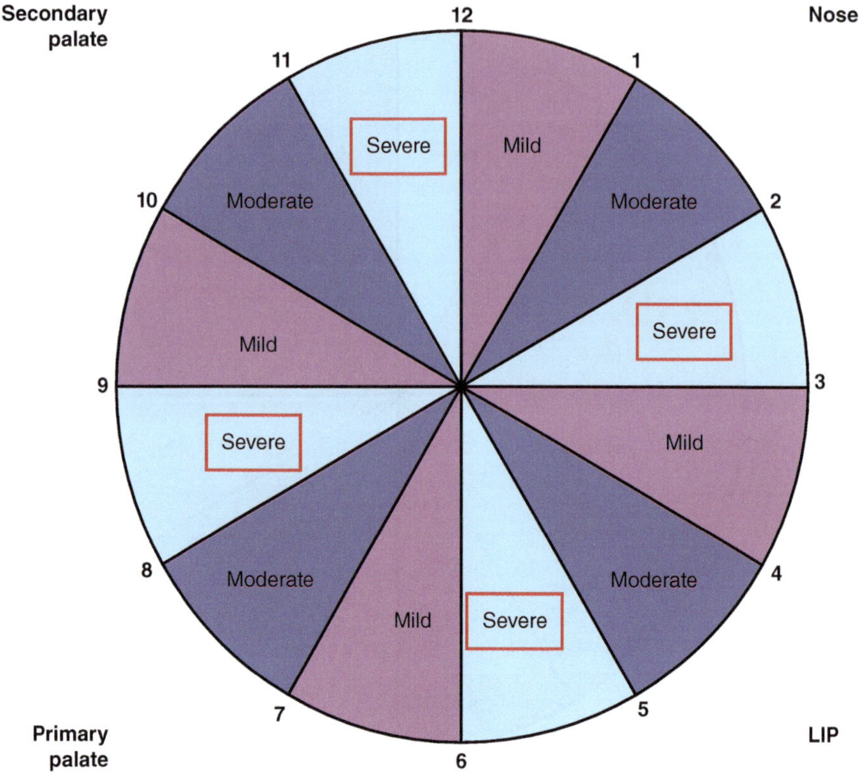

Fig. 3.5 Unilateral cleft lip and palate description using the clock diagram

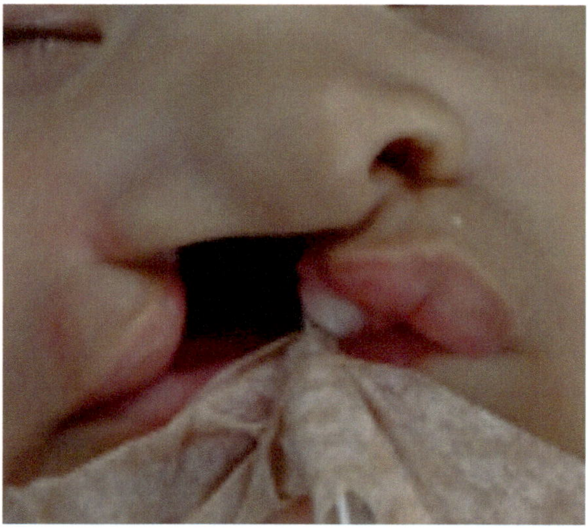

Fig. 3.6 Unilateral cleft lip and palate described in Fig. 3.5 using the clock diagram (cleft code: 3–6–9–12)

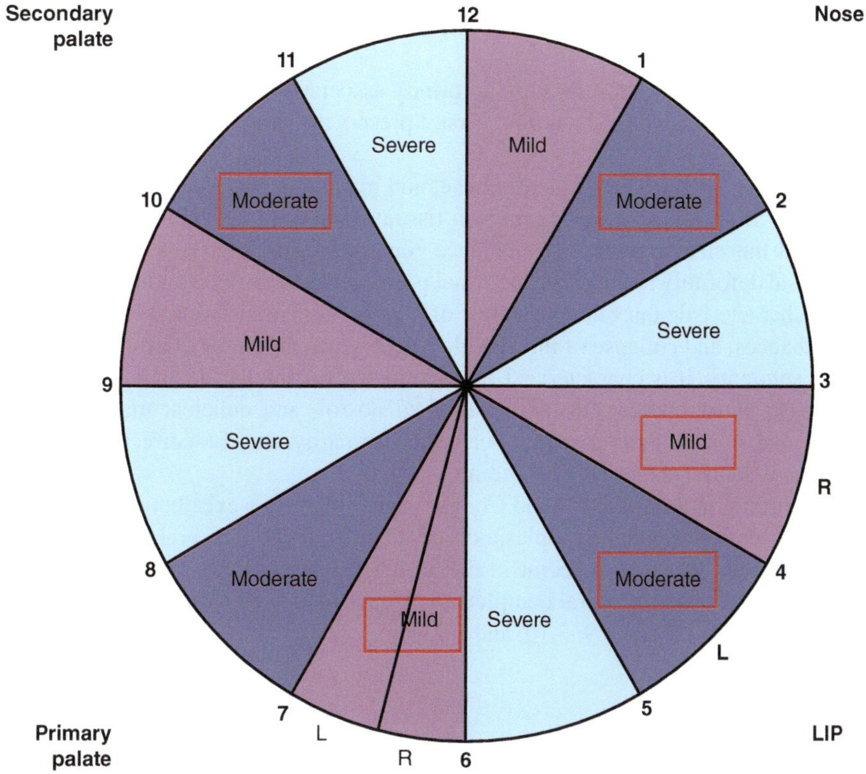

Fig. 3.7 Bilateral cleft lip and palate description using the clock diagram. R, right; L, left

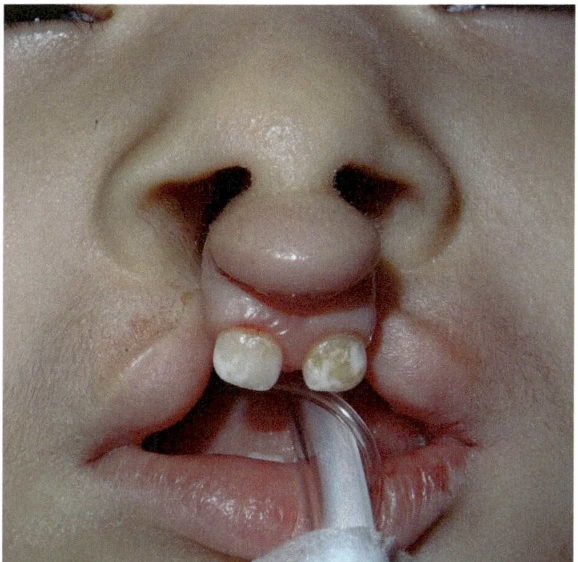

Fig. 3.8 Bilateral cleft lip and palate described in Fig. 3.7 using the clock diagram (cleft code: 2–4(5)–7–11)

Unilateral Complete Cleft Lip Nose

The author's classification for nose deformity associated with cleft lip and palate is the first description in the literature. First, I present the conventional description for cleft lip nose.

This type of cleft affects the lip, nose, and maxilla in one side and involves the structural framework as well as the soft tissue of the nose. The abnormal insertion of facial muscles produces an imbalance compounded by the skeletal hypoplasia, and nasal deformity includes an abnormal position of the nasal tip and septum creating a characteristic uneven appearance of the nostril in association with functional disturbances, and collapse of the maxillary arch worsens the nose deformity.

In summary, it is characterized by asymmetry, columellar deviation, displaced alar base wider and retrodisplaced affected nostril, and deficient maxilla. Even when total septal correction is not performed primarily, anterior correction appears to be an essential component according to Tse [6].

According to a study by David Chong, some differences exist between the right and left sides, with more hypoplasia observed in the right unilateral cleft lips. This condition may affect the outcome of the primary nose repair [7].

In summary, the unilateral complete cleft lip nose deformity is characterized by the following [8] (Figs. 3.9, 3.10, and 3.11):

Nose asymmetry
Columellar deviation
Cleft nostril buckle inward
Maxilla deficiency

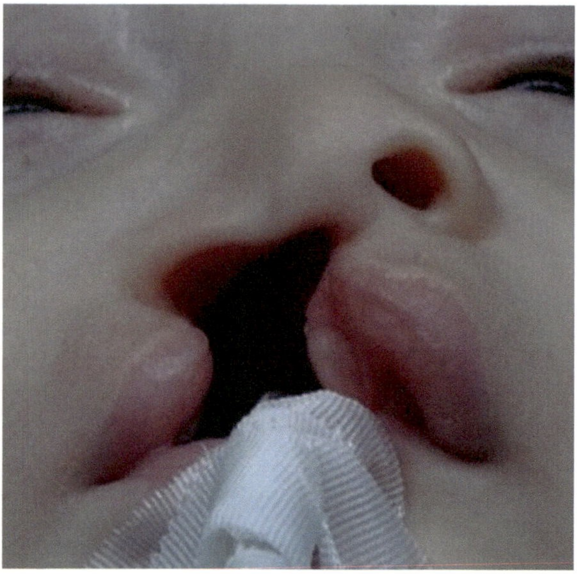

Fig. 3.9 Unilateral complete cleft lip nose deformity

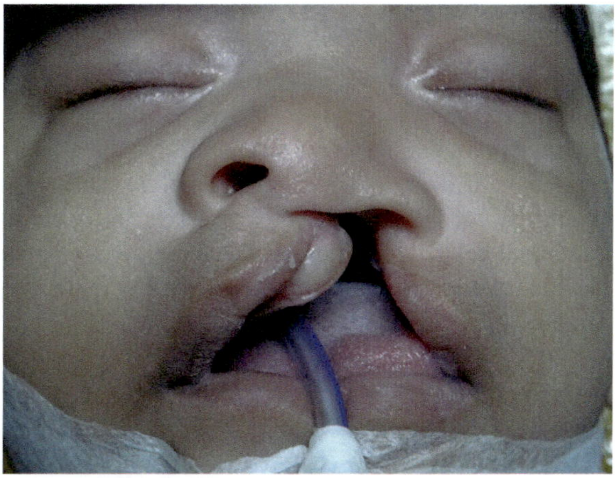

Fig. 3.10 Unilateral complete cleft lip nose deformity

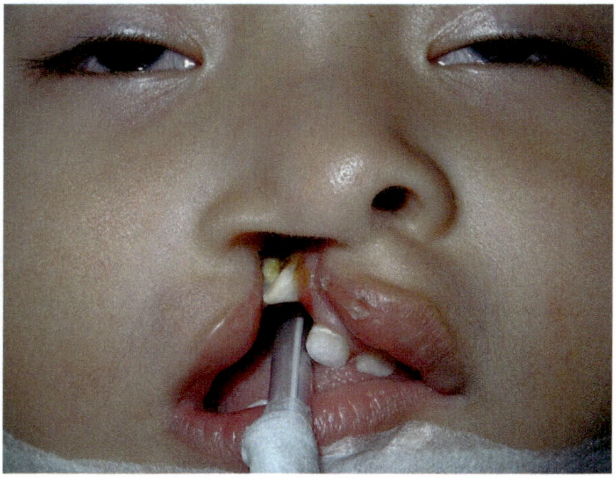

Fig. 3.11 Unilateral complete cleft lip nose deformity

Displaced alar base
Deviated caudal septum
Deviated premaxilla
Posterolaterally displaced alar base and pyriform aperture
Increased angle between medial and lateral crura
Shortened medial crus and lengthened lateral crus
Malpositioned upper and lower lateral cartilage

Unilateral Incomplete Cleft Lip Nose (Figs. 3.12, 3.13, and 3.14)

The incomplete form has a cleft affecting the white roll and vermillion associated with nose compromise characterized by downward displacement of the nasal ala and intact nasal sill. The nasal septum may be affected but in a mild form in comparison with complete forms. Incomplete cleft lip cases with a Simonart band should be considered as complete forms. In consideration of the findings of the author, all nose deformities associated with incomplete cleft lips should be treated, and the technique used for the nasal repair of an incomplete forms should not be the same as the methods used for complete forms.

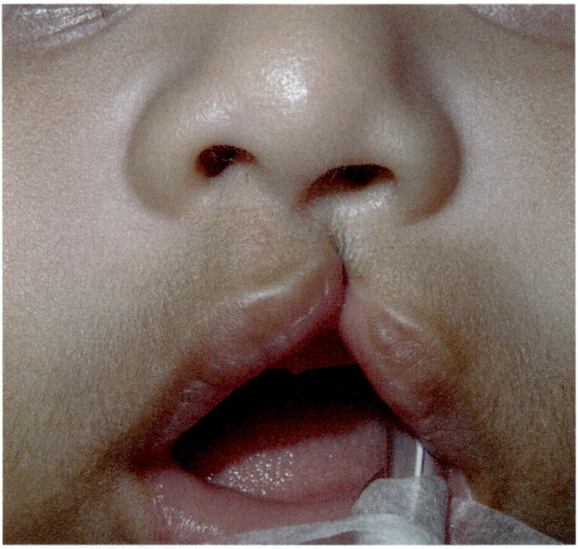

Fig. 3.12 Unilateral incomplete cleft lip nose deformity

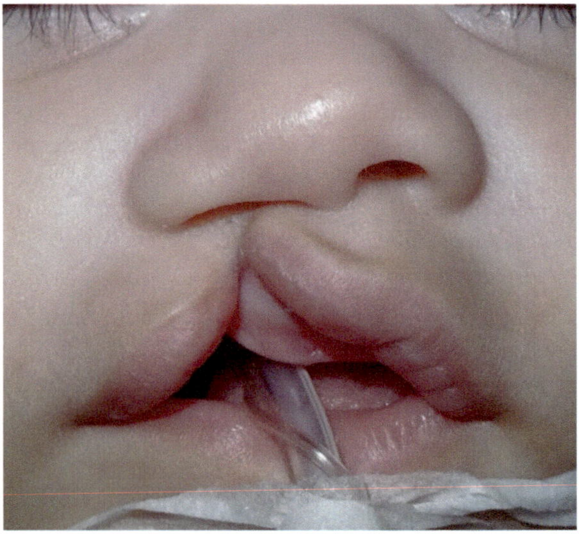

Fig. 3.13 Unilateral incomplete cleft lip nose deformity

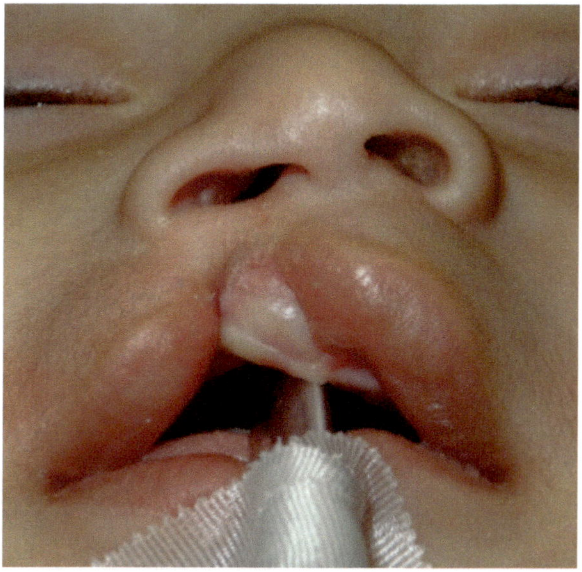

Fig. 3.14 Unilateral incomplete cleft lip nose deformity

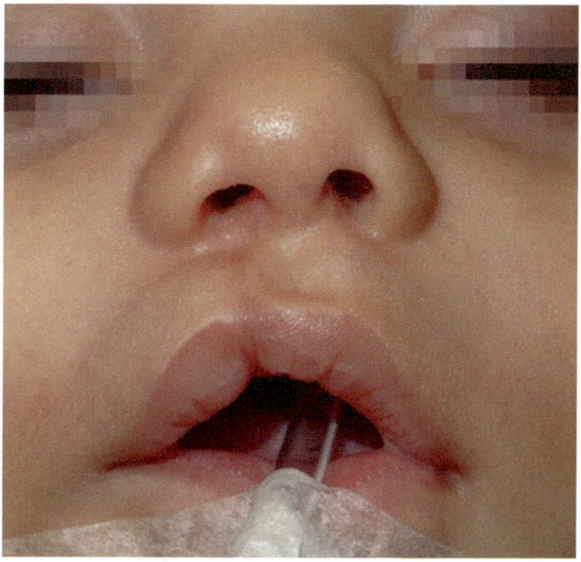

Fig. 3.15 Unilateral microform cleft lip nose deformity

Unilateral Microform Cleft Lip Nose (Figs. 3.15, 3.16, and 3.17)

This type of unilateral cleft lip is defined as a lip notch less than 3 mm above the normal peak. The characteristics of the microform cleft lip include the philtral groove, notched lip and vermillion-cutaneous junction, and a minor nasal deformity. Uncommonly, this type of cleft lip may affect the muscular component without an obvious cleft lip and associated with nose deformity, which is commonly minor in comparison with other types of unilateral cleft lip involving a depressed nasal sill, alar hooding, and alar base asymmetry, and its correction is sometimes limited to the nasal sill shortening.

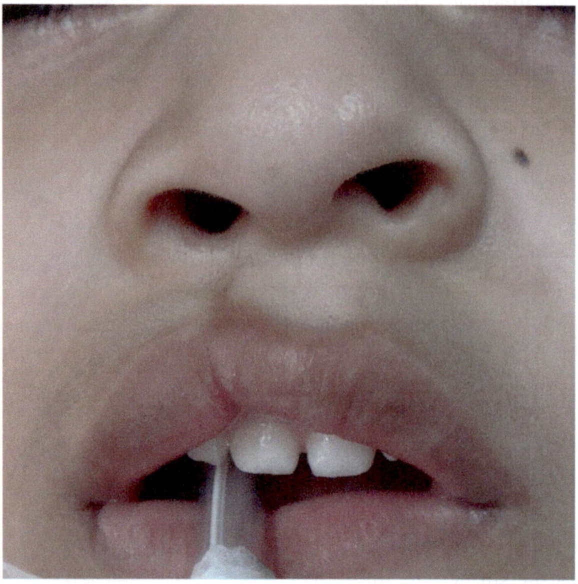

Fig. 3.16 Unilateral microform cleft lip nose deformity

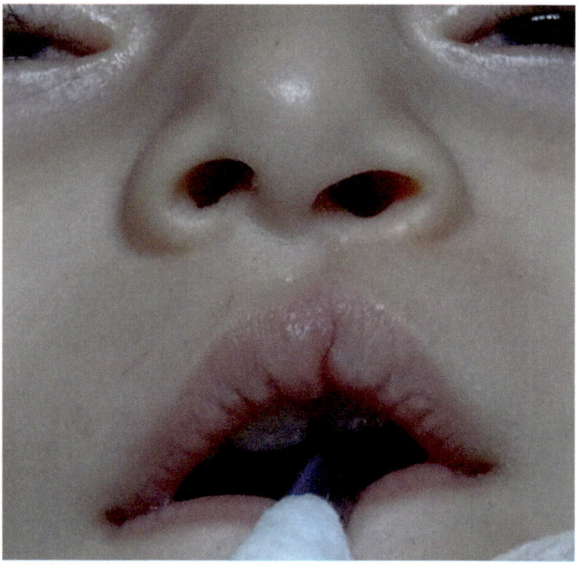

Fig. 3.17 Unilateral microform cleft lip nose deformity

Bilateral Complete Cleft Lip Nose

The bilateral form affects the lip, nose, and maxilla on both sides in association with protruding premaxilla and retropositioned lateral maxillary segments due to congenital hypoplasia.

The nose is characterized by a symmetric short columella (or absent), broad depressed nasal tip, and wide nose. The nasal septum is less commonly affected in comparison with unilateral forms and is usually observed in asymmetrical forms.

Adequate and early management of the skeleton is mandatory of the skeleton to provide good support for the soft tissue repair, and most of severe secondary deformities are caused by late treatment of the skeletal component. It is a common mistake that the performance of primary lip and nose repair with a severe skeletal malformation result in a sequel difficult to be repaired. It is accepted that skeletal component cannot be surgically corrected at early age because of the facial growth disturbance; therefore, early use of presurgical orthopedics or lip adhesion is essential in order to produce skeletal segment alignment to facilitate soft tissue repair. The use of presurgical orthopedics is indicated during the first weeks of life for skeletal alignment, but the efficacy of nasal molding is under debate actually because of the lack of supporting scientific evidence [9–14].

In summary, the bilateral complete cleft lip nose deformity is characterized by the following [8] (Figs. 3.18, 3.19, and 3.20):

Grossly symmetric
Wide nose and depressed tip
Short columella
Wide nostrils
Flared alae and vestibular webbing
Displaced alar domes
Increased angle between alar cruras
Protrusive premaxilla
Bilateral hypoplastic maxilla
Inferiorly displaced nasal septum
Absent nasal floor

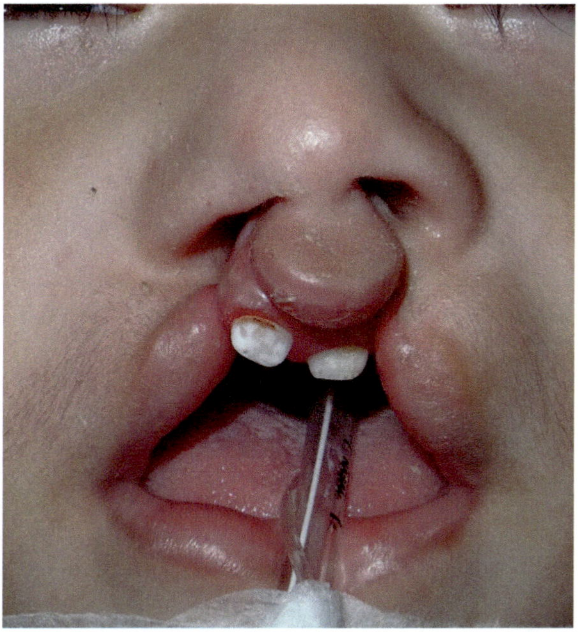

Fig. 3.18 Bilateral complete cleft lip nose deformity

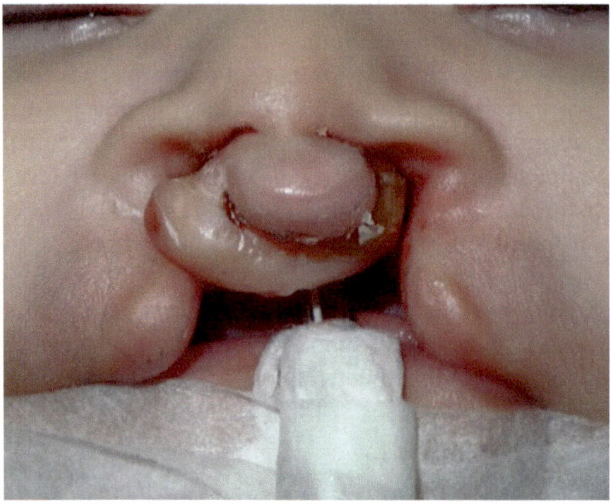

Fig. 3.19 Bilateral complete cleft lip nose deformity

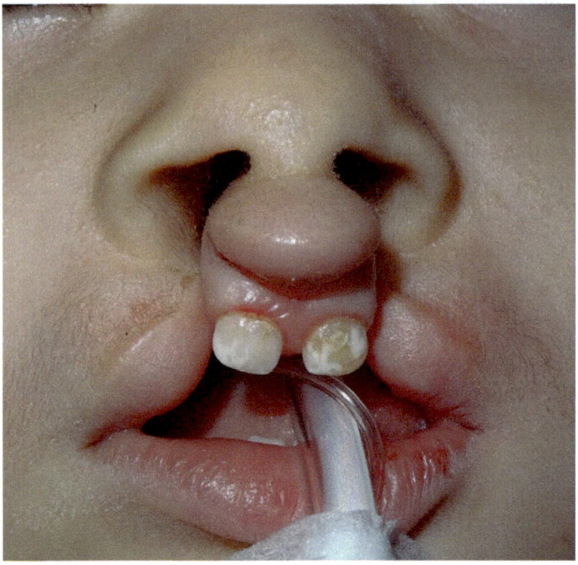

Fig. 3.20 Bilateral complete cleft lip nose deformity

Bilateral Incomplete Cleft Lip Nose (Figs. 3.21, 3.22, and 3.23)

The incomplete bilateral cleft lip involves the lip tissues and preserves the nasal sills. The skeletal deformity is preserved or affected in a mild form and may include incomplete cleft palate. A nasal sill is present but the columella is short and the nasal tip has a poor projection. Associated nasal deformities are usually more symmetric than complete nasal deformities. The presence of bilateral microforms is rare, and usually they are usually combined with complete or incomplete forms. The use presurgical orthopedics is not indicated for these forms.

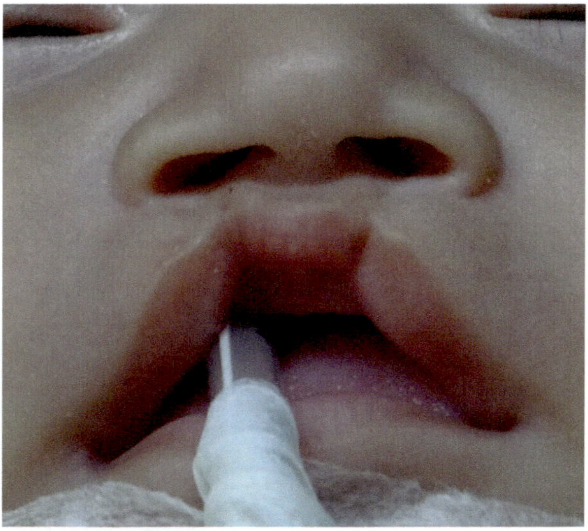

Fig. 3.21 Bilateral incomplete cleft lip nose deformity

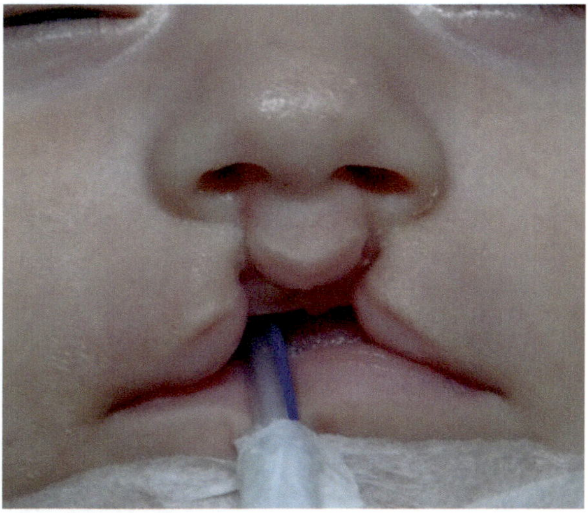

Fig. 3.22 Bilateral incomplete cleft lip nose deformity

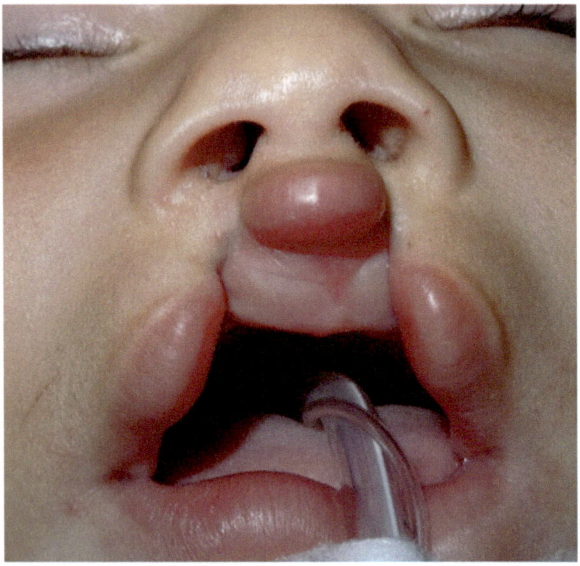

Fig. 3.23 Bilateral incomplete cleft lip nose deformity

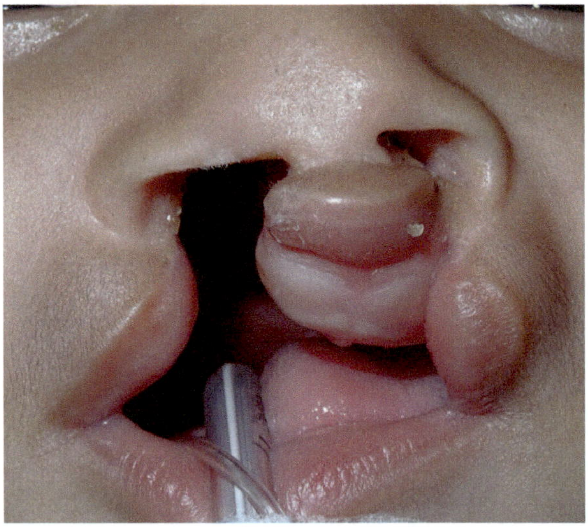

Fig. 3.24 Bilateral combined cleft lip nose deformity

Bilateral Cleft Lip Combined Forms (Figs. 3.24, 3.25, and 3.26)

Bilateral cleft lips are not always symmetric and may present a combination of complete, incomplete, and microforms; nasal deformities are asymmetric and require different treatments for each side. This type of cleft lip has difficulty achieving nose symmetry after the surgical repair. Presurgical orthopedics are an alternative for treating complete deformities on one side.

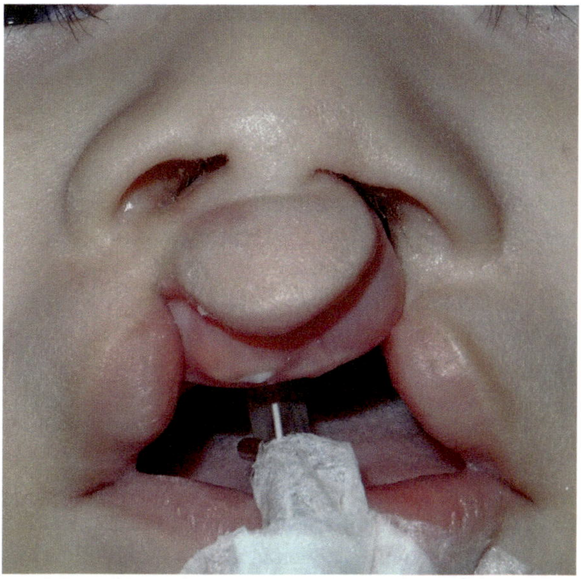

Fig. 3.25 Bilateral combined cleft lip nose deformity

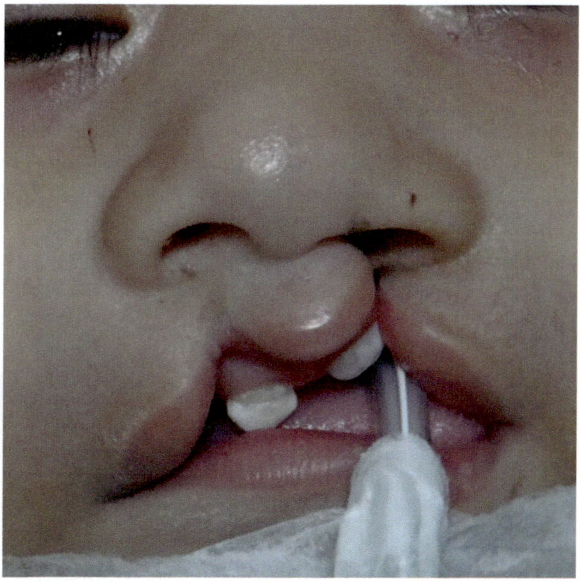

Fig. 3.26 Bilateral combined cleft lip nose deformity

The treatment of the nose using the nasal molding also has uncertain effects, and the outcome is mostly related to the primary surgery. It is also important to mention also that the nasal molding used in presurgical orthopedics is always associated with primary cleft rhinoplasty; therefore, it is not possible to estimate whether the outcome is due to the molding, surgery, or both.

Lima Outreach Surgical Center Classification of Severity

A classification of cleft lip and palate severity was created by the author, including a descriptive diagram named the "clock diagram" [4], and four components were considered for the primary cases as follows:

Upper lip, the degree of severity is estimated based on differences in the height of the lip between the cleft and noncleft sides (unilateral) or between the right and left sides (bilateral). Three degrees may be observed:

Mild (difference is less than 3 mm)
Moderate (difference is between 3 and 6 mm)
Severe (difference is more than 6 mm)

Nose, in unilateral the degree of severity is estimated based on the angle of the columellar deviation, as follows:

Mild (columellar angle greater than 60°) (Figs. 3.27)
Moderate (columellar angle between 30° and 60°) (Figs. 3.28)
Severe (columellar angle is less than 30°) (Figs. 3.29)

In bilateral, the degree of severity is estimated based on columellar height as follows:

Mild (columellar height is equal or greater than 4 mm) (Figs. 3.30)
Moderate (columellar height is between 2 and 4 mm) (Figs. 3.31)
Severe (columellar height is less than 2 mm) (Figs. 3.32)

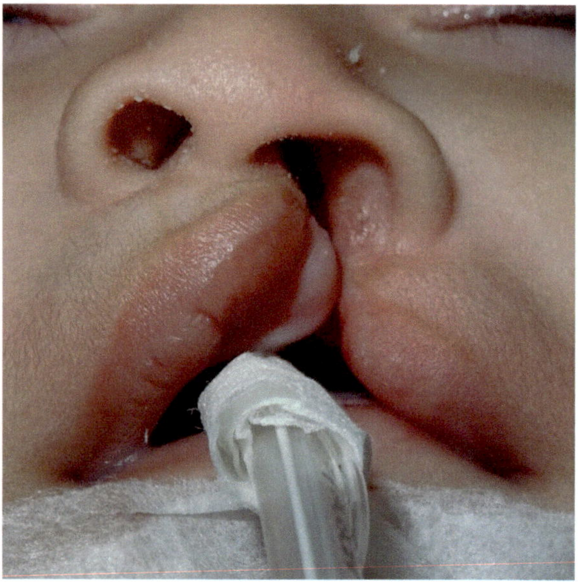

Fig. 3.27 Mild nose component unilateral cleft lip nose deformity

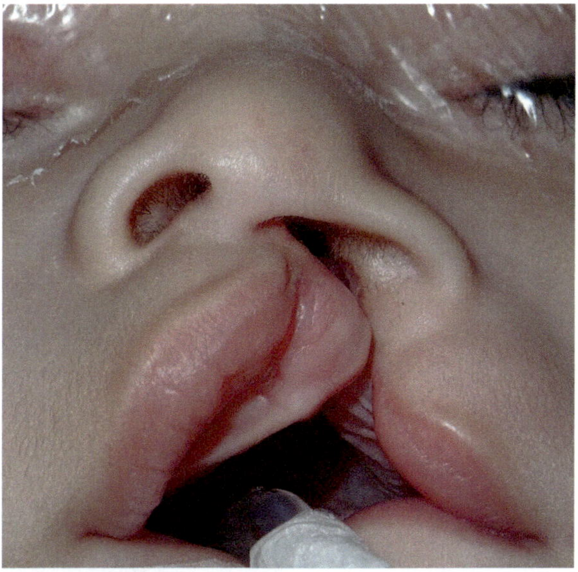

Fig. 3.28 Moderate nose component unilateral cleft lip nose deformity

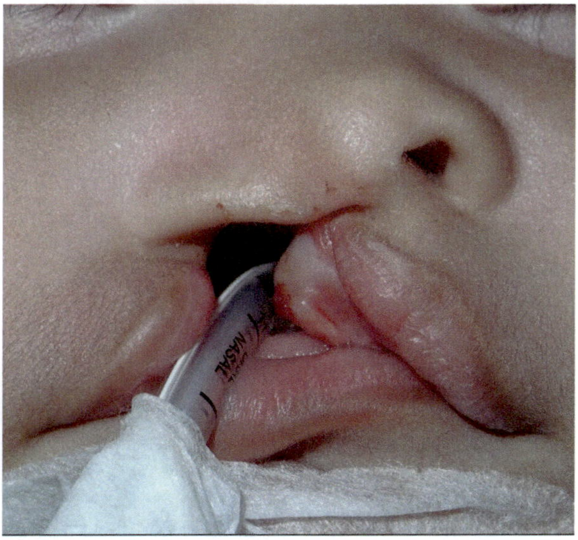

Fig. 3.29 Severe nose component unilateral cleft lip nose deformity

Primary palate, the cleft width is used to determine the severity of this component. In case of bilateral, the wider cleft side determines the type of cleft. The width of the alveolar gap is an important element for determining presurgical and surgical management of the cleft.

Unilateral:

Mild (alveolar gap less than 5 mm) (Fig. 3.33)
Moderate (alveolar gap between 5 and 10 mm) (Fig. 3.34)
Severe (alveolar gap wider than 10 mm) (Fig. 3.35)

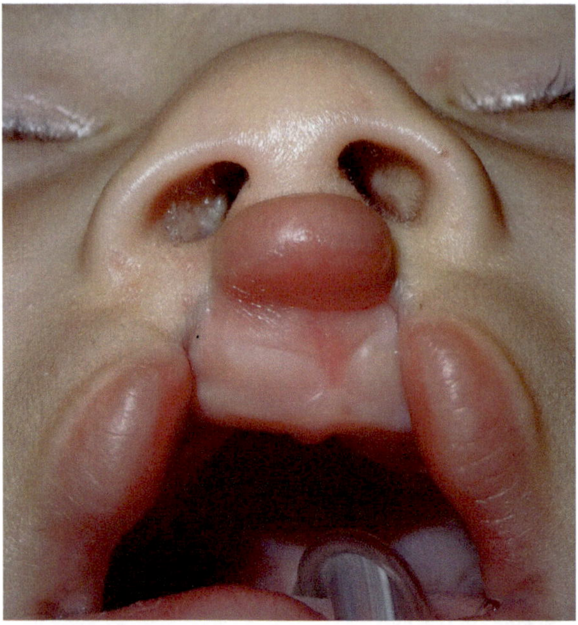

Fig. 3.30 Mild nose component bilateral cleft lip nose deformity

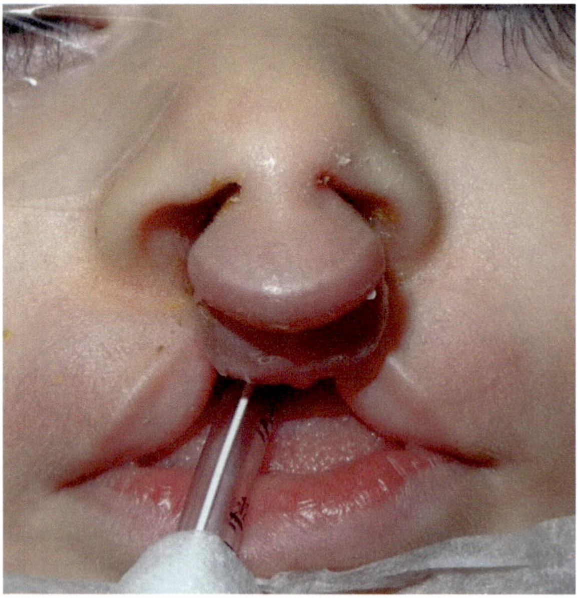

Fig. 3.31 Moderate nose component bilateral cleft lip nose deformity

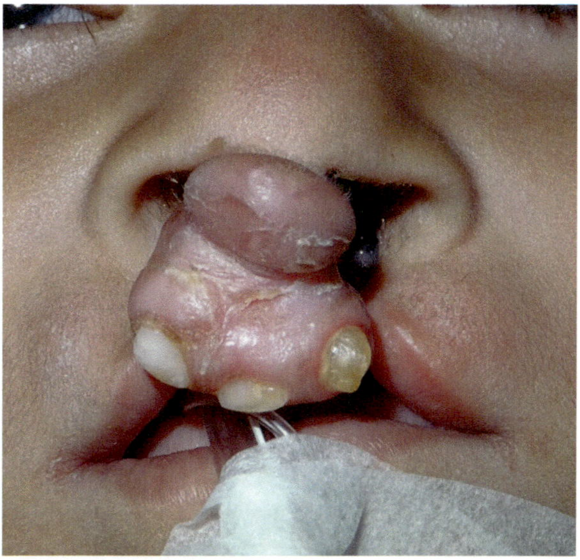

Fig. 3.32 Severe nose component bilateral cleft lip nose deformity

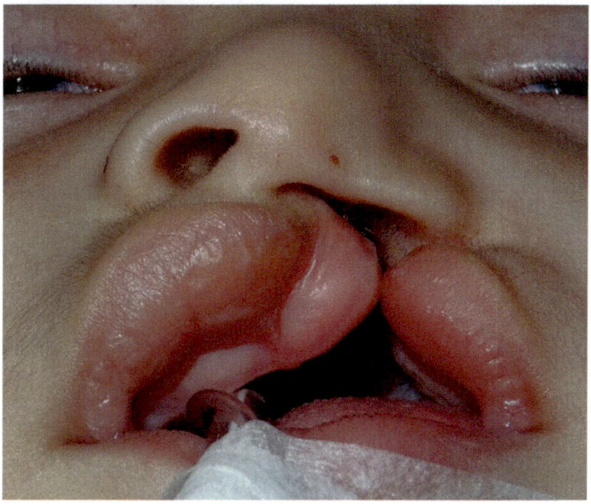

Fig. 3.33 Mild primary palate component unilateral cleft lip nose deformity

Bilateral:
Mild (wider gap less than 5 mm) (Fig. 3.36)
Moderate (wider gap between 5 and 10 mm) (Fig. 3.37)
Severe (wider gap wider than 10 mm) (Fig. 3.38)

Secondary palate, the estimation is done by comparing the cleft width and the sum of the width of the palatal segments. This proportion represents the cleft palate index.

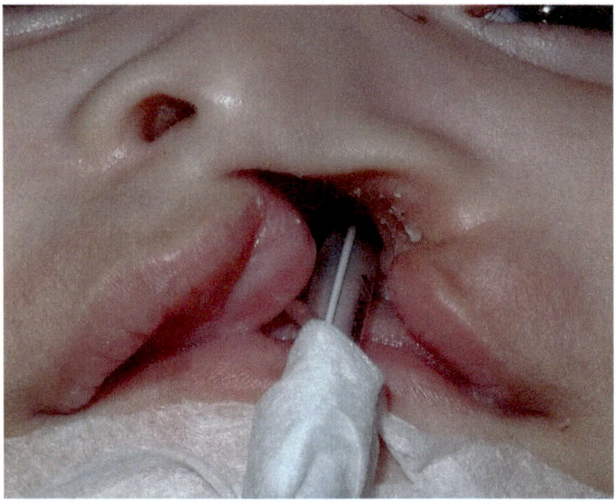

Fig. 3.34 Moderate primary palate component unilateral cleft lip nose deformity

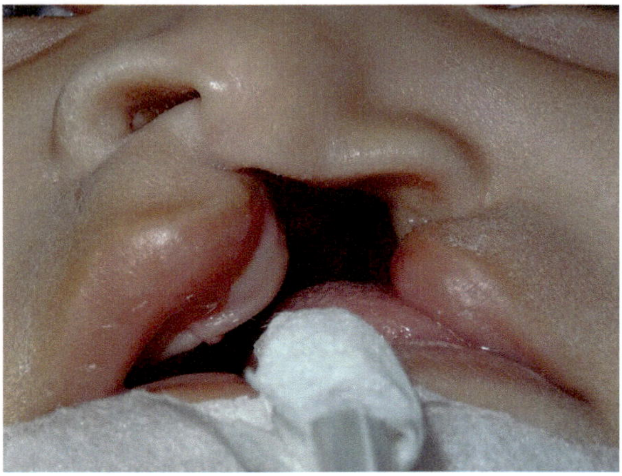

Fig. 3.35 Severe primary palate component unilateral cleft lip nose deformity

Mild: Cleft palate index less than 0.2
Moderate: Cleft palate index between 0.2 and 0.4
Severe: Cleft palate index greater than 0.4

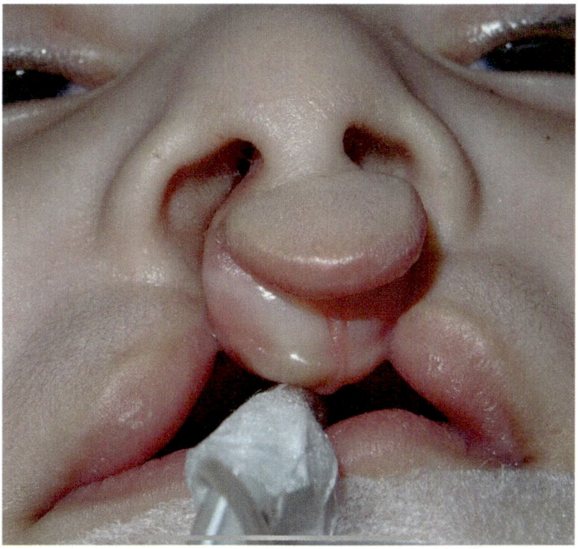

Fig. 3.36 Mild primary palate component bilateral cleft lip nose deformity

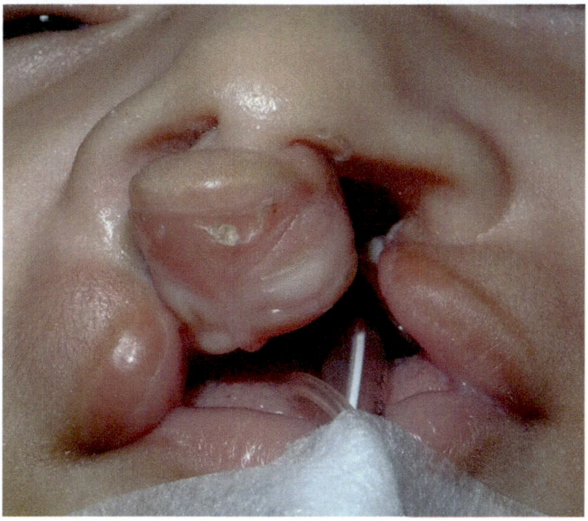

Fig. 3.37 Moderate primary palate component bilateral cleft lip nose deformity

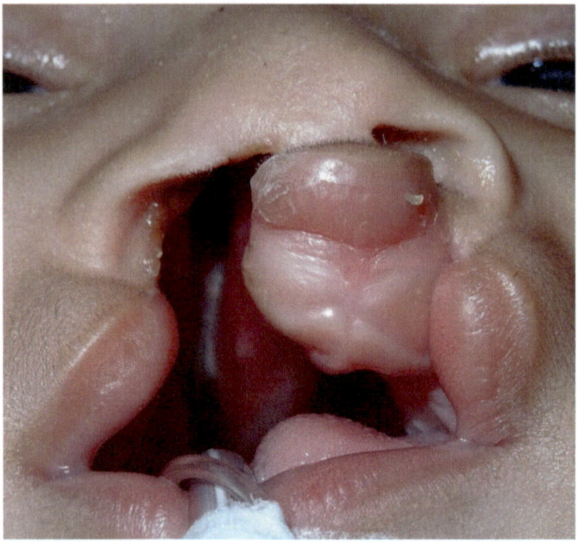

Fig. 3.38 Severe primary palate component bilateral cleft lip nose deformity

The Clock Diagram for Deformity Description

This diagram described by the author represents and illustrates cleft lip and palate deformities based on their severity. This is a circle divided into four quadrants, one for each cleft component; each one is subdivided into three segments (following the clock hours) representing three degrees of severity: mild, moderate, and severe (Fig. 3.4).

Numbers from 1 to 12 are assigned to each degree of severity as follows:

Right superior quadrant (lip component): mild (1), moderate (2), and severe (3)
Right inferior quadrant (nose component): mild (4), moderate (5), and severe (6)
Left inferior quadrant (primary palate component): mild (7), moderate (8), and severe (9)
Left superior quadrant (secondary palate component): mild (10), moderate (11), and severe (12)

The same diagram may be used for secondary deformity description considering the nose component as follows:

Mild (differences in nose measurements between both sides are less than 1 mm)
Moderate (differences in nose measurements between both sides are between 1 and 3 mm)
Severe (differences in nose measurements between both sides are greater than 3 mm)

Additional considerations such as columellar length should be included for secondary bilateral nose deformities.

Table 3.1 Surgical protocol for cleft lip nose based on Lima outreach surgical center classification of severity [23]

Age	Cleft lip and palate surgical protocol
Newborn	Presurgical orthopedics (PSO) for severe bilateral cleft lip and palate forms only
0–3 months	Surgical lip adhesion for severe bilateral cleft lip and palate forms if PSO fails
3–6 months	Primary cheilorhinoplasty
9–12 months	Primary cleft palate repair
18 months	Speech therapy
	Alveolar cleft closure
5 years	Velopharyngeal insufficiency surgery
	Intermediate cleft rhinoplasty
	Secondary cleft lip repair
7–9 years	Alveolar bone draft
16–18 years	Orthognathic surgery
	Secondary cleft rhinoplasty

The Cleft Code

This system is an easy-to-use system for cleft description and consists of four numbers representing an illustration of the cleft lip and palate deformity based on its degree of severity, as illustrated in the clock diagram [4] (Fig. 3.4).

Clock numbers (1–12) are assigned to each degree of severity of the four components. In comparison with conventional methods of description (such as Kernahan), this system provides a simple form to describe any cleft lip and palate because it is easy to understand and facilitates the communication between the members of the cleft team. Finally, this severity-based classification is related to the present cleft protocol used in our center (Table 3.1).

Surgical Timing

Another important criteria for classifying the cleft rhinoplasty is the surgical timing. Historically, surgeons have been influenced by experimental studies in animals that concluded that early rhinoplasty could produce long-term growth inhibition because of the disruption of growth centers. There is no consensus about when to perform the nose repair in patients with cleft lip, and different opinions exist. A recent study published by Jazayeri et al. [15] evaluated the contemporary practice of this surgery in different centers in the United States. It was a cohort study from 2000 to 2011 and included 4559 infants of whom only 1422 (31.2%) underwent primary cheilorhinoplasty. The number of patients receiving primary nose repair has been increased during the last years based on the findings of this study. Finally, there were no differences regarding rate of complications or length of stay between the groups. Another study published by Tan et al. [16] observed that more than half of cleft surgeons perform some type of primary rhinoplasty during infancy. Surgeons who are proponents of primary cleft rhinoplasty suggest that this early treatment may reduce the severity of the nose deformity and the number of subsequent secondary procedures; however, based on my personal perspective, the most important benefit is the reduction of the psychosocial impact of deformity during their development [17–19]. Actually, scientific evidence suggests that primary cleft rhinoplasty can be safely done without affecting nasal growth and improving long-term nasal tip symmetry, reducing the number of secondary procedures [19, 20]. Another debate in this field is the time of the surgery, and different proposals exist from early to late procedures. Based on these criteria, we may consider three types of cleft rhinoplasty.

Primary Cleft Rhinoplasty

This is the correction of the nose deformity during the primary lip repair (usually performed between 3 and 6 months of age). Early correction allows for the repositioning of the alar base, nasal sill, alar cartilage, and the improvement of nasal tip symmetry. It is important to mention that the primary repair can be considered independent of the age if the nose was not operated before. Based on my personal protocol, the type of cleft rhinoplasty is indicated according to the severity of the deformity. The rotational composite flap is mostly used to correct the nose in incomplete cleft lips and the V-Y-Z method; a more aggressive surgery is indicated to repair severe forms of complete cleft lips.

Intermediate Cleft Rhinoplasty

Conventionally, this term is assigned to any cleft rhinoplasty performed between 4 and 10 years of age. However, this definition is not accurate because the nose surgery was done previously or not. At this point, we must differentiate a primary repair from a secondary repair. To clarify this classification, we believe that the intermediate cleft rhinoplasty is a primary repair performed between 4 and 10 years of age. This period of time should be modified considering that the patient must be in the best conditions to face the school period; therefore, intermediate cleft rhinoplasty must be performed at approximately 5 years of age in combination with minor lip corrections if necessary. Some indications for intermediate cleft rhinoplasty are severe septal deviation with airway obstruction, severe nose deformity, and psychological distress. Associated psychological problems have been described around 8 years of age [21]. Finally, this type of cleft rhinoplasty may be divided in two optional times, the first during preschool age (ideally 5 years of age) and second during mixed dentition period in combination with alveolar bone graft. I prefer to indicate the intermediate cleft rhinoplasty at 5 years old even when this represents an additional surgical time. Finally, we have to differentiate the primary repair (unrepaired nose) from the minor secondary correction of the primary surgery previously performed. Also, the intermediate cleft rhinoplasty should be differentiated from the nose revision. An interesting study published by Murali et al. reported that long-term outcomes can be achieved after primary cleft rhinoplasty avoiding intermediate rhinoplasty [22].

Definitive Rhinoplasty

This is the time of final corrections (if needed) after addressing dentofacial proportions including alveolar bone grafts, orthodontics, and sometimes orthognathic surgery. It is usually performed around 16–18 years and 6 months after final correction of the skeletal deformity. Minor refinements may be included during this time; however, major defects can sometimes be observed in adult patients, and more complex strategies are required for their correction.

References

1. Veau V. Discussion on the treatment of the hare-lip. Proc R Soc Med. 1928;21(12):1868–88.
2. Spina V. A proposed modification for the classification on cleft lip and cleft palate. Cleft Palate J. 1973;10(3):251–2.
3. Kernahan D, Stark R. A new classification for cleft lip and cleft palate. Plast Reconstr Surg. 1958;22(5):435–41.
4. Rossell-Perry P. New diagram for cleft lip and palate description: the clock diagram. Cleft Palate Craniofac J. 2009;46(3):305–13.
5. Fisher D, Tse R, Marcus J. Objective measurements for grading the primary unilateral cleft lip nasal deformity. Plast Reconstr Surg. 2008;122:874–80.
6. Tse R, Mercan E, Fisher D, Hopper R, et al. Unilateral cleft lip nasal deformity: foundation based approach to primary rhinoplasty. Plas Reconstr Surg. 2019;144(5):1138–49.
7. Chong D, Somasundaram M, Ho E, Dhooghe NS, Fisher D. Comparison of presurgical anthropometric measures of right and left complete unilateral cleft lip and/or palate. Plast Reconstr Surg. 2022;149(2):248e–53e.
8. Cuzalina A, Jung C. Rhinoplasty for the cleft lip and palate patient. Oral Maxillofac Surg Clin North Am. 2016;28(2):189–202.
9. Yin J, Zhang S, Huang N, Shi B, Zheng Q, Yang C. Short-term surgical outcomes in patients with unilateral complete cleft lip and palate after presurgical nasoalveolar molding therapy: a three-dimensional anthropometric study. Front Pediatr. 2022;10:1101184.
10. Rossell-Perry P. The surgical nasoalveolar molding: a rational treatment for unilateral cleft lip nose deformity and literature review. Plas Reconstr Surg Glob Open. 2020;8(8):e3044.
11. Rossell-Perry P, Olivencia-Flores C, Delgado-Jimenez MP, Ormeño-Aquino R. Surgical nasoalveolar molding: a rational treatment for bilateral cleft lip nose and systematic review. Plas Reconstr Surg Glob Open. 2020;8(9):e3082.
12. Dalaserra M, Pantoja T, Salazar J, Araya I, Yanine N, Villanueva J. Effectiveness of presurgical orthopedics on patients with cleft lip and palate and meta análisis. J Stomatol Oral Maxillofac Surg. 2022. https://doi.org/10.1016/j.jormas.2022.02.004.
13. Hosseini H, Kaklamanos E, Athanasiou A. Treatment outcomes of presurgical infant orthopedics in patients with non-syndromic cleft lip and palate: a systematic review and meta analysis of randomized controlled trials. PLoS One. 2017;12:e0181768.
14. Maillard S, Retrouvery J, Ahmed M, et al. Correlation between nasoalveolar molding and surgical, aesthetic, functional and socio economic outcomes following primary repair surgery: a systematic review. J Oral Maxillofac Res. 2017;8:e2.
15. Jazayeri H, Lopez J, Pourtaheri N, et al. Clinical practice trends and postoperative outcomes in primary cleft rhinoplasty. Cleft Palate Craniofac J. 2022;59(8):1079–85.
16. Tan SP, Greene AK, Mulliken JB. Current surgical management of bilateral cleft lip in North America. Plast Reconstr Surg. 2012;129(06):1347–55.
17. Anderl H. Unilateral cleft lip nose. Plast Reconstr Surg. 1987;79(04):661–2.

18. Brussé CA, Van der Werff JF, Stevens HP, et al. Symmetry and morbidity assessment of unilateral complete cleft lip nose corrected with or without primary nasal correction. Cleft Palate Craniofac J. 1999;36(04):361–6.
19. Haddock NT, McRae MH, Cutting CB. Long-term effect of primary cleft rhinoplasty on secondary cleft rhinoplasty in patients with unilateral cleft lip-cleft palate. Plast Reconstr Surg. 2012;129(03):740–8.
20. McComb HK, Coghlan BA. Primary repair of the unilateral cleft lip nose: completion of a longitudinal study. Cleft Palate Craniofac J. 1996;33(01):23–30.
21. Volpicelli EJ, Pfaff MJ, Hakimi K, Bradley JP, Solem RC, Lee JC. Age-related differences in psychosocial function of children with craniofacial anomalies. Plast Reconstr Surg. 2017;140(04):776–84.
22. Murali S, Denadai R, Sato N, Lin H, Hsiao J, Pai B, et al. Long-term outcomes of primary rhinoplasty with overcorrection in patients with unilateral cleft lip: avoiding intermediate rhinoplasty. Plast Reconstr Surg. 2023;151:441e.
23. Rossell-Perry P, Luque-Tipula M. The lima surgical protocol for cleft palate repair. J Craniofac Surg. 2020;31(6):1533–8.

Presurgical Management

4

Martha Mejia, Juan Pablo Gomez Arango,
and Percy Rossell-Perry

Contents

M. Mejia
Department of Plastic Surgery, Nicklaus Children's Hospital, Miami, FL, USA

J. P. G. Arango
Department of Biomechanics, University of Manizales Colombia, Pereira, Colombia

P. Rossell-Perry (✉)
Health of Science Faculty, School of Human Medicine, Peruvian University Union (UpeU), Lima, Peru
e-mail: percy.rossell@upeu.edu.pe

P. Rossell-Perry (ed.), *Atlas of Primary Cleft Rhinoplasty*,
https://doi.org/10.1007/978-3-031-68012-0_4

Introduction

There is a wide spectrum of cleft lip and palate and the degree of severity may vary significantly; these complex forms require an interdisciplinary, advanced, and life-long management. The main limitation in complex cases is the skeletal deformity, specially bilateral cleft lip and palate cases. These patients may benefit from interdisciplinary treatment in advance of the cleft deformity to improve skeletal conditions via a process known as presurgical orthopedics. The term "orthopedic" comes from the Greek which means "straight" or "align" and the term "paideia" means "rearing of children." This word was initially used for the kind of treatment used for skeletal deformities in children. The presurgical techniques for cleft lip and palate management are classified as surgical or nonsurgical methods. Surgical method used for orthopedic treatment includes lip adhesion, and nonsurgical methods include tapes or elastic bandages and passive or active alveolar plates that can be used for the same purpose in combination with nasal stents.

These methods provide different treatments for repositioning of the maxillary segments and premaxilla (in bilateral) closer to each other, facilitating primary lip and nose surgery. In 1689, Hoffmann used a facial binding to narrow the cleft preventing postsurgical dehiscence, and later Desault used a similar method to retract the premaxilla segment in bilateral cleft lip and palate patients [1, 2].

Early intervention using presurgical treatments is extremely important, and these methods should be used during the first few weeks after birth prior to primary cleft lip and nose repair.

Reducing the severity of the anatomic defect as a means of facilitating corrective surgery has always been of interest to clinicians treating patients with nasoalveolar clefts. In the 1950s and 1960s, pioneers like McNeil and Burstone [3, 4] first published the idea that by stimulating the overlying soft tissues, using different acrylic appliances, the morphology of the maxillary structures could be modified, favoring growth, while reducing the width of the alveolar and palatal clefts. Within the same line of thought, Hotz et al used selective, periodic grinding (every 4–6 weeks) in specific areas of acrylic plates to modify the position of the greater and lesser maxillary segments and vomer [5].

Later, an important step in presurgical orthopedic method development was based on Matsuo's findings for treating congenital auricular deformities. He observed that during the first 3 months after birth, the elasticity and malleability of the auricular cartilage allowed him to correct it. Matsuo et al. offered a preliminary explanation for the mechanism behind the molding of the alar cartilages, claiming that during this short period, it was possible to presurgically modify these specific nasal structures, favoring results in shape and symmetry [6, 7]. The groundbreaking work done by Grayson and Cutting in the early 1990s provided the first thoroughly described nasoalveolar molding (NAM) protocol, accompanied by documented clinical results, demonstrating that alveolar and nasal structures could be rapidly and successfully modified toward their normal form and position, facilitating primary surgical correction [8, 9]. The use of this presurgical orthopedic method (in special the nasal molding) is a common debate in different cleft meetings actually, and some authors as Samuel Berkowitz believe that presurgical orthopedics may restrict the maxillary development after the molding process, creating a vomero-premaxillary synostosis and therefore affecting its growth and development [10, 11]. Finally, it looks like that the use of plates is not necessary for feeding or orthodontic reasons; therefore it may not improve feeding efficiency or child's growth [12]. All its described benefits are actually under scientific debate and questioning.

These challenges have motivated the advancement of novel alternatives, based on digitally devised strategies for designing and manufacturing NAM devices [13] increasing access to treatments by reducing the dependency on the proficiency of a small group of experts. This new generation of early treatment modalities is still often regarded primarily as a tool for facilitating initial cleft surgery. However, it serves a broader purpose, offering the opportunity to return the segments to a more physiological alignment without compromising the maxillary length, alignment of the occlusal plane, or straightening of the nasal septum, consequently enabling more normal functions such as breathing, swallowing, and feeding, with the potential benefits for future growth and development of the facial complex.

Another potential benefit of presurgical orthopedics is the gingivoperiosteoplasty (GPP), which requires alignment and approximation of the alveolar segments to narrow the alveolar cleft, reducing the need for concurrent dissections during primary repair [14, 15]. GPP is a contentious technique employed by some surgeons and developed to achieve bony fusion across the cleft at the time of primary lip repair. Originally, the aim was to raise flaps in the subperiosteal or supraperiosteal plane and close the alveolar defect to create sufficient bone stock for dental eruption, potentially obviating the need for secondary bone grafting and reducing the occurrence of anterior fistulas, which are complex complications, especially in bilateral cases. Uni- or bilateral GPP executed during primary lip repair address the anterior portion of the primary palate, nose, and lip during the same procedure, providing numerous advantages for bilateral cleft patients, particularly those with anterior fistulas [16]. Furthermore, this approach may reduce the need for a secondary alveolar bone graft or, if needed, enhance the success of such an intervention. In summary, the main objectives of these presurgical methods are to facilitate oral feeding, improving nasal deformity and maxillary growth, reposition the protruding premaxilla in bilateral clefts making easier the primary lip and nose surgeries and improve wound healing by reducing lip tension which benefits the quality of the lip scar. Importantly, all the described benefits are not supported by adequate scientific evidence, and many researchers question whether these short-term outcomes will have any beneficial long-term effects.

Despite of the lack of scientific support based on our experience, we believe that the use of presurgical orthopedics is essential for obtaining adequate outcomes after primary cleft rhinoplasty in patients with severe bilateral cleft lip and palate. This benefit is related to the skeleton remodeling and not necessarily to the nasal molding which is currently under discussion actually.

Types of Presurgical Orthopedics

Nonsurgical Orthopedics

Lip Taping

This is a widely used presurgical orthopedic method because of its low cost and availability. The use of lip taping was initially described by Hullihen in 1844 stressing the importance of the presurgical preparation of clefts using an adhesive tape binding [2]. In 1905, Brown described the method as follows: "production of narrowing effect stretching the lip muscles and skin on each side whenever the patient cries or laughs" reducing the need for soft tissue undermining and establishing a continuity of the orbicularis oris muscle [17].

In 1922, Federspiel reported that the use of adhesive tape after birth lessened the impact of the deformity on the parents and aided in reducing the maxillary cleft [18].

Later, the use of lip taping was well described and reported in the literature by Pool in 1994 as presurgical management for primary cleft lip repair [19]. His method was based on the use of tape strips across the cleft before the primary cleft lip repair. Like other presurgical orthopedic methods, the age of the start of the treatment is essential and should be done during the first week of life in order to achieve this objective. Its use at a later age is ineffective, especially for protruding premaxilla management. The main effect is over the maxillary segments, molding the alveolar segments and making the primary lip repair easier. The main limitation of the method is that it has little effect on nasal correction. Skeletal changes may help with primary cleft rhinoplasty making this procedure easier, but this has not yet been demonstrated.

Observed complications are skin reactions to the tapes and treatment failure. A recent modification of this method was described as Dynacleft and used in combination with nasal elevators to mold nasal cartilages. It is a self-adhesive tape that helps to align skeletal and soft tissues in patients with cleft lip and palate [20] (Fig. 4.1).

Dynacleft nasal elevators are plastic hooks that lift and support nasal tissues from a tether strip. A gentle adhesive placed against the child's forehead pulls it. The hook repositions the nasal structures; however, there is a lack of scientific evidence supporting this method. Different studies on its efficacy have been published; however, they have not yet demonstrated better lip and nose outcomes using this method and well-designed studies are needed. Monasterio et al. compared the Dynacleft with NAM and observed similar changes after using them but the outcome after primary surgery was not studied [21]. Most of the published studies regarding the efficacy of lip taping show skeletal changes after its use (preoperatory outcomes), but they do not present lip and nose outcomes.

Therefore, after surgery, there is no evidence of whether the outcome is the result of the surgery or the combination of both methods. A recent randomized controlled trial study published by Abd El-Ghafour et al. [22] studied the effect of using taping alone and reported good outcomes. The technique of presurgical orthopedic lip taping described by Pool is detailed here. Treatment starts during the first week of life

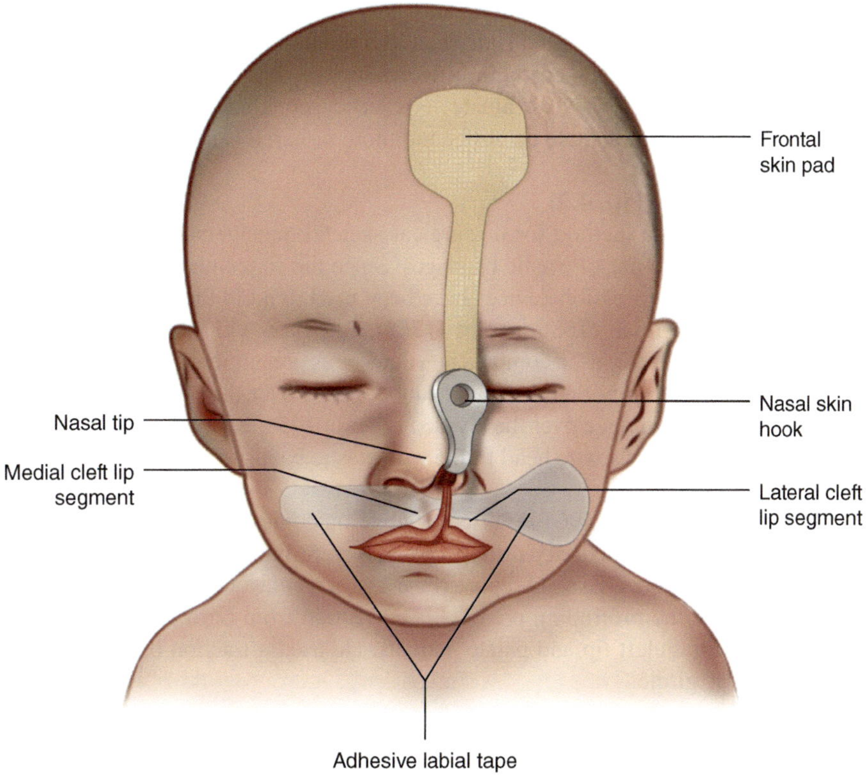

Fig. 4.1 Dynacleft system for presurgical orthopedic treatment of unilateral cleft lip and palate

(a key point of the success) when the use of presurgical orthopedics is indicated (mostly severe forms of bilateral cleft lip and palate) and is accomplished over a 6-week period, on average, and surgical repair of the lip is performed at an average age of 12 weeks.

During early phases, the tape must be reapplied daily; however, when skin irritation occurs, a recess of several days is mandatory. Adherent skin is applied, followed by three or four narrow strips of tape.

It is important that the parents should be instructed in applying the tapes to make them feel participatory in their child's treatment. Long strips of tape should be applied first to the cheek, and then after the alveolar gap is improved, shorter strips are applied to the lip on either side of the cleft.

The objective to be achieved is to move the alveolar segments within 5 mm to each other recontouring the lip and nose soft tissues.

The forces at work from lip taping have a functional effect on maxillary growth due to the action of the orbicularis muscle.

This is a simple and low-cost procedure that facilitates lip and nose repair and protects the maxillary growth molding maxillary arches and mobilizes lip and nose soft tissues. Finally, we must consider that this method requires compliance from the parents with regular and costly in-office visits.

A recent meta-analysis to evaluate its efficacy concluded that there are not enough studies to demonstrate its utility and more research is needed [23].

Elastic Bandages (Fig. 4.2)

Another widely used method for presurgical skeletal management in cleft lip and palate patients is the use of elastic bandages. Since the sixteenth century, bandages and mechanical compression devices have been used to mold the maxillary arch in these patients. Hoffman (1686), Louis (1768), Chaussier (1776), Desault (1790), and Von Esmarch (1892) used compression devices as presurgical treatments [2, 24].

In 1875, Thiersch reported the use of rubber bands over the premaxilla using an adhesive butterfly bandage over the cheeks. Later in 1954, Mc Neil [3] used a combined device including a wire head frame with elastic bands to apply pressure to the protruding premaxilla.

Brauer and Cronin in 1964 reported positive outcomes using a combination of elastic bandages and maxillary orthopedics in severe bilateral cleft lip and palate patients [25]. In 1966, Griswold reported the use of an elastic band system to apply compression for the protruding premaxilla correction from birth until 6–12 weeks of age in bilateral cleft lip and palate patients. He used a traction band made of a piece of elastic girdle.

Alveolar Molding Using Plates

Basically, there are two types of presurgical orthopedic plates: active and passive. Active maxillary devices produce controlled forces to move the alveolar segments in a predetermined manner.

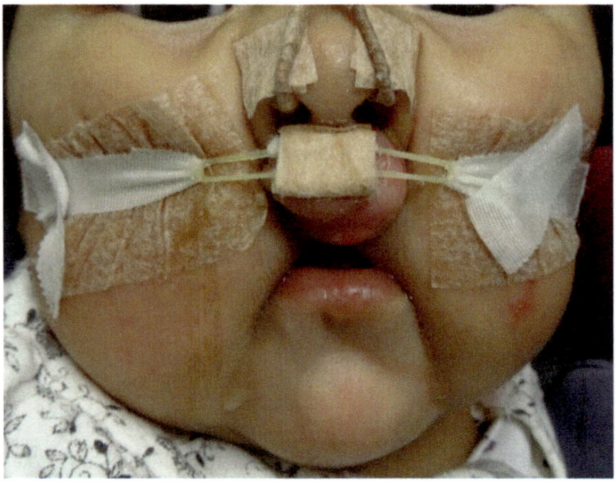

Fig. 4.2 Presurgical orthopedics using elastic bandages in the bilateral cleft lip and palate

Passive orthopedic plates act as a fulcrum upon which the forces with the forces generated by surgical lip closure enhance the alveolar segment molding in a predictable position.

In 1954, starting in the modern school, Mc Neil, a Scottish prosthodontist, used active plate series to gradually mold the alveolar segments into the desired position. He assumed that each successive plate under worn pressure would stimulate growth of the underlying bone, thus reducing the width of the cleft palate. Interestingly, changes in the width of the cleft palate are observed after cleft lip closure, and the use of active plates is not necessary. This is the concept proposed by the author as the “surgical nasoalveolar molding” [26].

In 1975, Giorgiade and Latham used another active appliance to retract the premaxilla and expand the maxillary segments in bilaterals [27] (Figs. 4.3 and 4.4).

Later in 1987, Hotz in Zurich, Switzerland, described the use of a passive orthopedic plate to align cleft segments. They devised an alveolar molding plate made of acrylic [28]. The surface of the plates was gradually modified such that the alveolar segments were pressed to mold into the desired shape and position.

All of these devices failed to address the nose deformity associated with the cleft lip and palate.

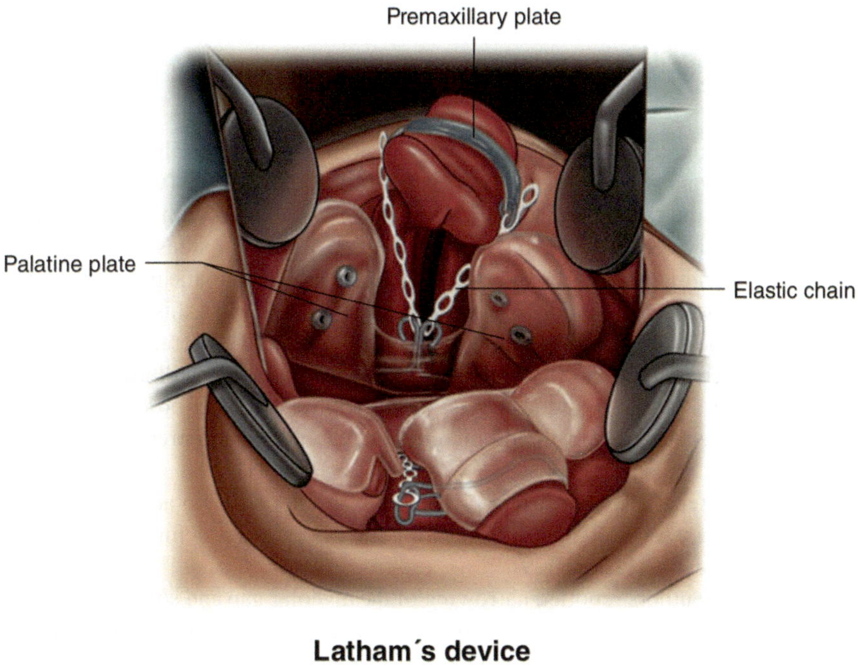

Fig. 4.3 Presurgical orthopedics based on the Latham device for bilateral cleft lip and palate treatment

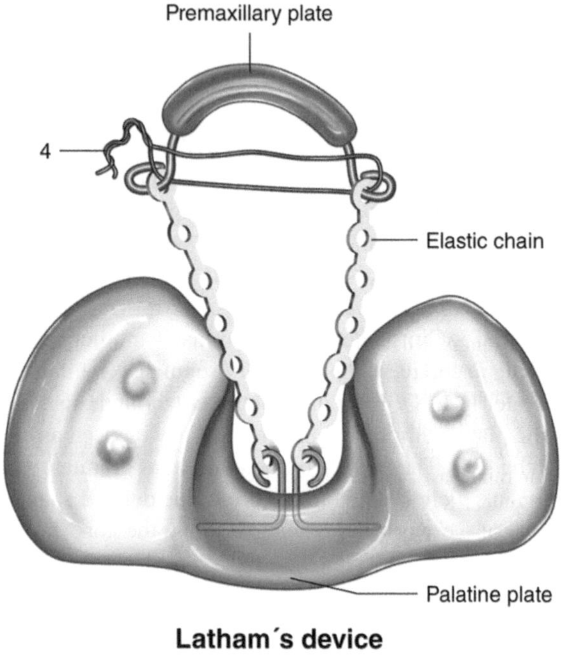

Fig. 4.4 Latham's device

Surgical Orthopedics

In fact, this method is not a presurgical treatment; however, it should be considered for pre-primary surgical orthopedics. This preliminary procedure (when it is properly applied) reduces the cleft size allowing the primary repair with less undermining and a greater of growth disturbances. The effect of extensive soft tissue mobilization on maxillary growth can be deleterious; therefore, the use of presurgical orthopedics may prevent these potential complications. First, this technique was described in the literature by Johanson in 1961 and used for bilateral cleft lip repair by authors such as Millard in 1960 and Spina in 1964, and then Millard in the same year proposed a partial lip adhesion as presurgical treatment in order to facilitate definitive surgery achieving same outcomes as external elastic pressure or dental appliances [2].

In 1966, Peter Randall, a strong proponent of preliminary lip adhesion, used a full-length lip adhesion. This extra operation facilitates better definitive repair and prevents secondary revisions [29].

All of these authors reported narrowing of the alveolar gap and soft tissue expansion of the prolabium. Surgical lip adhesion reduces the need for soft tissue undermining and facilitates the repair in wide clefts; however, it has a minimal effect on nasal repair even when some authors have described nasal deformity treatment during lip adhesion ("lip nasal adhesion") which is not a conventional method [30, 31].

The main limitations of using this presurgical orthopedic method are the risk and cost of additional surgery.

To achieve optimal outcomes over the skeleton, an early lip adhesion is mandatory. Based on my personal experience, the lip adhesion should be performed before 3 months of age, and any adhesion later than this age produces minimal changes in the skeleton. Even when the soft tissues are expanded after surgical lip adhesion facilitating the primary lip closure and minimizing the risk of lip dehiscence, the premaxilla remains protruded and will require a premaxillary setback in combination with maxillary orthopedics later. The timing of primary lip repair after lip adhesion remains controversial and is recommended to be 3–6 months after adhesion. Personally, I recommend the following protocol for severe bilateral cleft lip and palate treatment (alveolar cleft wider than 1 cm):

Bilateral surgical lip adhesion (before 3 months of age)
One stage primary palatoplasty (9–12 months of age)
Primary cheilorhinoplasty (18–24 months of age)
Alveolar bone graft (mixed dentition period)

There is a risk of lip dehiscence after lip adhesion exists, and some authors have reported 24% for bilateral clefts [32]; however, other authors have reported 5% of total dehiscence [33].

Surgical Technique

The method described here is based on Randall's description.

Markings (Fig. 4.5)

Two flaps are designed at the central segment (prolabium and columellar base flaps), and three flaps are designed at the lateral segments (lateral mucosa, oral mucosa, and alar flaps). Flaps are elevated from the central and lateral segments, and then the upper lip muscles are freed from their abnormal insertion. Surgical repair starts with suturing of the prolabium flap to the oral mucosa via the oral mucosa flap from the lateral segment on both sides. Then, the muscles are attached to the subcutaneous tissue of the prolabium on both sides. Finally, the lateral mucosal flap is turned up medially and sutured to the skin of the prolabium; simultaneously the lateral alar flap is sutured to the medial columellar flaps. I like to add that a "cinch" suture of polypropylene is brought through the dermis of each alar base, which is passed beneath the nasal philtrum narrowing the interalar distance.

Premaxilla reposition and tissue expansion produced by the surgical lip adhesion help surgeons perform the primary bilateral cleft rhinoplasty under good conditions (Figs. 4.6 and 4.7).

The utility of primary premaxillary setbacks has been actualized recently; however, their safety and utility are under strong debate actually (Figs. 4.8, 4.9, 4.10 and 4.11).

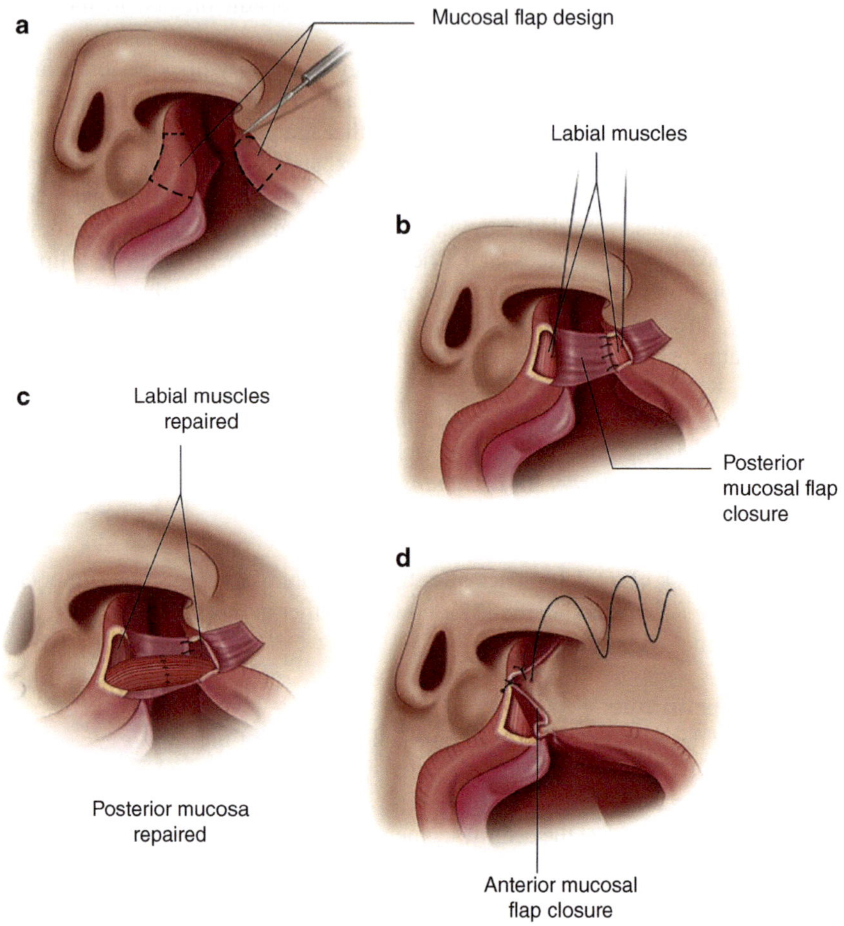

Fig. 4.5 Randall's technique for surgical lip adhesion

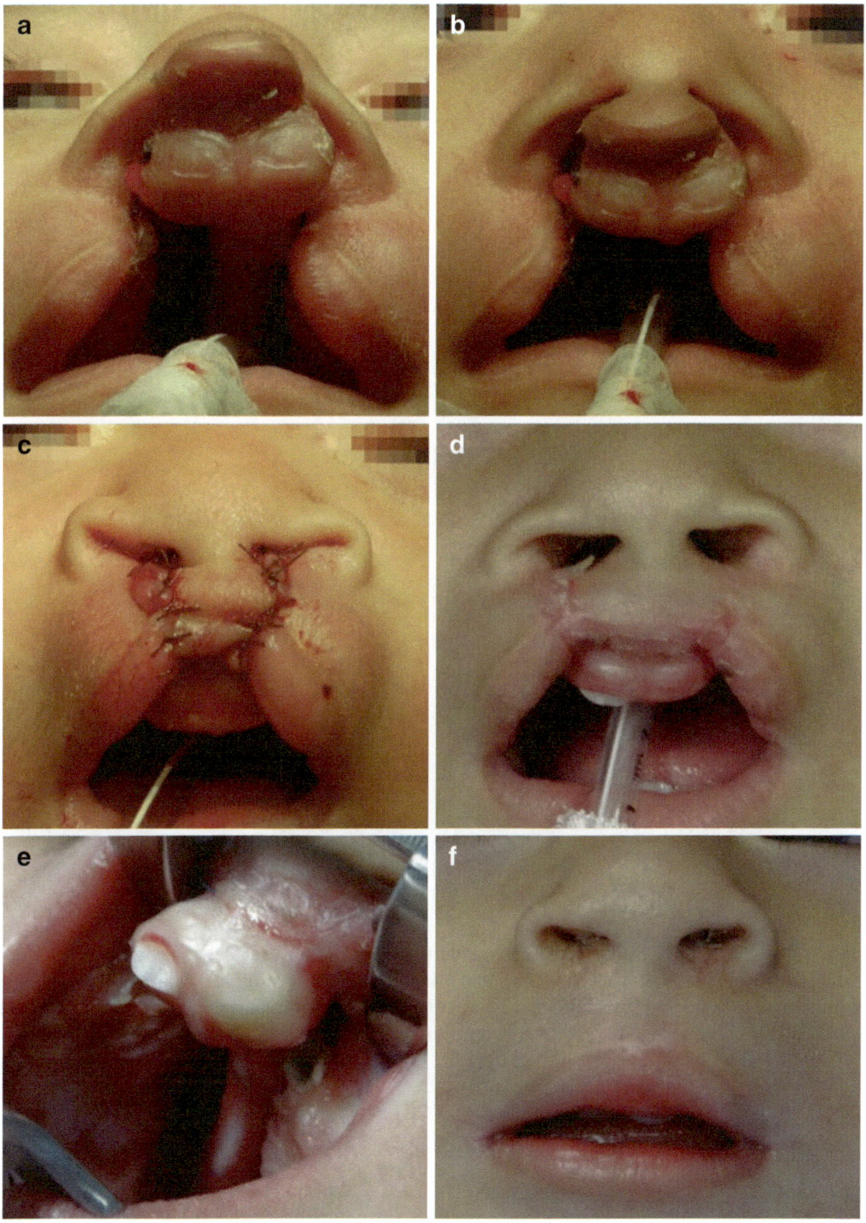

Fig. 4.6 Patients born with severe bilateral cleft lip and palate were treated using the surgical lip adhesion. (**a**) Worm eye view (alveolar gap 15 mm). (**b**) Frontal presurgical view. (**c**) Immediate postoperative view. (**d**) Postoperative view after 4 months. (**e**) New position of the premaxilla (alveolar gap 5 mm). (**f**) Postoperative view 1 year after primary cheiloplasty

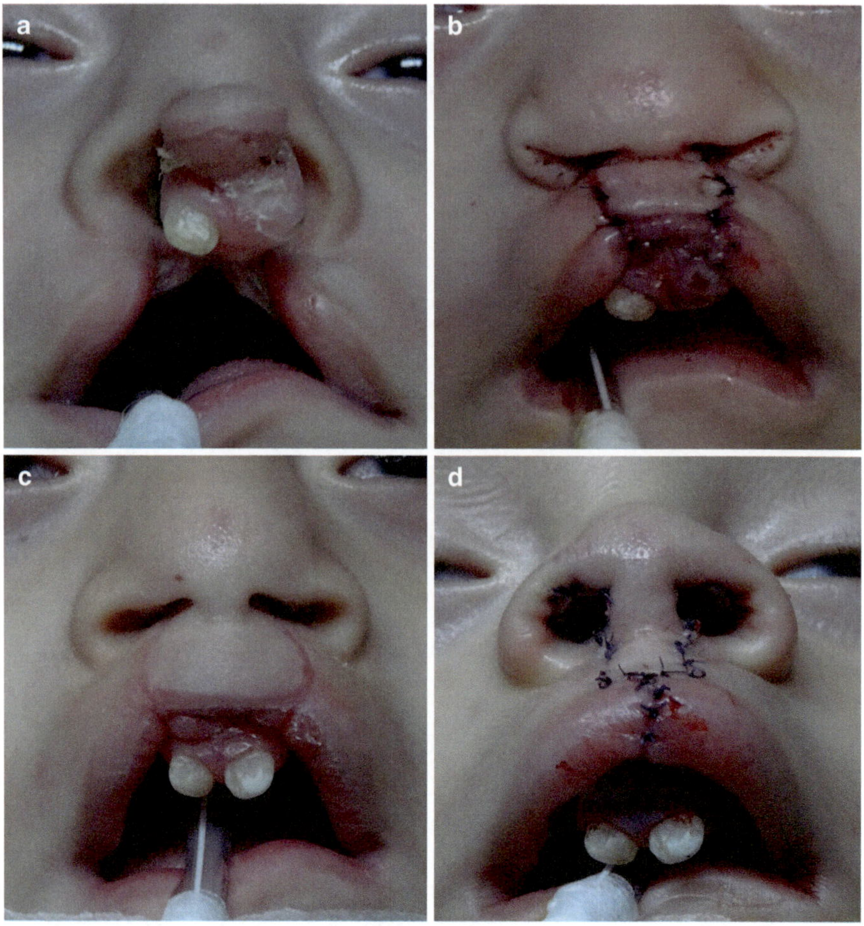

Fig. 4.7 Patients born with severe bilateral cleft lip and palate were treated using the surgical lip adhesion. (**a**) Worm eye view (alveolar gap 14 mm) (frontal presurgical view). (**b**) Immediate postoperative view. (**c**) Postoperative view after 6 months. (**d**) Immediate postoperative view after primary rhinoplasty using the rotational composite flap method

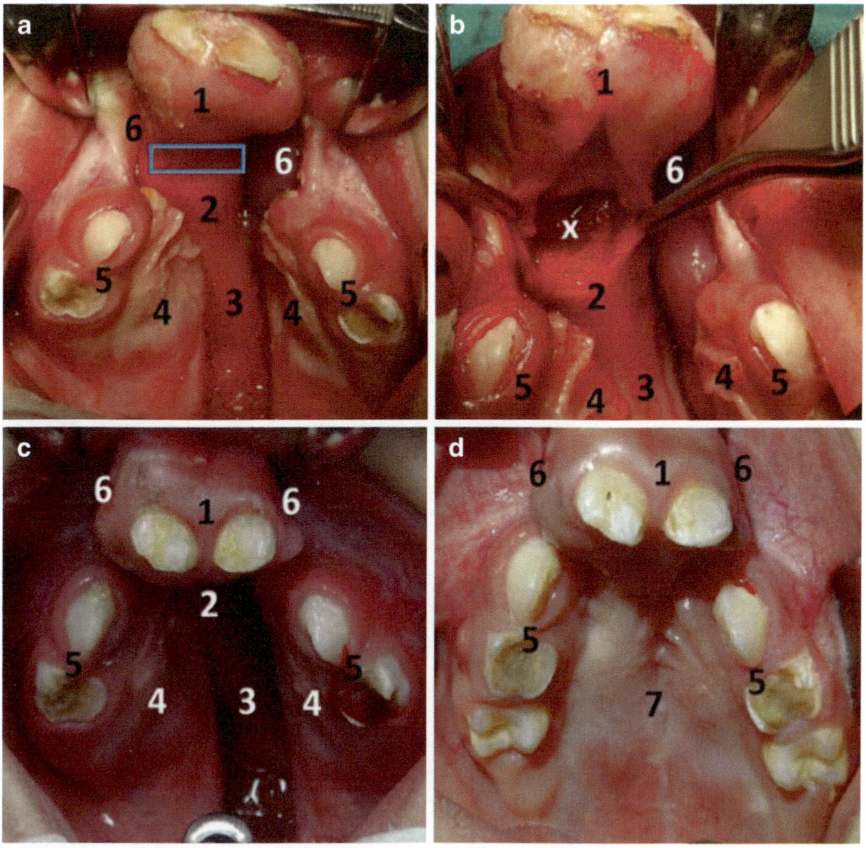

Fig. 4.8 Premaxillary setback surgical technique. (**a**) A 3-year-old patient with severe bilateral cleft lip and palate. (**b**) Vomer midline incision and ostectomy. (**c**) Premaxilla position after 6 months after surgical setback. (**d**) Premaxilla position 1 year after surgery. 1. Premaxilla. 2. Premaxillary-vomerine suture. 3. Vomer. 4. Cleft palate segments. 5. Maxillary arch. 6. Alveolar cleft. 7. Hard palate. x: Ostectomy

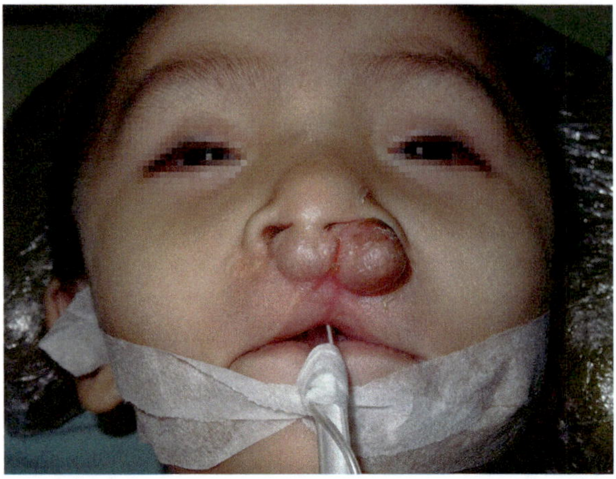

Fig. 4.9 A 1-year-old patient with cleft lip repair dehiscence due to protruded premaxilla

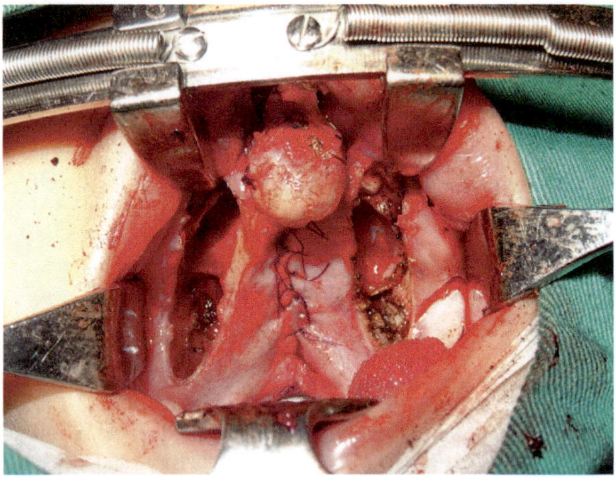

Fig. 4.10 Premaxilla setback combined with primary palatoplasty

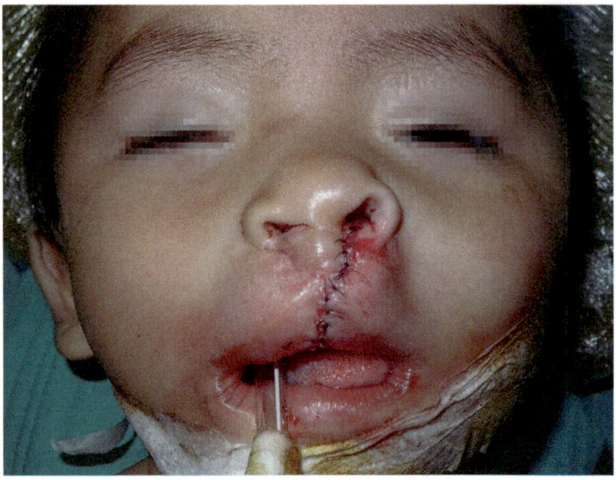

Fig. 4.11 Secondary cleft lip closure after premaxilla reposition. Nose requires secondary correction later

The Nasoalveolar Molding (NAM)

This is a well-known presurgical orthopedic method based on the concepts of presurgical orthopedics developed since the 1950s and the contributions of Matsuo to modeling congenital ear deformities using splints. This innovative concept was introduced by Grayson in 1993 [6, 8]. The device used for maxillary alignment and nasal molding was named as nasoalveolar molding (its acronym is NAM) and designed to correct skeletal discrepancies and nose deformities to a normal form and position during the neonatal period in patients with cleft lip and palate (Figs. 4.12, 4.13, 4.14, 4.15 and 4.16).

The best time to begin using the nasoalveolar molding is 1–2 weeks after birth. This technique utilizes wire and acrylic nasal stents attached to an intraoral denture, and its objective is to reduce the lip and nasal severity before primary surgery. Weekly visits are required to modify the molding plate to guide the alveolar segments into the desired position. Nasal stent molding is added when the alveolar cleft is reduced to 5 mm or less, and the phase can last between 3 and 6 months depending on cleft's severity.

The different advantages described by authors such as improved feeding, easier surgical procedures, better aesthetic outcomes, and reduced number and cost of revision surgical procedures were not demonstrated scientifically at this time. This is why this method is alternative and not the standard of care, and maxillary

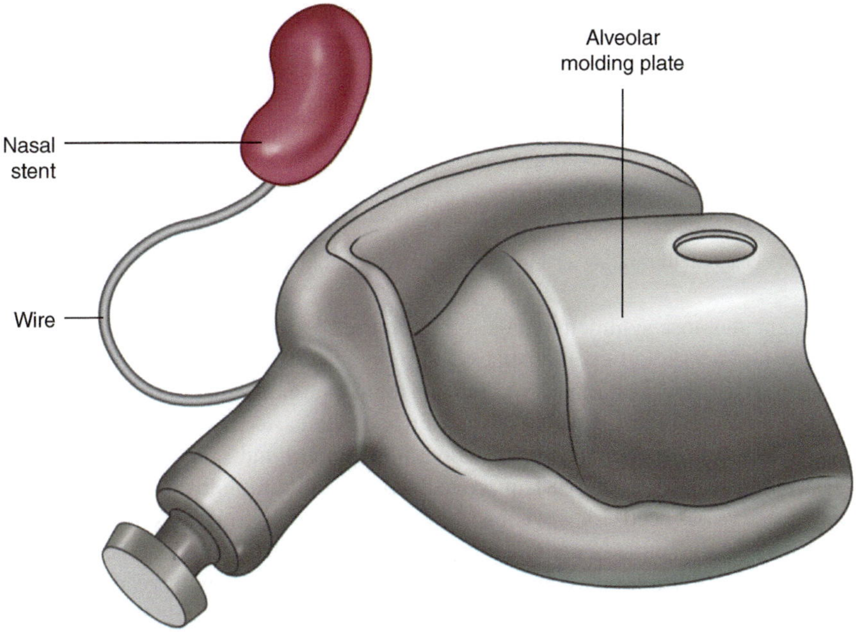

Fig. 4.12 Nasoalveolar molding device used for presurgical treatment of cleft lip and palate

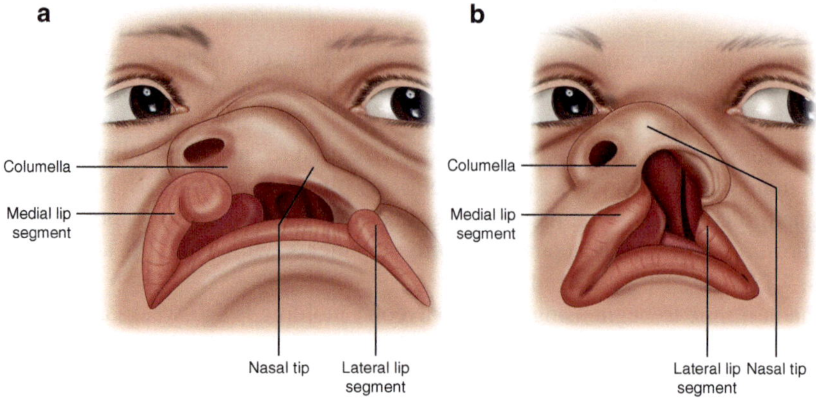

Fig. 4.13 Pre- and posttreatment condition of unilateral cleft lip and palate using NAM

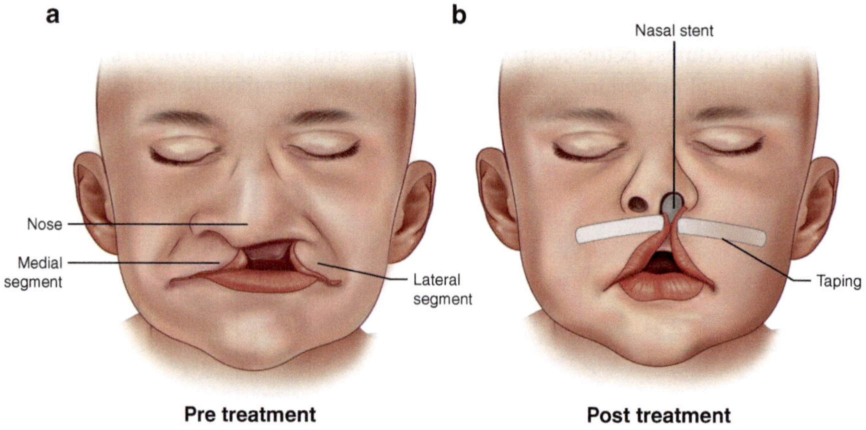

Fig. 4.14 Diagram illustrating a patient with unilateral cleft lip and palate using NAM device

alignment and nose symmetry can also be achieved properly by surgical techniques alone in unilateral cleft lip and palates [26].

At present, NAM is considered part of the presurgical treatment protocols for patients with bilateral and unilateral cleft lip and palate. According to previous studies, NAM has been shown to improve nasal symmetry and shape [34–36], reduce the size of the cleft gap [37, 38], improve the premaxilla-midline deviation [39], and may reduce the need for revision surgery and the associated costs [40, 41]. Nevertheless, the implementation of NAM therapy protocols requires the coordination of an interdisciplinary team of therapists and technicians with years of experience, as well as highly trained and motivated caregivers, along with other practical requirements that can make the technique difficult to implement.

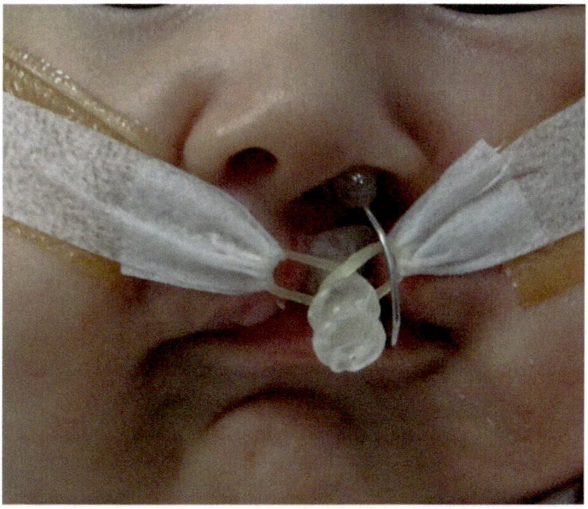

Fig. 4.15 Patient with unilateral cleft lip and palate using NAM device

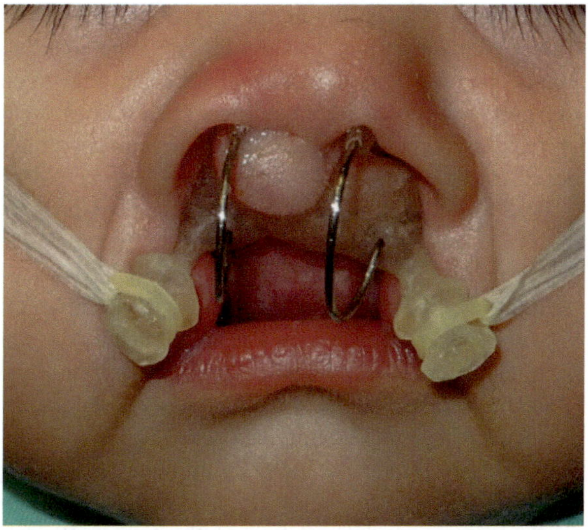

Fig. 4.16 Patient with bilateral cleft lip and palate using NAM device

The protruded premaxilla in the bilateral cleft lip and palate can also be corrected by any other presurgical orthopedics. A study published by Monasterio in 2013 compared NAM versus the lip taping method (specifically Dynacleft) and revealed no difference between these two techniques regarding cleft width and nasal symmetry [21].

The author (PR) developed an innovative concept based on nasal vestibule elongation (as a nasal stent of NAM produced) using the VYZ rhinoplasty and maxillary alignment as a result of muscular action after lip repair, this method has been named "the surgical nasoalveolar molding" [26, 42].

The Three-Dimensional CAD-CAM Presurgical Orthopedics

Computer-aided design (CAD) and computer-aided manufacturing (CAM) technologies have impacted all areas of medicine in which complex devices are needed, becoming safer, faster, less expensive, and easily accessible, allowing highly accurate fabrication of digitally designed appliances [43, 44]. The level of digitalization of current NAM protocols range from the implementation of direct intraoral scanning to the replacement of traditional impression techniques [45] progressing toward the digital manipulation of digital models that are subsequently three-dimensional printed and used for appliance manufacturing [46]. At present, the most advanced protocols start out with a digital model that is then modified to produce sequential treatment stages that are finally used to design and directly three-dimensionally print the actual devices [47].

The currently available literature offers studies that simultaneously support and discourage presurgical orthopedic intervention. This contradiction results from the unfortunate lack of high-quality randomized clinical trials, in which the efficacy of PSIO has not been sufficiently demonstrated. Heterogeneity of study designs and treatment methods, difficulty in the repeatable localization of anatomic landmarks, deficient data reporting, and the difficulty encountered in the standardization of the highly operator-dependent manual appliance adjustments required in most intervention protocols, especially in multicentered studies, are the main barriers to obtaining more reliable evidence-based results to validate clinical efficacy and guide further development.

This technology and its application involve the following steps:

1. Appliance manufacturing: Traditional PSIO techniques involve the labor-intensive fabrication of therapeutic devices, which rely on manual craftsmanship, years of experience, and a high degree of manual dexterity. This approach often results in significant interoperator variability. In contrast, digital appliance manufacturing workflows effectively eliminate this variability, facilitating standardization and reducing dependence on individual clinician expertise.
2. Treatment implementation: By utilizing sequentially delivered appliance kits as opposed to one consecutively modified device that requires manual adjustments, the clinical implementation of the treatment protocol becomes simpler. This approach relieves both patients and healthcare professionals of the burden of executing complex adjustments and activations that can be challenging for many.

The method designed by Dr. Juan Pablo Gomez and Dr. Martha Mejia proposes the development of a fully digitalized workflow for NAM, consisting of three independent interventions: Labial Taping, the Rhinoplasty Appliance System, and Sequential Alveolar Aligners System.

Labial Component (Lip Taping)

The clinical objectives of lip taping in patients with clefts are as follows:

1. The elongation of labial tissues reduces the width of the cleft, facilitating surgical correction.
2. Contributing to the elongation of the columella.
3. In unilateral cases, it contributes to correcting nasal and palatal asymmetries.
4. In bilateral cleft cases, it helps reposition the premaxilla and prolabium when they are displaced laterally and anteriorly. A downward force vector applied to the prolabium also contributes to the elongation of the columella (Fig. 4.17).

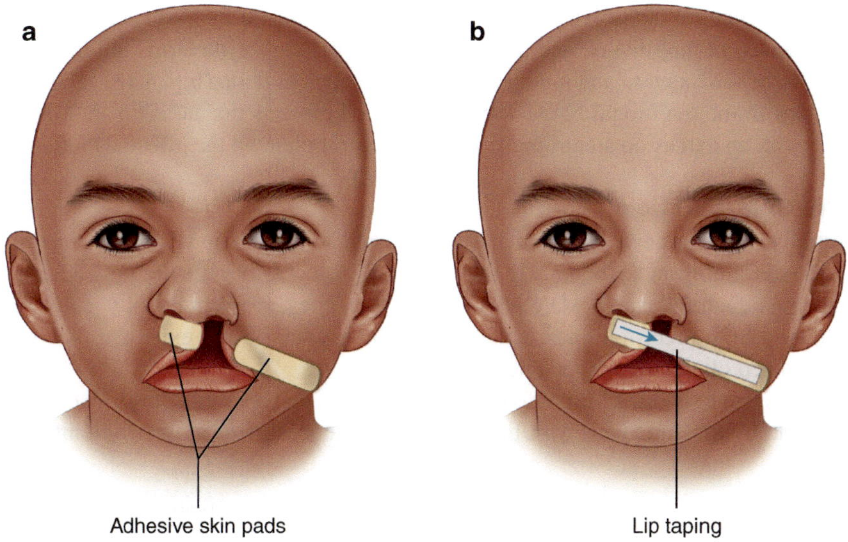

Fig. 4.17 The RAS labial component is composed of the following elements: protective pads on the lip and contralateral cheek (**a**). Adhesive tape, tensing the prolabium, and philtrum DOWNWARDS toward the cleft side, partially closing the cleft gap (**b**). To protect the delicate skin of the newborn patient from the repetitive removal and placement of tapes, protective pads are positioned on the surfaces that will accommodate the tapes. To apply the technique, first the short (2 cm approximately) end of the tape was adhered to the lip opposite to the cleft. The long end of the tape (6 cm approximately) was then pulled in a downward—lateral direction, approximating the labial structures—and adhered to the opposite cheek

Rhinoplasty Appliance System (RAS) Nasal Component

The clinical objectives of the Rhinoplasty Appliance System are as follows [48]:

1. The vertical and transverse asymmetries of the nose were corrected, the septum and nostrils were displaced to a more physiological and esthetic positions before surgery, and the nasal cartilage was subsequently corrected to avoid collapse after surgery.
2. This contributes to the elongation of the columella, facilitating surgical correction.

With its intranasal extensions (Fig. 4.18), the device must be controlled to displace the cartilaginous structure of the nasal septum laterally in infants with unilateral and bilateral clefts. The therapeutic force is produced by elastics anchored at the cheeks, pulling the device from the hook at the end of the arms, allowing the nose to be relocated to and maintained in a corrected position (Fig. 4.18). This contrasts with the traditional NAM appliance, which projects the nasal tip anterolaterally, with an extension stemming from the intraoral plate on the affected cleft side.

CAD CAM Workflow

Initially, the RAS devices were manufactured and adjusted manually, requiring high levels of training and expertise. In the proposed protocol, they are digitally designed and manufactured via CAD/CAM technology. They are sequentially delivered, allowing high precision and reducing the dependency on the expertise of highly specialized clinicians and technicians (Fig. 4.19).

Our system requires a kit of four nasal appliances that are sequentially exchanged at home by the caregiver, with the help of remote treatment progress monitoring,

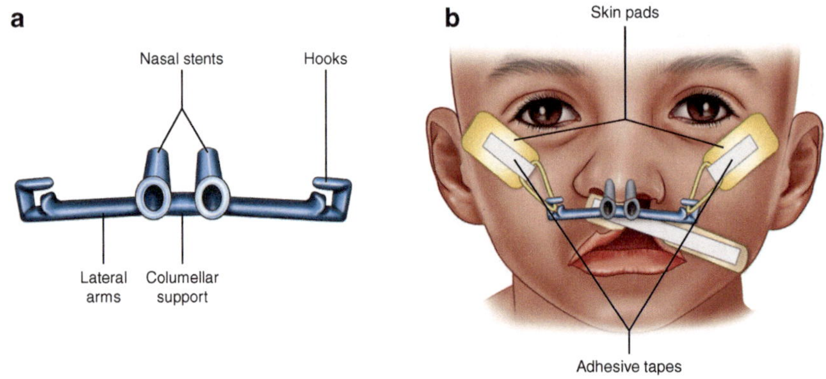

Fig. 4.18 The RAS nasal component is composed of the following elements: (**a**) nasal device consisting of intranasal extensions (stents) inserted into the nostrils, united by columellar support and two lateral arms ending in hooks (**a**). Two protective pads that avoid direct contact between the adhesive tapes that sustain the elastic elements of the patient's skin (**b**). Two adhesive tapes that sustain the elastic elements providing orthopedic forces (**b**)

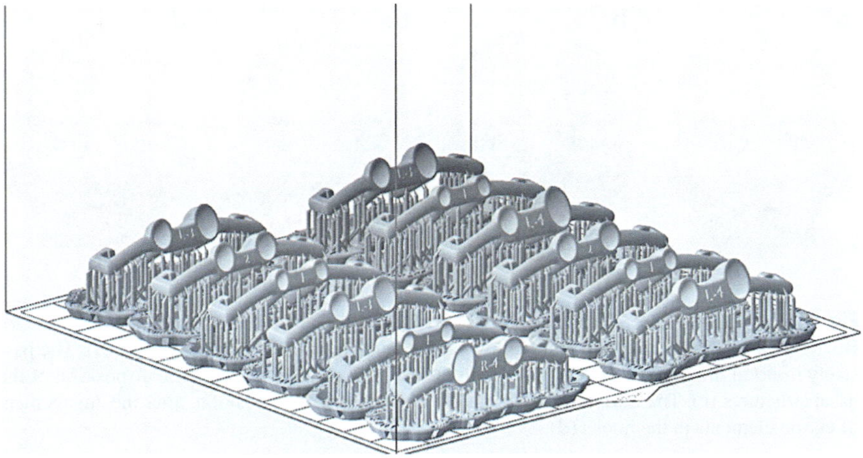

Fig. 4.19 RAS KIT digital manufacturing workflow. Digitally designed sets of appliances distributed on the virtual printing platform (**a**). Three-dimensional printed, four-step RAS kit for a bilateral cleft lip and palate patient (**b**)

during the active phase of treatment. The smallest appliance is initially fitted and activated. Then it should subsequently be changed periodically, increasing the size to modify the nasal structures in preparation for primary lip repair surgery. The kits are available for bilateral and right and left unilateral CLP and can be delivered at home by the caregiver, with the help of cellphone-based, remote treatment progress monitoring, in cases where travel to the treatment center constitutes a burden for patient and family.

For bilateral cleft lip and palate cases, each device presents a symmetrical sequential increase in the intranasal extensions to achieve the goal of elongating the columella and projecting the nasal tip. Each size is applied based on the degree of deformity. In typical cases, each sequential device should be used for 2 weeks, totaling 8 weeks of nasal molding. In more severe cases, in which the columella is markedly shortened, the appliances should be changed every 3–4 weeks, extending the nasal molding duration to 12–16 weeks. The kits for managing unilateral cleft lip and palate (right and left unilateral) are asymmetric, preserving the size of the healthy nostril while actively addressing the affected nostril. Progression to subsequent stages is implemented according to the severity of the defect. If the nasal deformity was minor, the conformer was switched every 2 weeks, and if it was more substantial, it was switched every 3–4 weeks. The overall nasal molding period ranged from 8 to 16 weeks.

Only after the labial component (lip tape) has been installed is the nasal component delivered, following the steps described in Fig. 4.20.

Once properly delivered and activated, the device produces a unique force system (Fig. 4.21) that is biomechanically independent of the alveolar molding device, favoring the resolution of the fundamental morphologic discrepancies found in newborn patients with CLP.

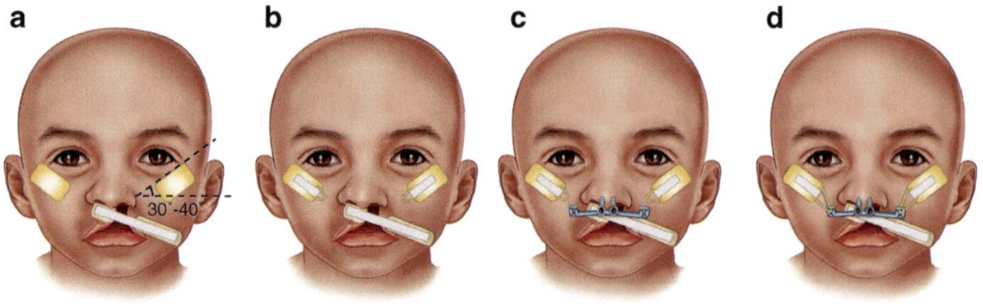

Fig. 4.20 Step-by-step RAS setup procedure: Protective pads placed at a 30–40-degree angle (**a**). Bilateral tapes with elastic elements, following the angulation of the protective pad (**b**). The passively inserted rhinoplastic device was slightly tilted, following the asymmetric disposition of the nasal structures (**c**). The device was activated in a more horizontal position, after the engagement of elastic elements in the hooks (**d**)

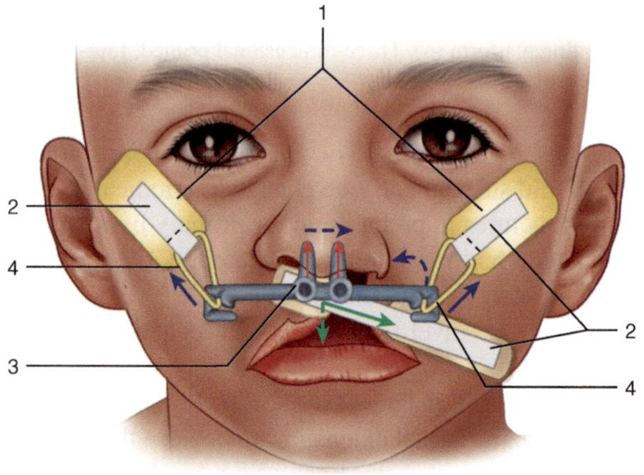

Fig. 4.21 The RAS force system (unilateral left CLP): Asymmetric upward-outward forces (continuous blue arrows) that displace the deviated nasal septum toward the midline (dotted red arrow). Counterclockwise rotation (dotted blue curved arrow) was used to elevate the nasal ala of the cleft side. The downward force component (dotted green arrow) of the diagonal traction force applied by the lip tape (continuous green arrow). Upward force produced by the elastic force at the columellar support (continuous red arrows)

When adequately installed, mild ischemia should appear on the nasal dome of the cleft side, resulting from the pressure applied by the prominence incorporated into the specific intranasal extension (Fig. 4.22), favoring the projection of the nasal tip and remodeling of the alar cartilage.

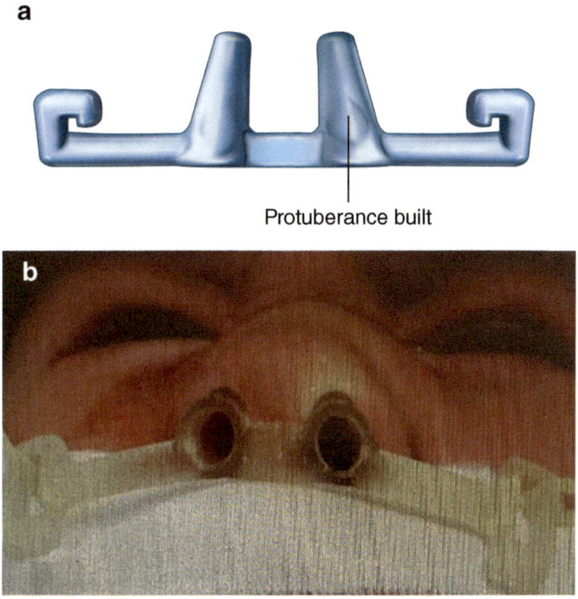

Fig. 4.22 The protuberance built into the appliance is intended to apply pressure in specific areas. (**a**) Nasal device. (**b**) Patient using the nasal device

Alveolar Component (SAAS)

The clinical objectives of modifying the morphology ("molding") of the alveolar segments using palatal plates in patients with clefts are as follows:

1. The approximation of the borders of the alveolar processes, facilitating surgical correction
2. Improvement of support for alar base
3. Restoration, to variable extent, the normal anatomy of the palate:
   - Allowing more normalized function, favoring growth
   - Avoiding early posterior crossbite
4. Avoiding the positioning of the tongue within the cleft
5. Facilitation of feeding and reduction of risk of aspiration
6. In bilateral cases, three-dimensional repositioning of the premaxilla

Our method proposes the development of a fully digitalized workflow for alveolar molding that includes the virtual modification of three-dimensional scanned models from bilateral and unilateral CLP newborn patients, generating a series of sequential, three-dimensional printed devices (alveolar aligners). By providing the patient with the complete set of aligners for at-home administration, coupled with the possibility of remotely monitoring treatment progress through a cellphone-based application, we can significantly reduce the burden of travel associated with conventional PSIO protocols.

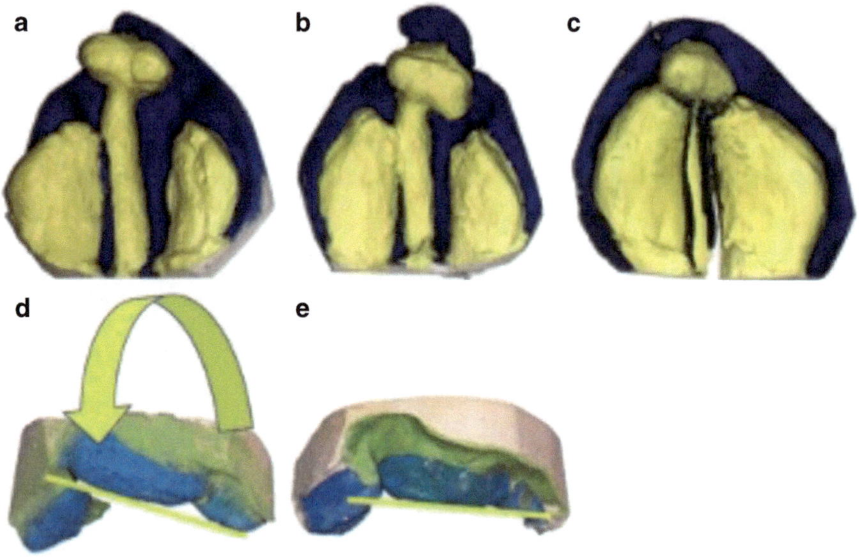

Fig. 4.23 Repositioning of the premaxilla in the transverse and sagittal planes, reconfiguring the palatal arch form (**a–c**). Counterclockwise rotation of the premaxilla improved the vertical discrepancy (**d**, **e**)

CAD Phase In the initial digital design phase (CAD), the patient digital model of the maxillary arch (Fig. 4.23a) is processed by a specialized software (AcuuCleft) (Fig. 4.23b), which delivers a series of sequential digital models (Fig. 4.23c) in the form of data sets that serve as the blueprint for designing successive devices (Fig. 4.23d) for the different stages of anatomical correction. In addition to its parametric alveolar molding algorithm, the software incorporates the normal three-dimensional growth of the newborn palate during the initial months during which the intervention is undertaken.

CAM Phase The resulting set of individual digital appliances is then used in the subsequent digital manufacturing phase (CAM) which relies on rapid additive prototyping (three-dimensional printing) to produce high-precision, sequential palatal molding devices, without the limitations that come with conventional handmade acrylic appliances which require highly trained clinicians and technicians for manufacturing and weekly adjustments (Figs. 4.24 and 4.25).

The parametric nature of the treatment software allows for adjustment in the incremental amount of alveolar modification applied by each individual device/stage. The number of sequential devices/stages employed in each individual case will depend on the severity (width) of the cleft defect, the frequency of aligner changes, and the amount of modification per stage defined by the clinician. A typical example of treatment planning possibilities for the closure of a 10 mm alveolar cleft could be as follows:

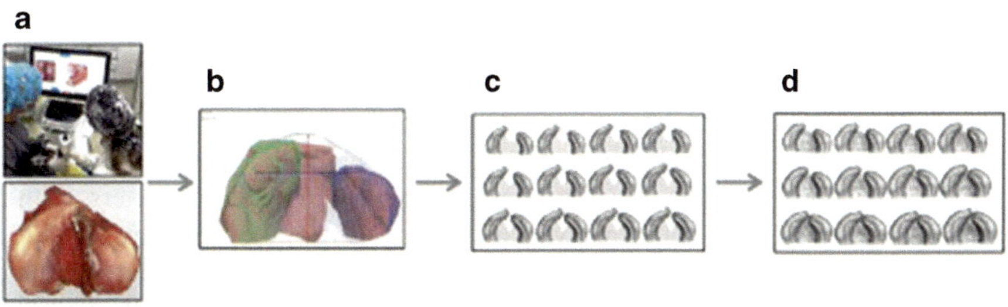

Fig. 4.24 The CAD phase of the digital workflow proposed for designing and manufacturing sequential alveolar aligners for presurgical infant orthopedics begins with the direct intraoral scanning of the infant's palate (**a**), followed by AccuCleft sequential treatment stage simulation (**b**), and the individualization of sequential treatment stages (**c**), which are used to design each individual sequential aligner (**d**)

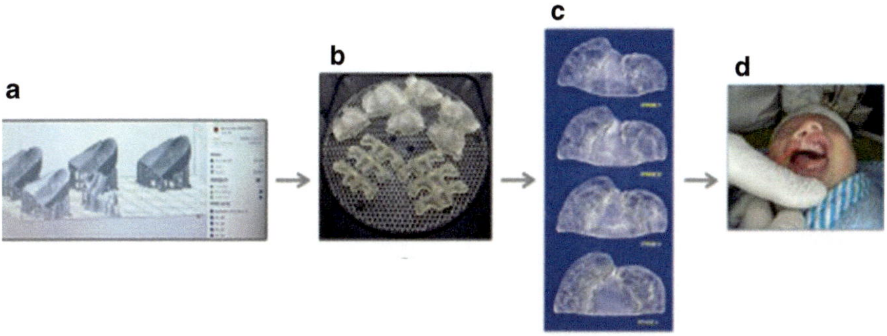

Fig. 4.25 The CAM phase of the digital workflow begins with the preparation of the digital aligner models on the virtual three-dimensional printing platform, with their corresponding supports (**a**). Once printed, they must undergo a strict washing and post curing protocol (**b**), and final removal of printing supports and finishing and sterilization (**c**), before being delivered to the patient's mouth (**d**)

#1: Ten alveolar aligners with 0.5 mm increments (at each alveolar border)
#2: Five alveolar aligners with 1 mm increments (at each alveolar border)

The fundamental implication of duplicating the extent of modification per stage (from 0.5 to 1.0 mm, in this case) is that the frequency of appliance change can be proportionately reduced (from 10 to 20 per stage, for example). This adaptability provided by the digital nature of the system offers clinicians the possibility of tailoring the biomechanical capabilities of the devices to different clinical circumstances, in a repeatable and precise manner.

Caregivers are instructed in the proper delivery and care of the devices, as well as the sequential appliance substitution regime, which is specifically formulated for each patient, usually ranging between 1 and 4 weeks per stage.

Clinical Cases RAS

Complete Unilateral Cleft Lip and Palate

Patient #1: A 2-week-old male patient with a complete unilateral-right cleft lip and palate in which a severe collapse of the right nasal ala and deviation of the nasal septum were observed. The initial interlabial gap measured 20 millimeters, with a 16-millimeter separation between alveolar segments (Fig. 4.26). PSIO was initiated with alveolar molding devices with the objective of descending the occlusal plane to a better position, rotating the greater process toward the midline, and approximating the alveolar segments. After 3 weeks of alveolar molding, the patient began with the RAS protocol to address nasolabial asymmetry and reduce the columellar dimension. After a total PSIO treatment of 16 weeks, substantial improvement was attained in nasal symmetry, columellar length and deviation, morphology of the nasal ala, width of intralabial gap, and projection of the nasal tip (Fig. 4.27).

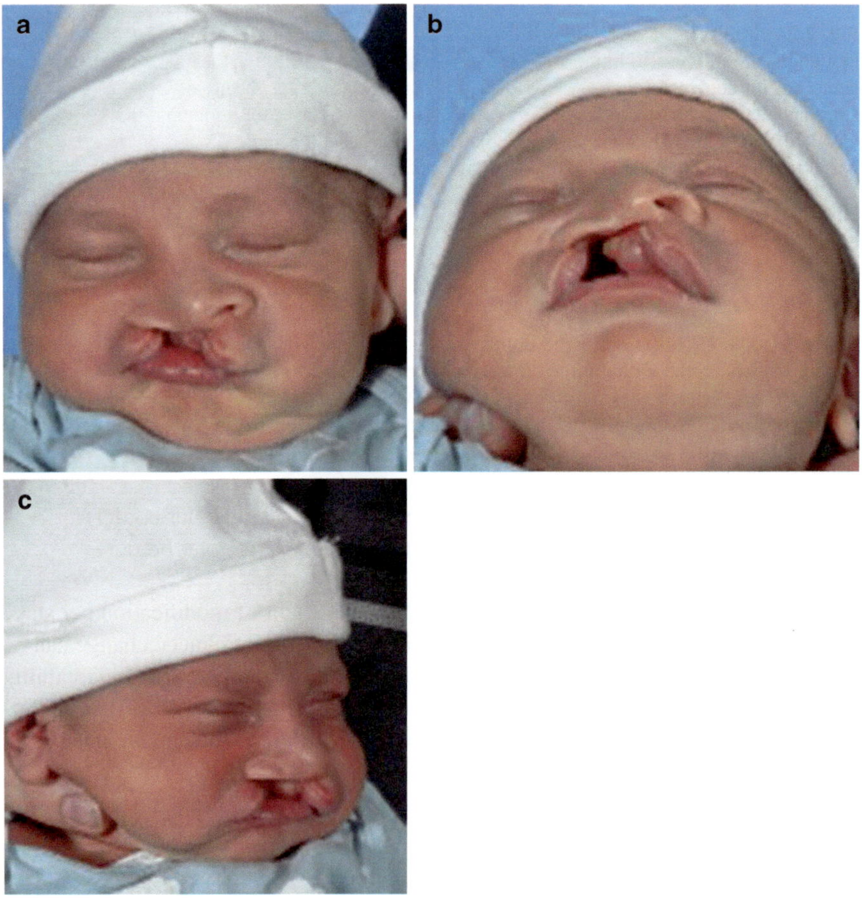

Fig. 4.26 Case #1: Pretreatment photographs

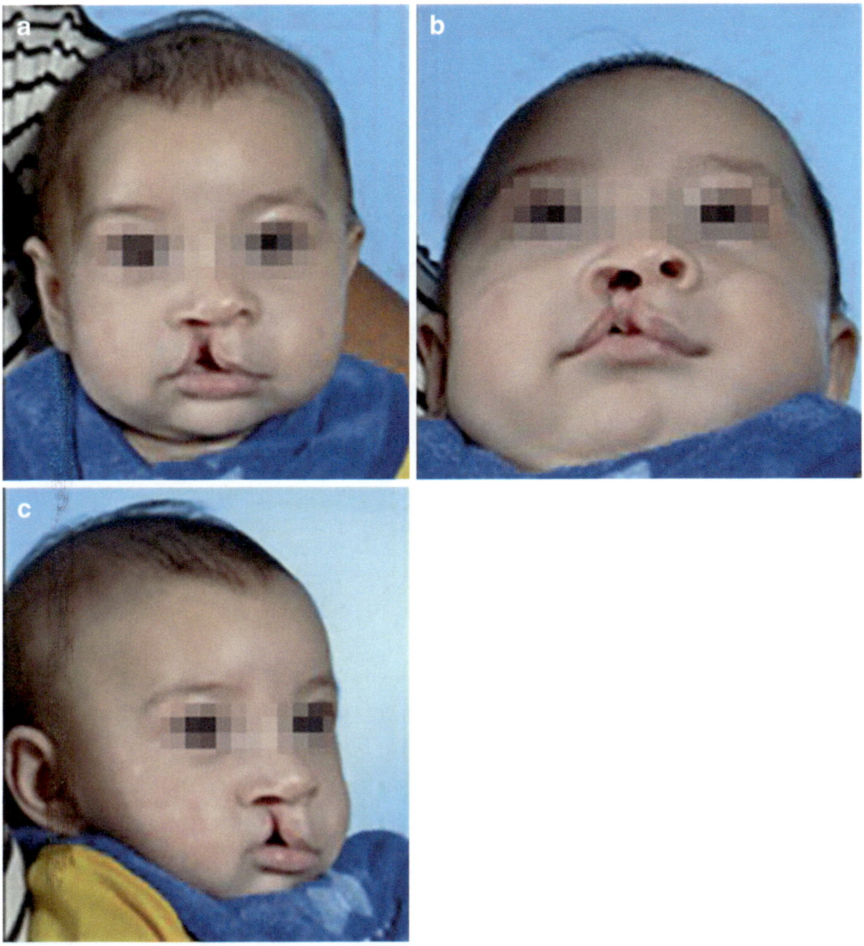

Fig. 4.27 Case #1: Posttreatment photographs

Complete Bilateral Cleft Lip and Palate

Patient #2: A 3-week-old patient with a complete bilateral cleft, accompanied by a deviation of the nasal septum and premaxilla toward the left side (Fig. 4.28). The right-sided cleft lip and alveolus had an initial width of 18 mm, while the left side measured 17 mm. Treatment was initiated to align the premaxilla with the alveolar arch and bring the nasal septum to the midline. This initial treatment was carried out using alveolar aligners for 3 weeks, followed immediately by the bilateral RAS protocol. Correction of the premaxillary deviation was achieved, as well as elongation of the columella and elevation of the nasal tip and improvement of nasal al morphology (Fig. 4.29). At 5 months of age, upon completion of the presurgical treatment, the patient was able to undergo surgery, which included primary palate closure with gingivoperiosteoplasty, lip surgery, and nasal correction.

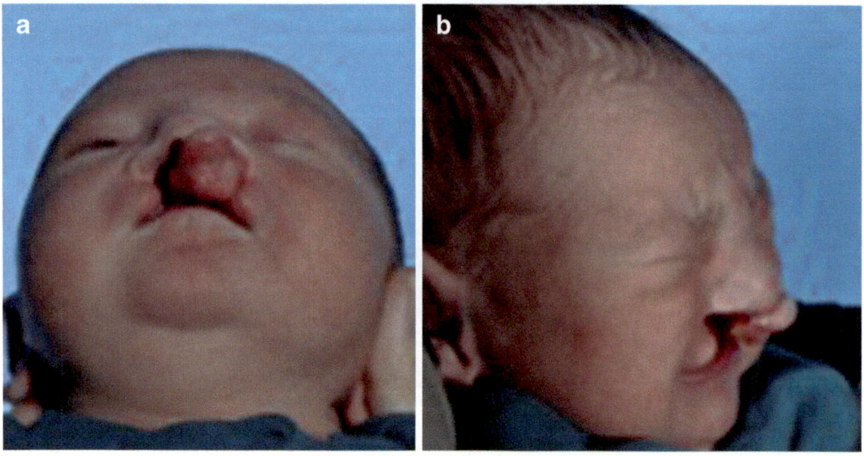

Fig. 4.28 Case #2: Pretreatment photographs

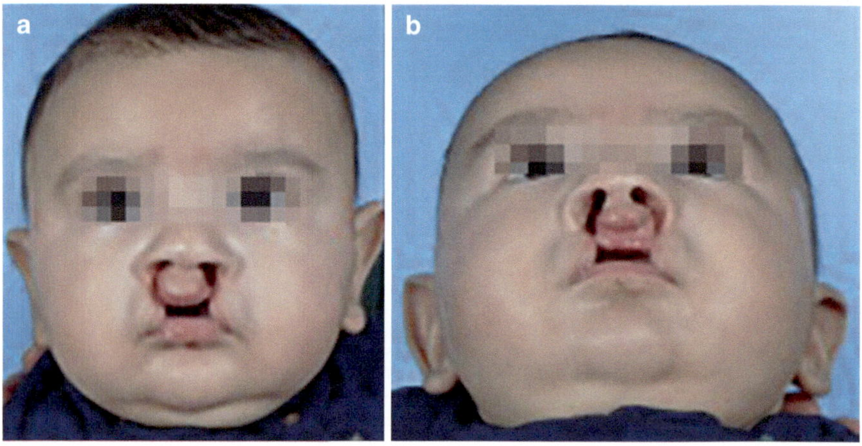

Fig. 4.29 Case #2: Posttreatment photographs

Complete Bilateral Cleft Lip and Palate

Patient #3: Premature male infant with a complete bilateral cleft lip and palate with a prominent premaxilla on the midline (Fig. 4.30). PSIO was initiated at 2 months of age with alveolar aligners, after which the RAS protocol was implemented for 16 weeks. Posterior repositioning of the premaxilla and its alignment with the alveolar arch were achieved. The columellar length, nasal tip projection, and improvement in alar curvature were significantly improved (Fig. 4.31). Corrective primary surgery was performed at 6 months of age.

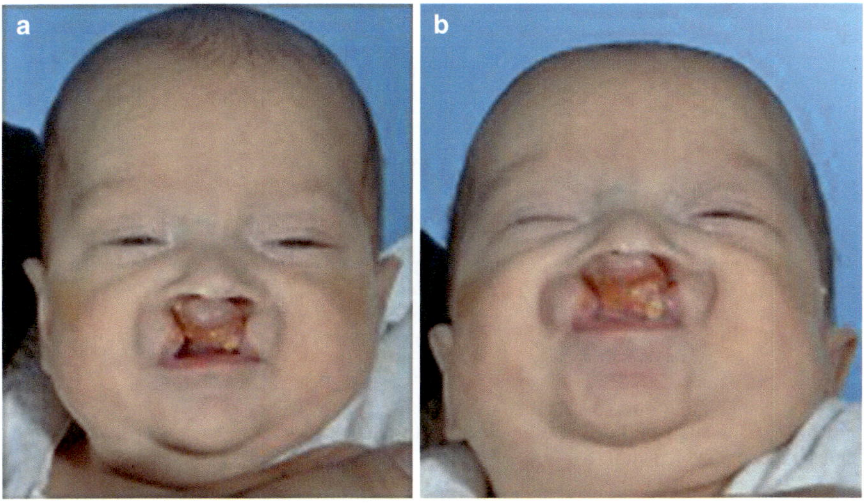

Fig. 4.30 Case #3: Pretreatment photographs

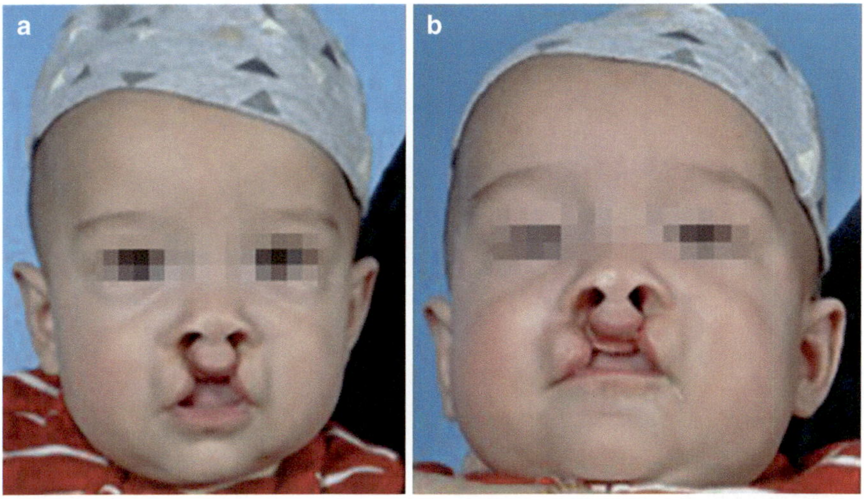

Fig. 4.31 Case #3: Posttreatment photographs

Complete Unilateral Cleft Lip and Palate (SAAS)

Patient #4: A 3-week-old patient with a complete unilateral left cleft, with significant deviation of the nasal septum and flattening of the left nasal ala. The initial anterior width of the cleft was 9.74 mm. Alveolar aligners were initiated simultaneously with the RAS at 4 weeks of age for a total of 12 weeks. A reduction in anterior and posterior cleft width was achieved, along with sagittal and transverse development of the alveolar arch (Figs. 4.32, 4.33, 4.34 and 4.35).

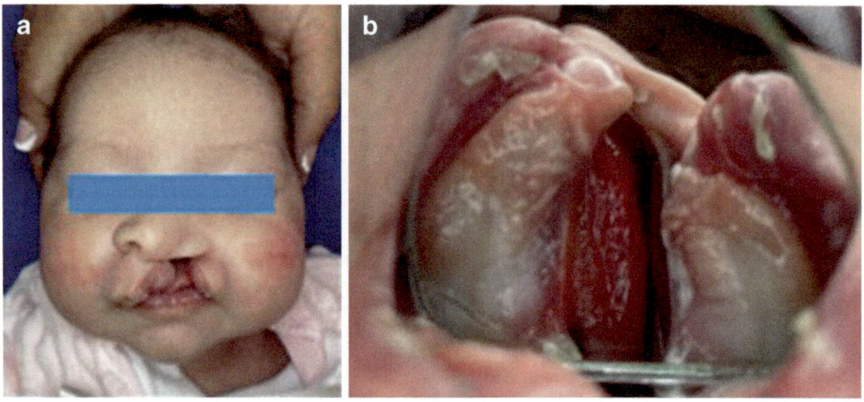

Fig. 4.32 Clinical case: Initial presurgical facial (**a**), and occlusal photographs of a patient with a unilateral complete left cleft (**b**)

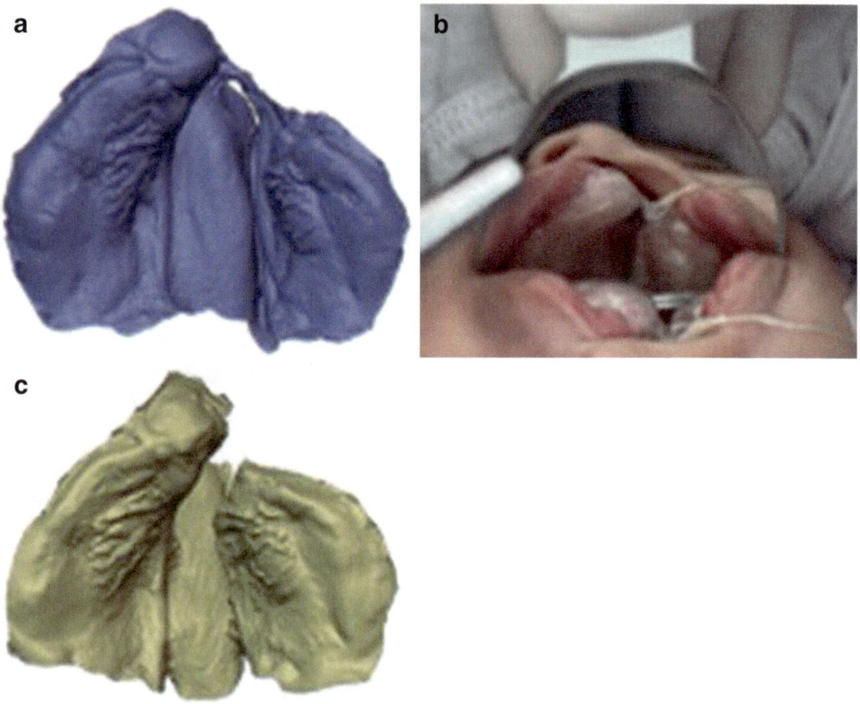

Fig. 4.33 Clinical case: The pretreatment digital model portrays the morphology of the left unilateral complete cleft (**a**). Intermediate occlusal image with the aligner properly inserted (**b**). Posttreatment digital model revealing the favorable change in palatal anatomy (**c**)

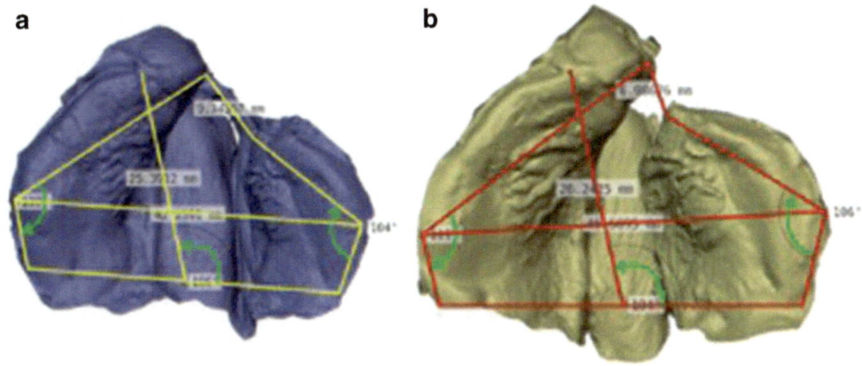

Fig. 4.34 Clinical case: Accurately scaled digital models of a unilateral left cleft of the palate, before (blue) and after (yellow) alveolar molding (**a**, **b**) with sagittal and transverse linear and angular measurements

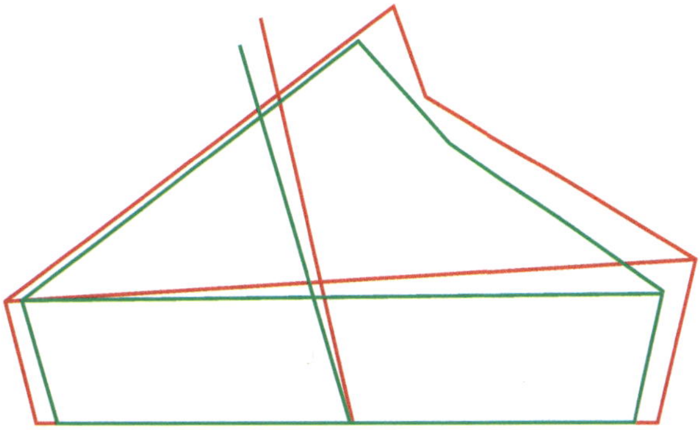

Fig. 4.35 Evaluation of treatment effect using superimposition of pretreatment (green) and posttreatment (red) polygons. A reduction of cleft width, improvement in sagittal/transverse dimensions, and midline deviation can be observed, as well as favorable clockwise rotation of the greater palatal segment

Associated Poor Outcomes and Complications

The main problem associated with the use of presurgical orthopedics is the compromise of the final aesthetic treatment outcome. Based on the Levy-Bercowski et al.'s study [49], we may consider two types of complications associated with presurgical orthopedics (specifically NAM): soft and hard tissue complications. These undesirable outcomes may be the result of inadequate use of the orthopedic device or individual reactions of the patients to the foreign material.

Soft Tissue Complications Soft tissues (skin and mucosa) may be affected by contact or pressure with the foreign material used for orthopedic purposes. It is not rare to observe skin and mucosa ulceration or irritation (reported in more than 10% of cases), bleeding, and infection during the use of these devices [49].

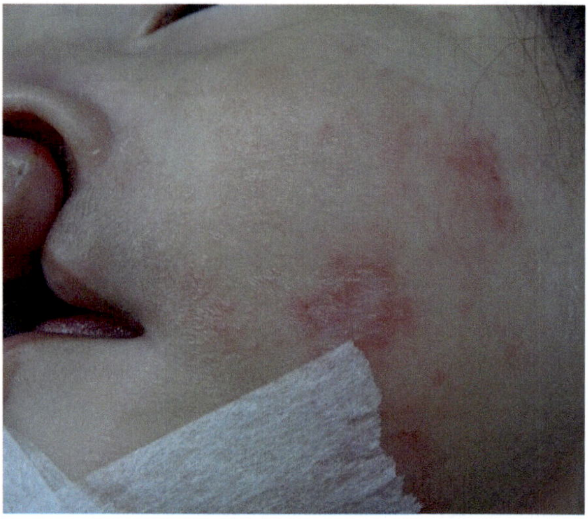

Fig. 4.36 Contact dermatitis produced by adhesives during nasoalveolar molding treatment in a cleft lip and palate patient

Skin irritation (contact dermatitis) is commonly observed in relation to the use of tapes and bandages which require temporal suspension of its use and local treatment. If the patient is hypersensitive to the material used, the treatment should be finished, and another alternative should be used (Fig. 4.36).

Ulceration is a more severe complication and may leave permanent scars with cosmetic and/or functional sequels. It is produced by contact of the acrylic material with the oral mucosa or skin.

Parents must identify these problems early in order to alert the healthcare provider and proceed with an adequate treatment. Any delay will worsen the complication resulting in permanent sequels that complicate surgical procedures later.

Infections (in special fungal infections) are mostly associated with *Candida albicans*. The molding plate should be removed and cleaned regularly in order to prevent this problem. They should be treated using Nystatin or Amphotericin ointment.

In relation to the nasal soft tissues, ulcers, bleeding, and irritation are also observed. Bleeding produced by a rough nasal stent may be avoided by deactivating the device for approximately 1 week to allow for tissue recovery, after which the stent can be reactivated with reduced force.

Personally, I observed nasal soft tissue thinning after molding; this condition affects the performance of surgical techniques involving cartilage dissection and may produce more poor outcomes and complications.

Hard Tissue Complications These complications are related mostly to incorrect mobilization of the cleft segments. Adequate approximation of the segments is crucial, to facilitate an adequate alignment of the maxilla.

Another important poor outcome is the secondary maxillary hypoplasia. This was described by Samuel Berkowitz, and it is related to vomeropremaxillary junction synostosis as a consequence of premaxilla retrusion by the action of an alveolar molding device [10]. Finally, another complication is the premature eruption of the premaxillary incisors as a result of the pressure exerted by the molding plate. Their extraction may be indicated if the erupting tooth is mobile or interferes with activation of the device.

References

1. Hoffman W, Lierle D. Studies on the pathologic anatomy of the unilateral harelip nose. Plast Reconstr Surg. 1949;4:225–34.
2. Millard DR. A rhinoplasty tetralogy: corrective, secondary, congenital, reconstructive. Little Brown & Company; 1996.
3. McNeil CK. Orthodontic procedures in the treatment of congenital cleft palate. Dent Record. 1950;70:126–32.
4. Burston WR. (1960). The pre-surgical orthopaedic correction of the maxillary deformity in clefts of both primary and secondary palate. In: Wallace AB, editor. Transactions of the International Society of Plastic Surgeons, Second Congress, London. Edinburgh/London: E&S Livingston Ltd.; 1959. p. 28–36.
5. Hotz M, Gnoinski W. Comprehensive care of cleft lip and palate children at Zürich University: a preliminary report. Am J Orthod. 1976;70(5):481–504.
6. Matsuo K, Hirose T. Nonsurgical correction of cleft lip nasal deformity in the early neonate. Ann Acad Med Singap. 1988;17(3):358–65.
7. Matsuo K, Hirose T, Tomono T, Iwasawa M, Katohda S, Takahashi N, Koh B. Nonsurgical correction of congenital auricular deformities in the early neonate: a preliminary report. Plast Reconstr Surg. 1984 Jan;73(1):38–51.
8. Grayson BH, Cutting C, Wood R. Preoperative columella lengthening in bilateral cleft lip and palate. Plast Reconstr Surg. 1993;92(7):1422–3.
9. Grayson BH, Cutting CB. Presurgical nasoalveolar orthopedic molding in primary correction of the nose, lip, and alveolus of infants born with unilateral and bilateral clefts. Cleft Palate Craniofac J. 2001;38(3):193–8.
10. Berkowitz S. The facial growth pattern and the amount of palatal bone deficiency relative to cleft size should be considered in treatment planning. Plast Reconstr Surg Glob Open. 2016;4:e705.
11. Berkowitz S. Why hasn't Cutting and Grayson done a longitudinal study to show why nasoalveolar molding should not be used? Cleft Palate Craniofac J. 2019;56(1):141.
12. Freitas R, Lopes A, Douat H, Moraes N, Nakakogue T, et al. Weight gain in children with cleft lip and palate without use of plates. Plast Surg Int. 2012;2012:973240.
13. Batra P, Gribel BF, Abhinav BA, Arora A, Raghavan S. OrthoAligner "NAM": a case series of Presurgical Infant Orthopedics (PSIO) using clear aligners. Cleft Palate Craniofac J. 2020;57(5):646–55.
14. Mejia M, Wolfe E, Murphy B, Rothenberg L, Tejero A, Bauer M, et al. Gingivosupraperiosteoplasty following presurgical maxillary orthopedics is associated with normal midface growth in complete unilateral and bilateral cleft patients at mixed dentition. Plast Reconstr Surg. 2021;148(6):1335–46.
15. Park J, Kaira A, Parsael Y, Rochlin D, Verzella A, Grayson B, et al. The effects of gingivoperiosteoplasty and cleft palate repair on facial growth. Plast Reconstr Surg J. 2023;153:1110. https://doi.org/10.1097/PRS.0000000000010681. Epub ahead of print. PMID: 37184473.
16. Wolfe S, Podda S, Mejia M. Correction of nostril stenosis and alteration of nostril shape with an orthonostric device. Plast Reconstr Surg J. 2008;121(6):1974–7.
17. Brown G. A system for the surgical correction of harelip and cleft palate. JAMA. 1905;44:848–59.

18. Federspiel M. Hare lip and cleft palate. Laryngoscope. 1922;32:909–28.
19. Pool R, Farnworth TK. Preoperative lip taping in the cleft lip. Ann Plast Surg. 1994;32(3):243–9.
20. Vinson L. The effect of DynaCleft® on cleft width in unilateral cleft lip and palate patients. J Clin Pediatr Dent. 2017;41(6):442–5.
21. Monasterio L, Ford A, Gutiérrez C, Tastets ME, García J. Comparative study of nasoalveolar molding methods: nasal elevator plus DynaCleft® versus NAM-Grayson in patients with complete unilateral cleft lip and palate. Cleft Palate Craniofac J. 2013;50(5):548–54.
22. Abd El-Ghafour M, Aboulhassan M, El-Beialy A, et al. Is taping alone an efficient presurgical infant orthopedic approach in infants with unilateral cleft lip and palate? A randomized controlled trial. Cleft Palate Craniofac J. 2020;57(12):1382–91.
23. Singhal R, Namdev R, Kumar A, Dayma C, Rani A. Treatment outcomes of lip taping in patients with non-syndromic cleft lip and/or palate. A systematic review and meta analysis. Cleft Palate Craniofac J. 2024. https://doi.org/10.1177/10556656241249822.
24. Thabitha S, Rajendra R, Manjula M, Sreelakshmi N, Rajesh A. Diversities in presurgical orthopedics: a review. J Adv Clin Res Insights. 2015;2:94–9.
25. Brauer R, Cronin T. Maxillary orthopedics and anterior palate repair with bone grafting. Cleft Palate J. 1964;1:31–42.
26. Rossell-Perry P. The surgical Nasoalveolar molding: a rational treatment for unilateral cleft lip nose deformity and literature review. Plast Reconstr Surg Glob Open. 2020;8(8):e3044.
27. Georgiade NG, Latham RA. Maxillary arch alignment in the bilateral cleft lip and palate infant, using pinned coaxial screw appliance. Plast Reconstr Surg. 1975;56(1):52–60.
28. Hotz MM, Gnoinski WM. Effects of early maxillary orthopaedics in coordination with delayed surgery for cleft lip and palate. J Maxillofac Surg. 1979;7(3):201–10.
29. Randall P. A lip adhesion operation in cleft lip surgery. Plast Reconstr Surg. 1965;35(4):371–6.
30. Millard DR Jr, Latham RA. Improved primary surgical and dental treatment of clefts. Plast Reconstr Surg. 1990;86:856–71.
31. Vander Woude DL, Mulliken JB. Effect of lip adhesion on labial height in two-stage repair of unilateral complete cleft lip. Plast Reconstr Surg. 1997;100:567–72.
32. Hamilton R, Graham W, Randall P. The role of the lip adhesion procedure in cleft lip repair. Cleft Palate J. 1971;8:1–9.
33. Nagy K, Mommaerts MY. Lip adhesion revisited: a technical note with review of literature. Indian J Plast Surg. 2009;42(2):204–12.
34. Moetamedi AK, Feizbakhsh M, Mortazavi M, Derakhshanfar H, Hasheminasab M. Nasoalveolar molding in cleft lip and palate, a review of literature. Asian J Chem. 2014;26(12):70–3. https://doi.org/10.1093/jae/ejp002.
35. Patel PA, Rubin MS, Clouston S, Lalezaradeh F, Brecht LE, Cutting CB, et al. Comparative study of early secondary nasal revisions and costs in patients with clefts treated with and without nasoalveolar molding. J Craniofac Surg. 2015;26(4):1229–33.
36. Rubin MS, Clouston S, Ahmed MM, Lowe KM, Shetye PR, Broder HL, et al. Assessment of presurgical clefts and predicted surgical outcome in patients treated with and without nasoalveolar molding. J Craniofac Surg. 2015;26(1):71–5.
37. Sischo L, Chan JW, Stein M, Smith C, Van Aalst J, Broder HL. Nasoalveolar molding: prevalence of cleft centers offering NAM and who seeks it. Cleft Palate Craniofac J. 2012;49(3):270–5.
38. Bauer FX, Schönberger M, Gattinger J, Eblenkamp M, Wintermantel E, Rau A, Güll FD, Wolff KD, Loeffelbein DJ. RapidNAM: generative manufacturing approach of nasoalveolar molding devices for presurgical cleft lip and palate treatment. Biomed Tech. 2017;62(4):407–14.
39. Barenghi L, Barenghi A, Cadeo C, Di Blasio A. Innovation by computer-aided design/computer-aided manufacturing technology: a look at infection prevention in dental settings. Biomed Res Int. 2019;2019:5–13.
40. Miyazaki T, Hotta Y, Kunii J, Kuriyama S, Tamaki Y. A review of dental CAD/CAM: current status and future perspectives from 20 years of experience. Dent Mater J. 2009;28(1):44–56.
41. Dalessandri D, Tonni I, Laffranchi L, Migliorati M, Isola G, Bonetti S, Visconti L, Paganelli C. Evaluation of a digital protocol for pre-surgical orthopedic treatment of cleft lip and palate in newborn patients: a pilot study. Dent J (Basel). 2019;7(4):111.

42. Rossell-Perry P, Olivencia-Flores C, Delgado-Jimenez MP, Ormeño-Aquino R. Surgical naso-alveolar molding: a rational treatment for bilateral cleft lip nose and systematic review. Plast Reconstr Surg Glob Open. 2020;8(9):e3082.
43. Schiebl J, Bauer FX, Grill F, Loeffelbein DJ. RapidNAM: Algorithm for the Semi-Automated Generation of Nasoalveolar Molding Device Designs for the Presurgical Treatment of Bilateral Cleft Lip and Palate. IEEE Trans Biomed Eng. 2020;67(5):1263–71.
44. Yu Q, Gong X, Shen G. CAD presurgical nasoalveolar molding effects on the maxillary morphology in infants with UCLP. Oral Surg Oral Med Oral Pathol Oral Radiol. 2013;116(4):418–26.
45. Abd El-Ghafour M, Aboulhassan MA, Fayed MMS, El-Beialy AR, Eid FHK, Hegab SE, El-Gendi M, Emara D. Effectiveness of a novel 3D-Printed Nasoalveolar Molding Appliance (D-NAM) on improving the maxillary arch dimensions in unilateral cleft lip and palate infants: a randomized controlled trial. Cleft Palate Craniofac J. 2020;57(12):1370–81. https://doi.org/10.1177/1055665620954321. Epub 2020 Sep 10.
46. Zheng J, He H, Kuang W, Yuan W. Presurgical nasoalveolar molding with 3D printing for a patient with unilateral cleft lip, alveolus, and palate. Am J Orthod Dentofacial Orthop. 2019;156(3):412–9. https://doi.org/10.1016/j.ajodo.2018.04.031. PMID: 31474271.
47. Ahmed MK, Ahsanuddin S, Retrouvey JM, Koka KS, Qureshi H, Bui AH, Taub PJ. Fabrication of nasoalveolar molding devices for the treatment of cleft lip and palate, using stereolithography additive manufacturing processes and computer-aided design manipulation software. J Craniofac Surg. 2019;30(8):2604–8.
48. Alvarez M, Escobar D, Castillo T, Gonzales-Hernandez E, Chaurasia A, et al. Preliminary results for a three dimensional printer novel approach in nasal molding for infants with unilateral cleft lip and palate. J Cleft Lip Palate Craniofacial Anomalies. 2024;11(1):30–6.
49. Levy-Bercowski D, Abreu A, DeLeon E, Looney S, Stockstill J, Weiler M, Santiago PE. Complications and solutions in presurgical nasoalveolar molding therapy. Cleft Palate Craniofac J. 2009;46(5):521–8.

The Unilateral Cleft Lip Nose Deformity

5

Percy Rossell-Perry

Contents

Introduction

Nasal deformity associated with the unilateral cleft lip can vary from minor to severe (Figs. 5.1, 5.2, and 5.3). This is a three-dimensional deformity, and its components include the tip and columella, caudal septum, the vestibule, nasal floor, muscular components, and the skeleton. The nasal tip is displaced and asymmetric in association with short and deviated columella, and the fibers of the orbicularis oris muscle do not develop across the midline and produce unnatural lifting of the mouth with distortion of the lip and nose.

In addition, the skeletal distortion produces outward rotation of the primary palate and the simultaneous malposition of the lateral maxillary segment to different degrees. Even if the skeleton is not significantly affected, these discrepancies are responsible for nasal asymmetry.

The nasal septum plays an important role in nose deformity associated with the unilateral cleft lip. Due to the skeletal distortion, the caudal septum tilts over the cleft, exiting the vomerine groove. This abnormal position may be responsible for

P. Rossell-Perry (✉)
Health of Science Faculty, School of Human Medicine, Peruvian University Union (UpeU), Lima, Peru
e-mail: percy.rossell@upeu.edu.pe

P. Rossell-Perry (ed.), *Atlas of Primary Cleft Rhinoplasty*,
https://doi.org/10.1007/978-3-031-68012-0_5

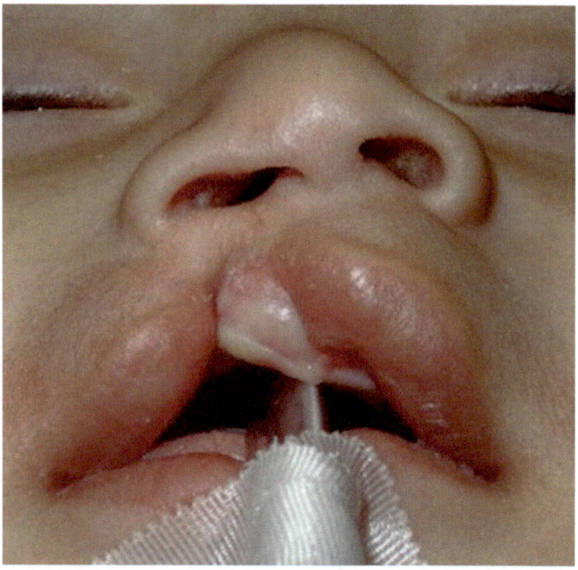

Fig. 5.1 Mild unilateral cleft lip nasal deformity

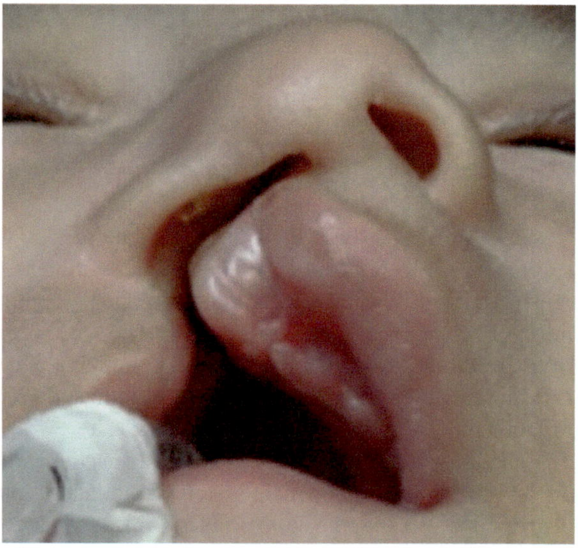

Fig. 5.2 Moderate unilateral cleft lip nasal deformity

the nasal tip appearance in unilateral cleft lips. In addition, septal malpositioning produces a decrease in the vertical height of the columellar defection to different degrees (Figs. 5.4, 5.5, and 5.6). Another associated finding may be lower turbinate hypertrophy and maxillary hypoplasia. The nasal floor may vary depending on the complete or incomplete nature of the cleft lip, from a wide gap to a nasal floor within a millimeter of the normal width. Regarding the alar cartilage, the affected lower lateral cartilage is dislodged from its natural position in the dome of the tip. The medial crus appears to be spread and stretched at an obtuse angle. The alar base

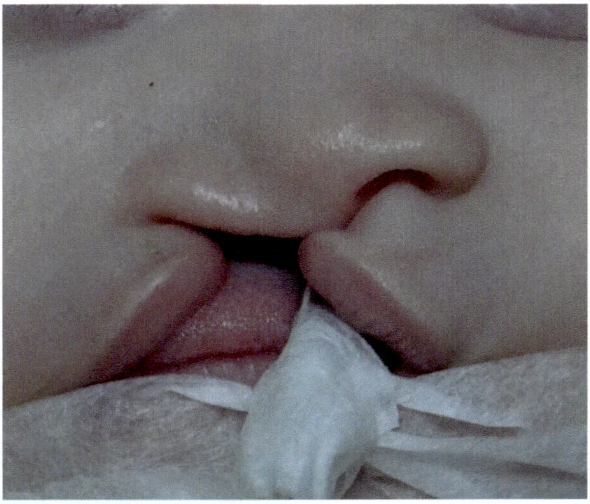

Fig. 5.3 Severe unilateral cleft lip nasal deformity

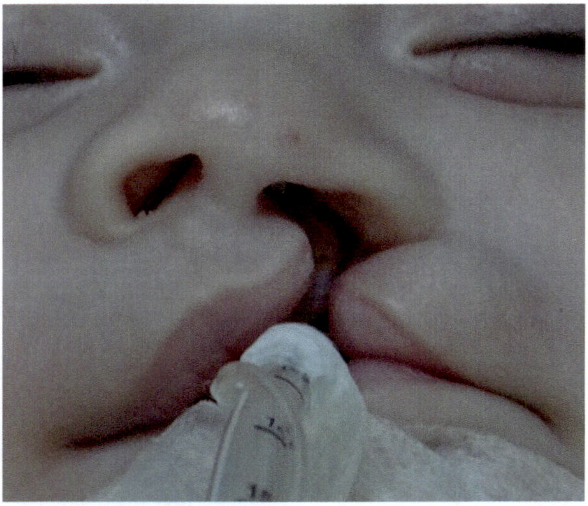

Fig. 5.4 Mild nasal tip and columellar deformity in unilateral cleft lip

is characteristically wider and rotated outwardly in a flare (Figs. 5.7, 5.8, and 5.9). The importance of the vestibular lining increases according to the type of surgical technique proposed by the author. These techniques produce lengthening of the stretched vestibule in order to normalize the position of the cartilages of the tip of the nose. The effect of this method reproduces the temporal effect of nasal molding using presurgical orthopedics; therefore, the author named this technique "surgical nasoalveolar molding" [1]. The vestibule of the nose seems to be stretched in comparison with the normal side; however, this concept is under debate since the normal appearance of the nasal tip can be achieved after releasing of the lateral crus from its lateral attachment to the pyriform aperture. At this point, it is important to mention that the nose distortion described here may be found in normal lips or relatively

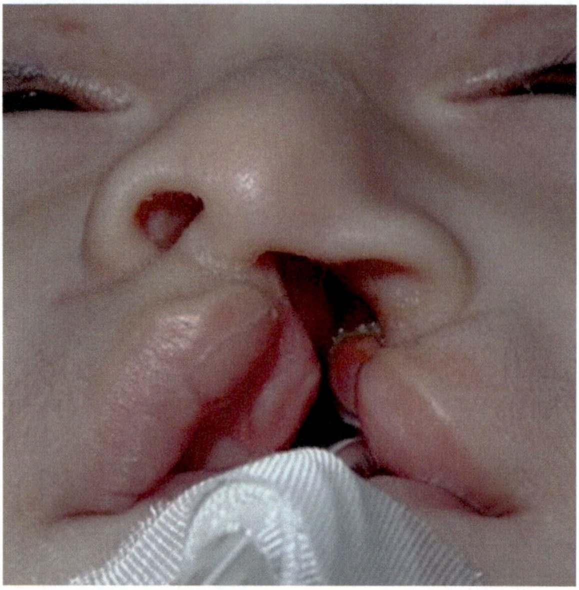

Fig. 5.5 Moderate nasal tip and columellar deformity in unilateral cleft lip

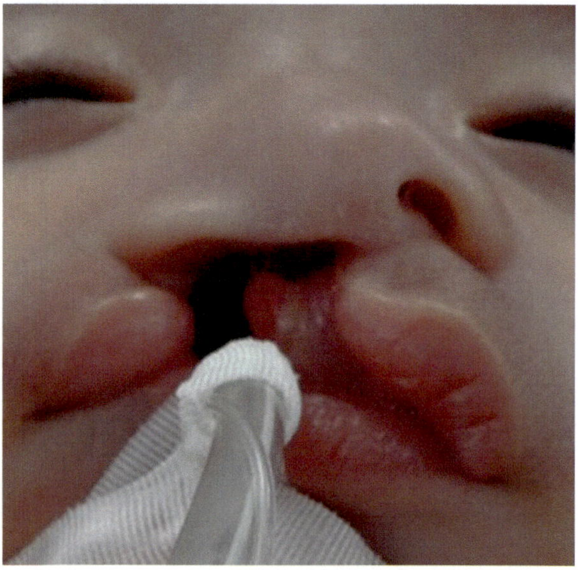

Fig. 5.6 Severe nasal tip and columellar deformity in unilateral cleft lip

small lip deficiencies as Ralph Millard Jr. mentioned in his book [2]. Considering that facial asymmetry is normal in the population, minor differences before or after surgery may be considered as normal, and any surgical indication should be well discussed with patients and their parents.

The following four basic types of unilateral cleft lip have been described: complete, complete with Simonart's band, incomplete, and microform. For surgical

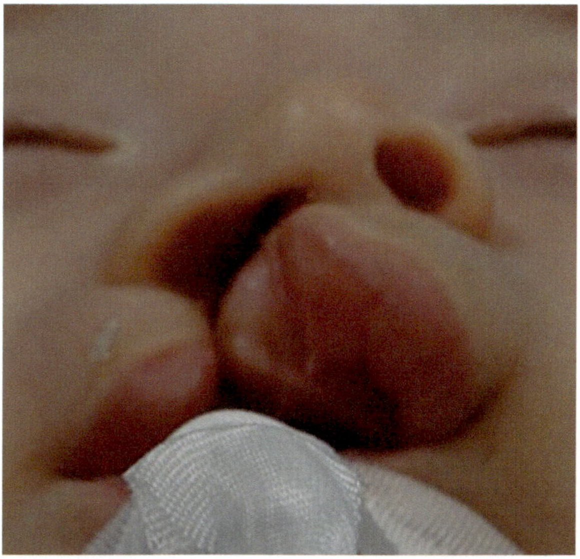

Fig. 5.7 Mild alar base deformity in unilateral cleft lip

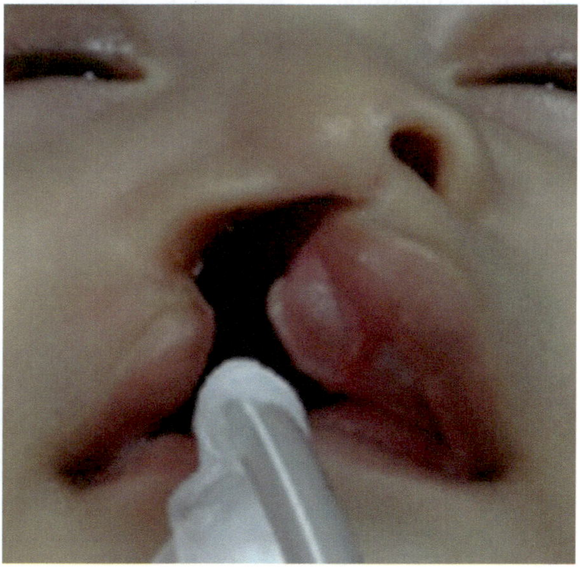

Fig. 5.8 Moderate alar base deformity in unilateral cleft lip

purposes, the complete form including a Simonart's band is managed as a complete form; therefore, they may be considered a single type. Nasal deformity associated with a unilateral cleft lip correlates well with these three types of deformity.

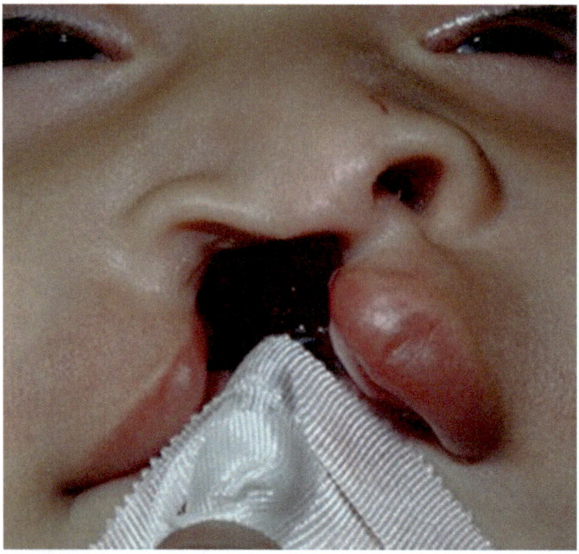

Fig. 5.9 Severe alar base deformity in unilateral cleft lip

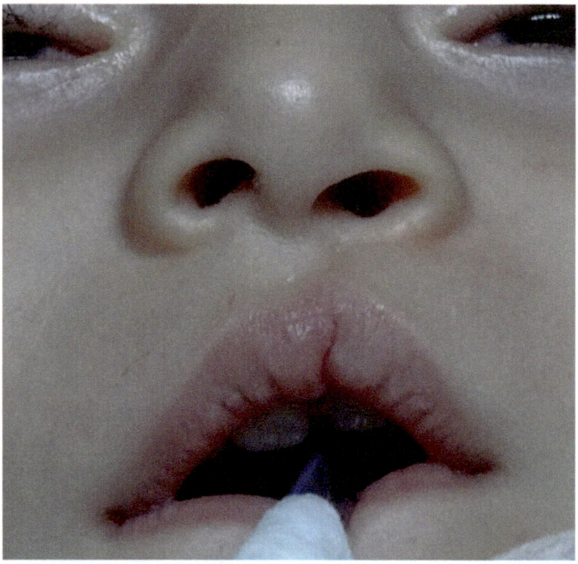

Fig. 5.10 Left microform unilateral cleft lip nose deformity

The Microform Unilateral Cleft Lip Nose Deformity (Figs. 5.10, 5.11, and 5.12)

Microforms are characterized by minor deficiencies in lip height (less than 3 mm), and nose deformity is often associated even in the absence of an obvious cleft lip (a muscular cleft may exist without skin or mucosa deficiencies). These nasal abnormalities may vary in their presentation; however, they are mostly characterized by alar base and nostril asymmetry and medial crus foreshortened. Septal and skeletal deficiencies are rare to be associated.

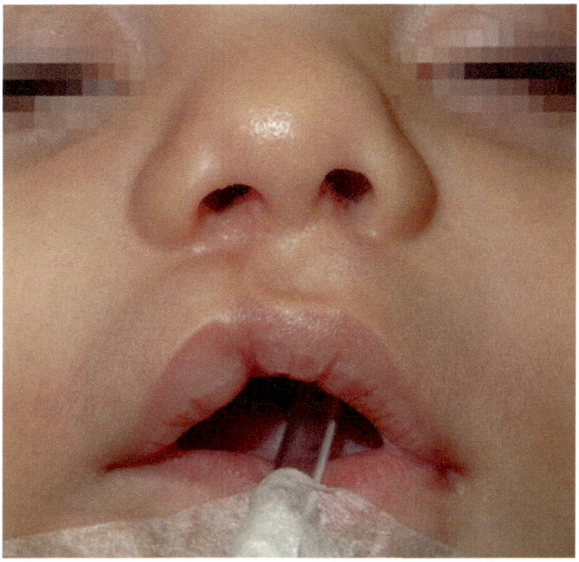

Fig. 5.11 Right microform unilateral cleft lip nose deformity

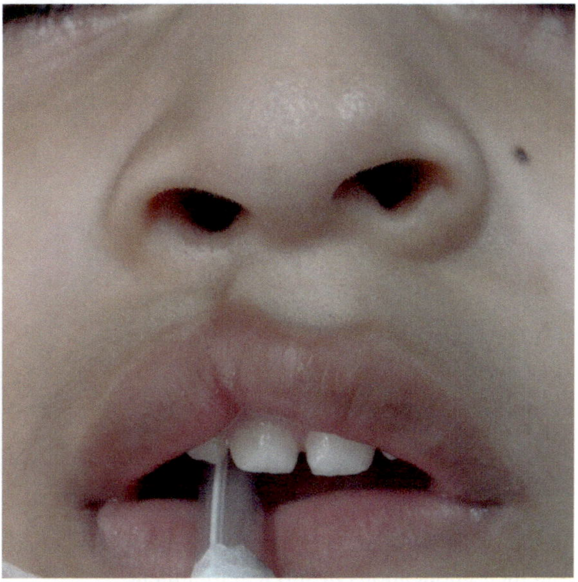

Fig. 5.12 Right microform unilateral cleft lip nose deformity

Incomplete Unilateral Cleft Lip Nose Deformity (Figs. 5.13, 5.14, and 5.15)

The spectrum of incomplete cleft lips may vary from microforms to extended incomplete clefts. Nose deformity usually correlates with the severity of an incomplete cleft lip. Sometimes the parents are unaware of their minimal malformations in their children, especially when they have microforms. Based on the components

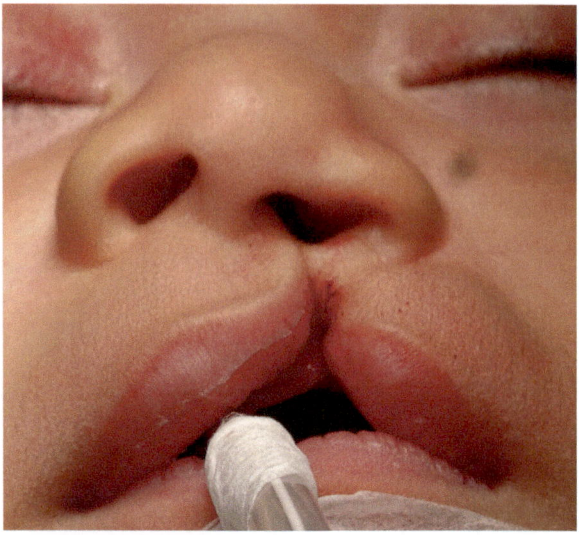

Fig. 5.13 Left incomplete unilateral cleft lip nose deformity

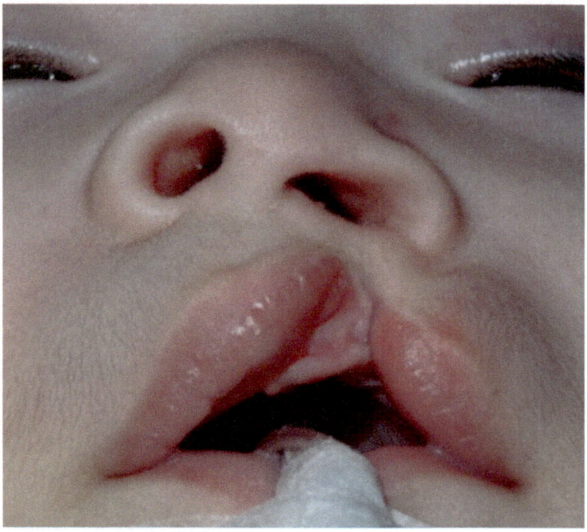

Fig. 5.14 Left incomplete unilateral cleft lip nose deformity

of the nose, we may describe the characteristics of incomplete unilateral cleft lips and their applications in surgical treatment.

Nasal floor The nasal floor has four sections as follows: nostril sill, primary palate (alveolus), secondary palate (hard palate), and soft palate. The nostril sill and primary palate may be partially or not affected in this type of cleft lip.

Columella Even when the columellar component looks "short," it is obliquely malpositioned and requires repositioning instead of lengthening. This concept is

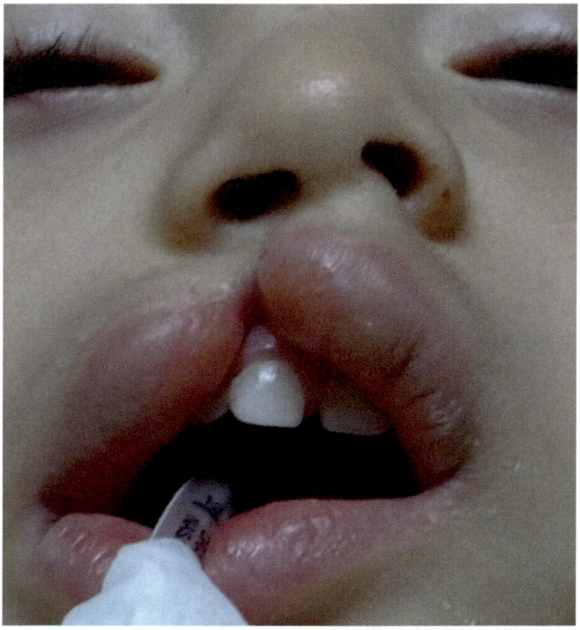

Fig. 5.15 Right incomplete unilateral cleft lip nose deformity

opposed to the traditional Millard's philosophy that promotes the lengthening of the columella using lip tissues.

Alar base Alar base distortion in incomplete cleft lips is characterized by alar base asymmetry with alar hooding. In addition, nostril asymmetry, inward buckling of the cleft side ala, and retrodisplacement of the cleft side alar dome may be observed. Therefore, the need for alar base repair is conditional on the severity of the incomplete form.

Nasal tip Even in small deficiencies of the lip, some abnormal changes can be observed, as follows: the tip of the nose may be deflected and the dome at the cleft side is retrodisplaced resulting in decreased projection. The angle between the medial and lateral crura is obtuse, and there may be some associated bone deficiency of the maxilla on the clef side.

Nasal septum The nasal septum often deviates but not to the same extent as the complete forms. The anterior nasal spine and the caudal septum are displaced to different extents to the noncleft side.

Alar cartilage An obtuse angle exists between the medial and lateral crura on the cleft side. In addition, inward buckling of the ala and retrodisplacement of the alar dome on the cleft side affect the form and extension of the nasal vestibule. It is important to mention that this structure may be congenital hypoplastic and may play an important role in the quality of surgical outcomes.

Nostril This component is asymmetric in comparison with the noncleft side. A wider nostril is observed on the cleft side.

Maxilla The existence of a cleft may vary among patients with incomplete cleft lips. Sometimes it exists as simple notch or as an alveolar cleft. Commonly, all of these variants have an aligned maxillary arch. It is not rare to observe the association between incomplete cleft lip and incomplete cleft palate.

Complete Unilateral Cleft Lip Nose Deformity (Figs. 5.16, 5.17, and 5.18)

This complex deformity involves distortion of the skeleton and soft tissues of the nose. The existence of a hypoplastic segment (cleft side) limits lip and nose reconstruction. Even when clear evidence exists regarding the hypoplasia of the lateral segment of the lip, there is not evident deficiency of the cartilage structures of the nose; therefore, total reconstruction of the nose is possible despite of the severity of the cleft. Based on the nose components, we may describe characteristics of complete unilateral cleft lips and their applications to the surgical treatment. They include the following:

Grossly asymmetric nose
Columella deviated toward the noncleft side
Nostril wider and retrodisplaced on the cleft side
Nostril margin buckles inward on the cleft side. This is because of bowing by the internal vestibular web.
Maxilla deficiency on the cleft side
Posterolaterally displaced alar base and piriform aperture on cleft side
Deviated caudal septum, premaxilla, and columella toward noncleft side

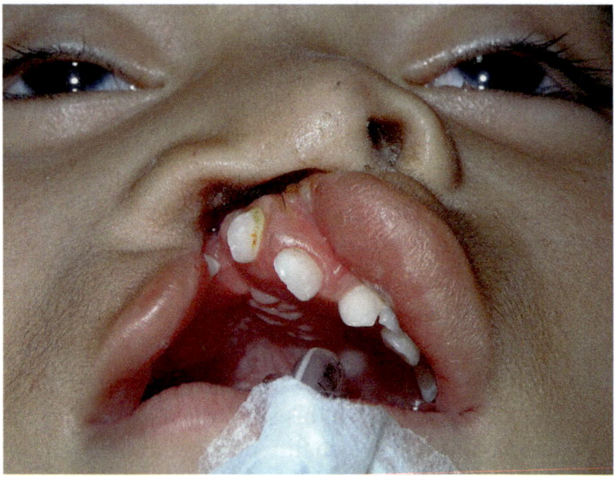

Fig. 5.16 Right complete unilateral cleft lip nose deformity

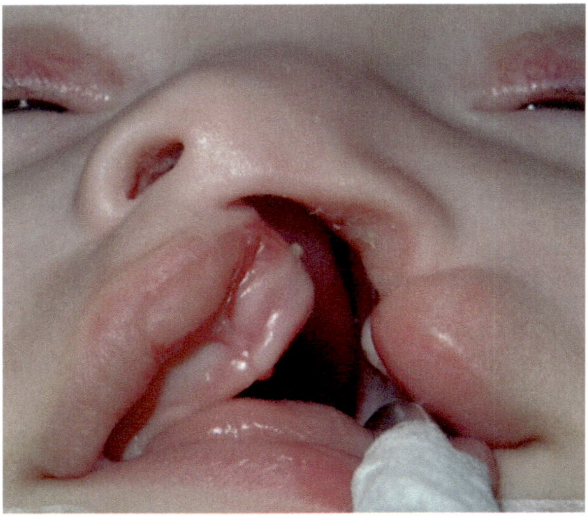

Fig. 5.17 Left complete unilateral cleft lip nose deformity

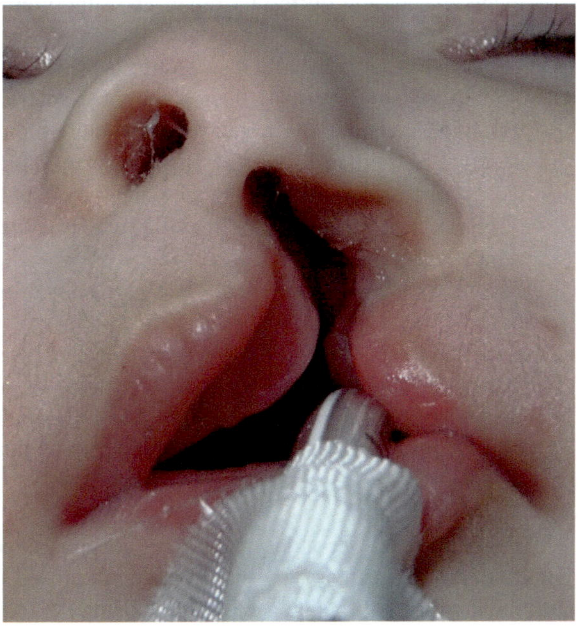

Fig. 5.18 Left complete unilateral cleft lip nose deformity

Posterolaterally displaced alar dome
Increased angle between the medial and lateral crura
Shortened medial crus and lengthened lateral crus
Malpositioned upper and lower lateral cartilage

Nasal floor The nasal floor has four sections as follows (Figs. 5.19):

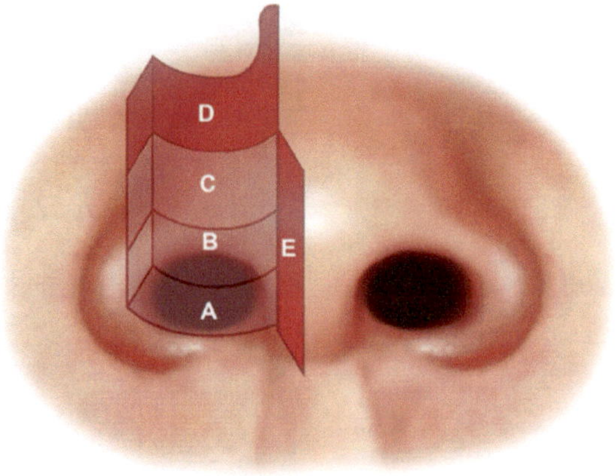

Fig. 5.19 The nasal floor in the unilateral cleft lip and palate. This is an intraoral view of a patient with unilateral cleft lip and palate illustrating the absence of segments of the nasal floor. (A) Nostril sill (nasal vestibule). (B) Primary palate (alveolus). (C) Secondary palate (hard palate). (D) Secondary palate (soft palate) (E) Nasal septum

(a) Nostril sill. This is the most anterior portion of the nasal floor and represents the nasal vestibule floor; this is repaired primarily using the lateral and medial elements of the cleft during lip repair and supported by the muscular reconstruction. The presence of Simonart's band is not relevant for reconstructive purposes, and it is usually resected during primary lip and nose repair.
(b) Primary palate (alveolus). This is the most anterior portion of the nasal skeleton. It is attached to the vomer (as the vomero premaxillary junction), the lower segment of the nasal segment. It is primarily repaired using the Oslo protocol [3]. A concern exists regarding the potential effect of the gingivoperiosteoplasty (GPP) on the growth of the maxilla, which is why it is not used in different protocols [4].
(c) Secondary palate (hard palate). It is represented by the posterior section of the nasal skeleton and is composed of two bones: the upper maxilla (palatine process) and the palatine bone (horizontal plate). This section is repaired during the primary palatoplasty and depends on the type of protocol used.
(d) Secondary palate (soft palate). This portion includes the palatine muscles covered by mucosa, is functional, and creates the anterior part of velopharyngeal sphincter.

The primary and secondary palates are repaired depending on the protocol used, for example, the primary and hard palate are closed together first using the Oslo protocol and the soft palate is closed first using the Goteborg protocol.

All these elements in complete unilateral cleft lip and palates are absent and should be repaired during primary surgery through the lip and palate surgery.

Alar base The lateral element of the cleft is attached to the skeletal structure (pyriform aperture of the maxilla). It should be released for proper alignment of alar bases during primary lip repair. Muscular repair is also important providing support for the nasal sill. Malposition of the alar base after primary cheilorhinoplasty is not related to a lack of skeletal support (a common misconception). In fact, this occurs because of a poor repair of the oral muscles.

Columella The concepts used for columellar repair are the same as those used for incomplete cleft lip repair. The columella should be repositioned instead of lengthened. The medial crus and dome medial repositioning (independent of the technique used) allowed us to correct the columellar position.

The columella should not be elongated using lip tissues as Millard proposed. The distal portion of caudal septum can be corrected by muscular action when it is properly done.

Nasal tip This structure is commonly affected in complete forms and to different degrees. Its distortion is related to maxillary collapse; however, maxilla correction is not necessary for nasal structure repositioning, and maxillary alignment occurs spontaneously as a consequence of nose and oral muscle reconstruction providing adequate support for the nose.

Nasal septum The nasal septum often deviates to different degrees and generates aesthetic and functional distortions of the nose. Even when some authors promote its primary correction as the key point of the primary cleft rhinoplasty, more studies are required to confirm its long-term effect in cleft lip patients.

Alar cartilage Between the medial and lateral crura on the cleft side, an obtuse angle exists depending on the severity of the nose deformity in unilateral cleft lips. Its role in the nasal vestibule determines the extent of the corrective surgery. The orthopedic nasoalveolar molding corrects the nasal vestibule but only temporarily which is why the primary surgery is always needed. The author creates the surgical nasal molding concept producing a surgical extension of the vestibule but without presurgical treatment.

Nostril This component is asymmetric in comparison with noncleft side, and wider nostril is observed on the cleft side; therefore, the objective of the primary repair is to create symmetric nostrils.

Maxilla Sometimes the surgical repair of the lip is sufficient to produce an alignment of the maxillary segments independent of the width of the cleft or maxillary collapse. The author named this effect as the "surgical nasoalveolar molding" which is evidence of the lack of need for plates. In addition, there is a lack of evidence supporting the effect of orthopedic devices for nasal and maxillary molding, and probably the best therapeutic molding is the one produced by repaired muscular action.

Surgical Protocol

Primary cleft rhinoplasty is an important step in cleft lip and palate reconstruction, and it is performed actually during the primary lip repair for all types of cleft lips; however, this complex deformity requires soft tissue and skeleton management at

Table 5.1 Unilateral cleft lip nasal repair surgical protocol

Age	Degree of severity	Surgery
3–6 months	Microform	Nasal base shortening
	Incomplete	Rotational composite flap technique
	Mild complete	Rotational composite flap technique
	Moderate complete	VYZ cleft rhinoplasty
	Severe complete	VYZ cleft rhinoplasty + septoplasty
5 years	All complete	Alveolar cleft closure
		Intermediate rhinoplasty or revision
7–9 years	All complete	Alveolar bone graft
16–18 years		Secondary rhinoplasty

different surgical times. Since the neonatal presurgical management to the secondary rhinoplasty refinement during the adulthood, the nose deformity associated with cleft lip requires different interventions from those of the interdisciplinary cleft team to achieve good functional and aesthetic outcomes. Management during the timeline of the patient's life is presented in Table 5.1. The presented protocol for primary unilateral cleft lip nose repair is indicated according to the type of unilateral cleft lip [5, 6].

References

1. Rossell-Perry P. The surgical nasoalveolar molding: a rational treatment for unilateral cleft lip nose deformity and literature review. Plast Reconstr Surg Glob Open. 2020;8(8):e3044.
2. Millard DR. A rhinoplasty tetralogy: corrective, secondary, congenital, reconstructive. Boston: Little Brown & Company; 1996.
3. Åbyholm FE, Borchgrevink HC, Eskeland G. Cleft lip and palate in Norway: III. Surgical treatment of CLP patients in Oslo 1954–75. Scand J Plast Reconstr Surg. 1981;15(1):15–28.
4. Berkowitz S. Gingivoperiosteoplasty as well as early palatal cleft closure is unproductive. J Craniofac Surg. 2009;20(8):1747–58.
5. Rossell-Perry P. Rotational composite flap technique for primary incomplete cleft nose deformity. Plast Reconstr Surg Glob Open. 2020;8(6):e2870.
6. Rossell-Perry P. Primary unilateral cleft lip nasal deformity repair using VYZ plasty: an anthropometric study. Indian J Plast Surg. 2017;50(02):180–6.

Surgical Techniques for Unilateral Cleft Lip Nose Repair

6

Percy Rossell-Perry

Contents

Supplementary Information The online version contains supplementary material available at https://doi.org/10.1007/978-3-031-68012-0_6.

P. Rossell-Perry (✉)
Health of Science Faculty, School of Human Medicine, Peruvian University Union (UpeU), Lima, Peru
e-mail: percy.rossell@upeu.edu.pe

P. Rossell-Perry (ed.), *Atlas of Primary Cleft Rhinoplasty*,
https://doi.org/10.1007/978-3-031-68012-0_6

Introduction

During long time, the primary treatment of the nose deformity associated with the unilateral cleft lip was delayed to later age because of the concern regarding growth disturbance; however, scientific evidence accumulated during the last years has been supported the utility and safety of the primary cleft rhinoplasty. Therefore it is including in most of the cleft protocols around the world [1, 2].

Different techniques have been published, and there is a lack of scientific evidence to determine which one is better than others. It seems that the surgeon's experience is more important than the surgical technique to guarantee good and long-term outcomes. During my personal experience, I used initially a more conservative method for nose repair during cleft lip surgery, specifically the Mc Comb's and later Salyer's methods [3, 4].

Based on these techniques, the structures of the tip of the nose were carefully dissected from the overlying skin and then repositioned using transcutaneous stitches, but the main issue during this time was the high rate of nose deformity relapse using this technique. Later during the appearance of the nasoalveolar molding devices (NAM), the method was included in our protocol but without any improvement in the quality of the nose outcomes. It is clear that the presurgical nasal molding is temporal, and only the surgical technique will provide long-term outcomes; lack of scientific evidence also confirms this statement [5, 6]. Looking for answers, I observed the effectiveness of techniques in secondary surgeries (some of these cases were not really secondary because the nose was not operated primarily; in fact they were primary cases). A combination of Potter's concept (the V-Y advancement) and Berkeley's method (lateral Z plasty) was used efficiently during long time for treatment of these "secondary" cases; therefore it may be useful for primary nose repair during lip closure [7–9]. The efficacy of this technique for primary cleft rhinoplasty was studied and included in our protocol for primary nose management; curiously, this method works well because of the expansion of the vestibule of the nose in a similar form that the orthopedic method (nasal molding) works; therefore, it was published as "surgical nasoalveolar molding" [10]. Finally, because of the observed differences of the nose deformity between the incomplete and complete cleft lips, a more conservative method was designed for incomplete cleft lips doing a rotational composite flap for alar cartilage reposition with good outcomes. The method was also studied and published to demonstrate its utility for incomplete cleft lip forms [11]. In this chapter, I describe these methods for primary unilateral cleft rhinoplasty in detail without the use of presurgical orthopedics and present well-illustrated long-term outcomes.

Presurgical Considerations

Age for primary lip cheilorhinoplasty seems to be under debate, and neonatal surgery is actually practiced in different centers; however, this is mostly applied to lip repair. In terms of nose and lip primary repair in patients with unilateral cleft lip, there is a consensus to schedule it around 3–6 months of age [2].

Preoperative Evaluation

Pediatric evaluation is essential to determine nutritional status and acute or chronic diseases, and patients qualified for primary surgery must have physical status class 1 or 2 based on parameters from the American Society of Anesthesiology (ASA) [12]. Syndromic cleft lip and palate cases must receive individual management and evaluation from the interdisciplinary team. The evaluation of primary nose repair should be outlined based on the "rule of ten" (10 pounds of weight, 10 g of hemoglobin per deciliter, and 10 weeks of life); however, this rule is only a combination of parameters easy to be remembered [13]. Recent reviews about the validation of these parameters as predictors of associated postoperative complications demonstrate that the most important parameter seems to be the weight of the child [14]. Presurgical evaluation should be completed with the following tests: full blood count, hemostasis, urine test, ECG, and cardiologic evaluation. The preoperative anesthesia evaluation should be performed the night before the surgery or even better the same day by pediatric anesthesiologist to identify if any active disease is present; in case of urinary or respiratory infection, the surgery should be delayed 2–4 weeks until the health status is improved. Presurgical instructions should include nothing per oral guidelines. The recommended fasting time is this: breast milk (4 h) and solids (6 h) and the surgical team should confirm this information from the parents [15]. Signed informed consent should be always obtained after enough information has been provided to the parents, and the surgical center must have a well-implemented postanesthetic care unit (PACU) and guaranteed access to pediatric intensive care unit (ICU).

Instruments

We have to consider that the cleft lip and nose surgery by definition is a microsurgery since we are working in a very small area, and adequate surgical instruments are recommended to perform this surgery. Surgical loupes are mandatory, and I prefer the 3.5 X magnification to be more precise during markings and surgical performance.

The surgical instrumental set for primary cleft rhinoplasty includes the following (Fig. 6.1):

Surgical pen marker. Scalpel round handle No 3. Surgical Blade No 15. Joseph double skin hook. Curved Iris supercut scissor. Straight Iris supercut scissor. Adson tissue forceps. Microsurgical needle holder. Stitch scissor.

They should be used in combination with proper surgical illumination during the procedure, and two types of light sources are commonly used. *Fixed light source*: they are operating room lamps (cialitic lamps). These lamps have more limitations to be adapted to difficult areas like nasal vestibule.

Mobile light source they are the headlights and more useful for primary cleft rhinoplasty purposes. Cephalic movements of the surgeon have proper illumination for

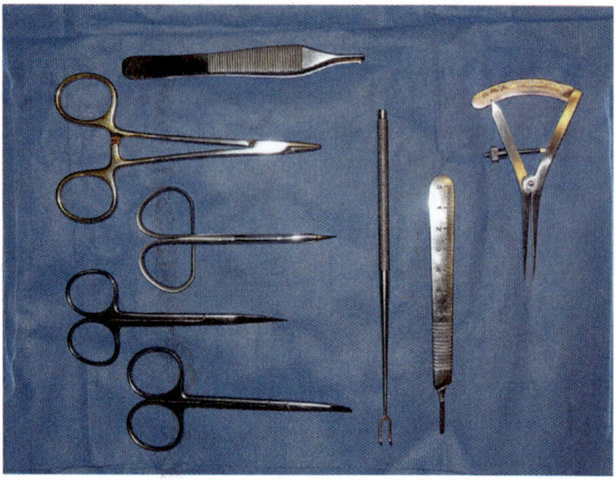

Fig. 6.1 Surgical instruments

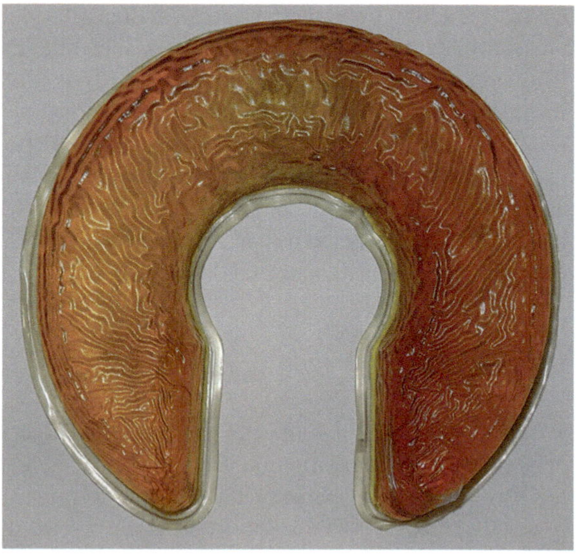

Fig. 6.2 Pediatric head positioning cushion

the different areas of the nose. The use of temperature monitors and warming devices is recommended during pediatric anesthesia, and the use of pediatric head positioning cushion is essential to limit any movement of the head during the surgery guaranteeing surgical precision and preventing neck injuries (Fig. 6.2). Surgical asepsis is performed using diluted iodine or chlorhexidine solutions, and fenestrated surgical drapes are commonly used in these surgeries. Throat packs are used to prevent aspiration of blood during cleft rhinoplasty surgery.

Anesthesia

The primary cleft rhinoplasty should be performed under general anesthesia provided by a pediatric anesthesiologist. Patient is intubated in supine position, and the endotracheal tube is centrally fixed using adhesive tapes. The use of local anesthetic is recommended to reduce the dose of general anesthesia and surgical bleeding during the procedure (because of the addition of vasoconstrictor). I personally like to perform lip markings before asepsis and anesthetic infiltration. Used amount of local anesthetic is 1 cc per Kg of xylocaine 1% or 0.5 cc per Kg of xylocaine 2%; in my practice, I use 1% solution, and then if the baby is 6 kg, I have 6 cc to be used for nerve block and local infiltration. A 0.1 ml of epinephrine (1:200,000) is added to the solution. Other local anesthetics like bupivacaine are not used because of the increased risk of side effects including cardiac arrest.

A combination of nerve block and local infiltration is used for nose anesthesia as follows.

Step 1. Infraorbital Nerve Block (Fig. 6.3)

The infiltration for infraorbital nerve block can be done through two different approaches using a fine needle (30-gauge needle). The first one is the external approach (through the skin) and the location of the infraorbital nerve is essential. Based on the literature, the mean distance from the base of the alae nasi to the infraorbital foramen is around 1 cm [16]. Another reference is considering a line drawn from the angle of the mouth to the midpoint of the palpebral fissure, and the nerve is situated approximately halfway along this line. The nerve block is performed only at the cleft side. If some bleeding is appearing after the injection, gentle pressure during few minutes is enough to stop it. The second approach (that I like to perform) is the internal (through oral mucosa), and the location of the infraorbital foramen is approximately 1 cm from the border of the pyriform aperture (Fig. 6.3). After location of the nerve position, using a syringe and fine needle, 1–1.5 cc of xylocaine 1% is infiltrated in the area to proceed with the nerve block. It is important that the surgeon should be advised to aspirate the needle before solution injection in order to prevent an intravascular access (infraorbital vessels).

Step 2. External Nasal Nerve Block (Fig. 6.4)

The nerve blocked in this procedure is the external branch of anterior ethmoidal nerve. This nerve arises from the nasociliary and exits between the border of the nasal bone and the upper lateral cartilage. It provides sensation to the nasal tip and medial aspect of the alae. The nerve approaches to the supraperichondral level from the notch conformed by the nasal bones (medially) and upper maxilla, more precise at the lowest point of the nasomaxillary suture. This point can be easily identified by palpation following the lower border of the nasal skeleton (Fig. 6.4). The nerve block can be done externally; however, this nerve is easily blocked during local infiltration of the nasal vestibule, and I recommend this option. After location of the nerve position, using a syringe and fine needle, 1 cc of xylocaine 1% is infiltrated in the area to proceed with the nerve block.

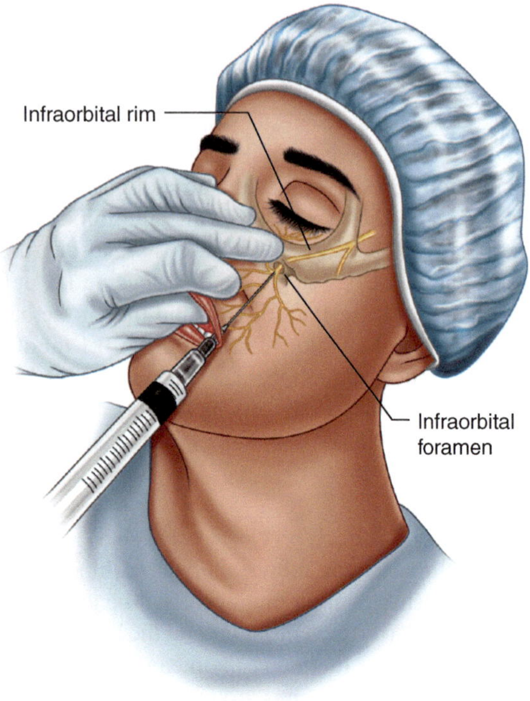

Fig. 6.3 Infraorbital nerve block internal approach

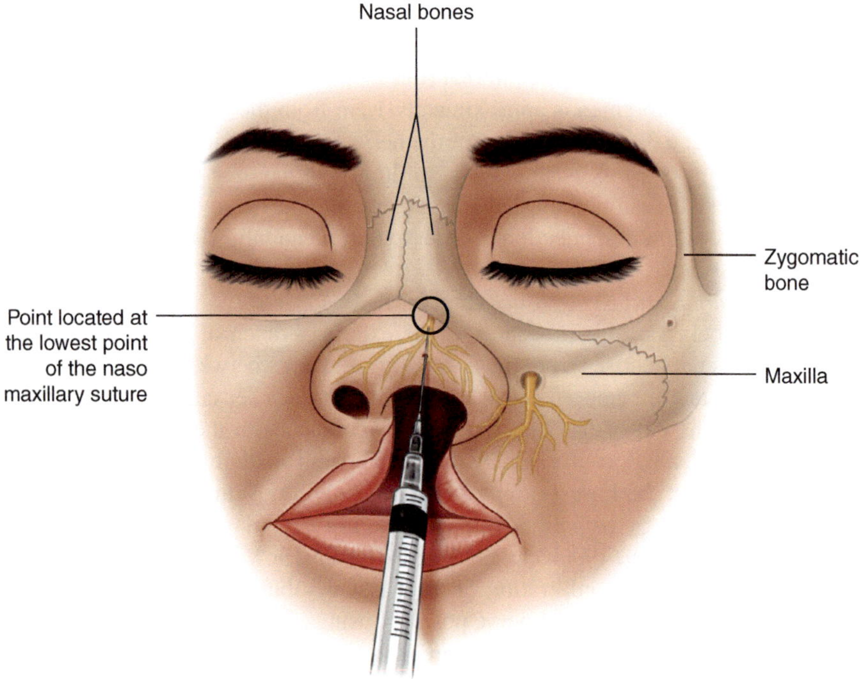

Fig. 6.4 External nasal nerve block procedure

Step 3. Nasal Tip Infiltration

Even when the infraorbital and external nasal nerve blocks are enough to produce local anesthesia for external nose, additional local infiltration is necessary for internal structures and the tip of the nose. Nasal tip is innervated by ophthalmic branches of the trigeminal nerve; specifically the external nasal nerve and the infiltration of this nerve may be enough for nasal tip anesthesia. However, additional infiltration to the nasal tip helps with dissection of the tip cartilages and reduces the surgical bleeding because of the vasoconstrictor effect. Approximately, 1 cc of xylocaine 1% is infiltrated over the supra perichondral level of the nasal tip. A fine needle is introduced through the nasal vestibule, specifically over the marginal border (lower border of alar cartilage).

Step 4. Vestibular Infiltration

Following the same concept applied to the nasal tip, infiltration of the nasal vestibule helps to the surgeon with the alar and dome cartilages of the nose developing a dissection of these structures. This maneuver makes easier the dissection of the nasal cartilages regardless of the used technique. Around 1 cc of xylocaine 1% is infiltrated using a fine needle following the marginal and the inter cartilaginous borders in both sides. In addition, the internal nasal valve (angle of medial intersection between the marginal and inter cartilaginous borders) infiltration let the surgeon block the nasal tip branches of the external nasal nerve.

Step 5. Caudal Septum Infiltration

The caudal septum is partially corrected during primary cleft rhinoplasty; therefore, the use of local anesthetic is necessary. Internal branches of anterior ethmoidal nerve provide sensation to the anterior portion of the caudal septum. Infiltration of the caudal septum helps to the surgeon with the dissection of this structure. Local infiltration of anesthetic in the subperichondrial area should be done in both sides of caudal septum and extended to the membranous septum and columellar base. We may confirm that the infiltration is successful by the mucosal blanching around the site of injection. One cc of xylocaine 1% may be necessary to be infiltrated in both sides. In general, around 5–7 min should be allowed after local anesthetic injection to obtain a proper effect.

Step 6. Postoperative Nerve Block

Multimodal anesthesia is actually used for pain control and includes nerve blocks, analgesics, and short-acting opioids. The main objective is the reduction of opioids use preventing its nondesirable side effects. The infraorbitary nerve block is commonly used in combination with other analgesics (NSAID) for postoperative pain control in cleft lip and nose repair. To proceed this nerve block, we may follow the same recommendations mentioned for cleft nose surgery [17].

Mc Comb Modified Technique

These techniques represent a group of conservative methods recommended to be used for nonexperienced surgeons preventing major complications as vestibular synechia. This technique may prevent the development of postoperative synechia because of the limited nasal incisions but not the development of lateral web which is created due to scar contracture and lateral incisions used for release of the alae from the lateral segment. It is described as a modification of Mc Comb description because of the use of different methods of nasal tissue suspension after its dissection and the inclusion of primary caudal septoplasty [18]. Mc Comb's and later Salyer's methods for primary cleft rhinoplasty were the first methods I used to address the nose deformity because of its simplicity to be practiced; however, the observed high rate of relapse and development of lateral webs made me decide to change the technique [3, 4]. Recently, Raymond Tse actualized a method in combination with primary caudal septum repair, and the nasal tip dissection is not performed. Only septoplasty, alar advancement, lateral sidewall repair, and floor closure produce the majority of the nasal correction using his method [19]. Comparative studies are required to estimate the utility of this conservative method.

Surgical Technique

The technique I performed initially uses an approach through extension of the lateral lip incision into the nose and partial degloving of alar cartilage to finally reposition them using transcutaneous stitches in combination with the medialization of caudal septum.

Nasal tip dissection Nose surgery starts after lip incisions, and the intranasal alar base incision (an extension of the lateral lip incision) is used to dissect the alar tissues from the skeletal base. Through this maneuver, we have access to the lower lateral cartilages to dissect them from the overlying skin leaving the alar cartilage attached to the dome. Then, the dissection is completed over the alar dome and onto the normal side freeing the skin to allow reposition of the displaced cartilages (Fig. 6.5). This is a degloving maneuver to release the cartilage structure from its abnormal position allowing its repositioning.

Caudal septum dissection The anterior nasal spine is accessed through the medial lip incision, and then an incision is performed through premaxillary periosteum detaching the anterior nasal spine, providing access to the caudal septum and allowing its reposition in bloc (including enveloping perichondrium and periosteum to the midline level) (Figs. 6.6, 6.7, and 6.8). The released caudal septum is repositioned using a transfixion suture (from periosteum to periosteum) (Fig. 6.9).

Nasal structure reposition (Fig. 6.10) The reposition of the dissected structures is done by placement of transcutaneous stitches from vestibular lining to skin across the cartilages into desired position. The alar dome is shifted at the genu providing optimal projection of the nasal tip. I prefer to use 5/0 PDS sutures. Several stitches are necessary to achieve optimal position and nasal shape.

Nasal floor repair Finally, the anterior nasal floor is repaired. The floor of the nasal vestibule is done by reposition of the alar base into proper position by the muscle

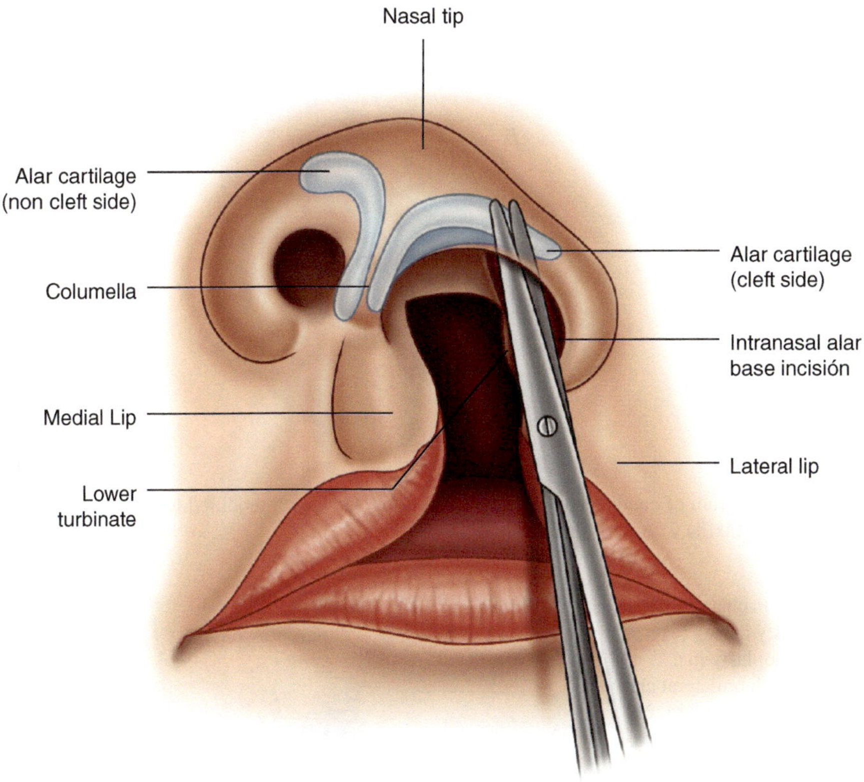

Fig. 6.5 Nasal tip dissection using the Mc Comb modified cleft rhinoplasty

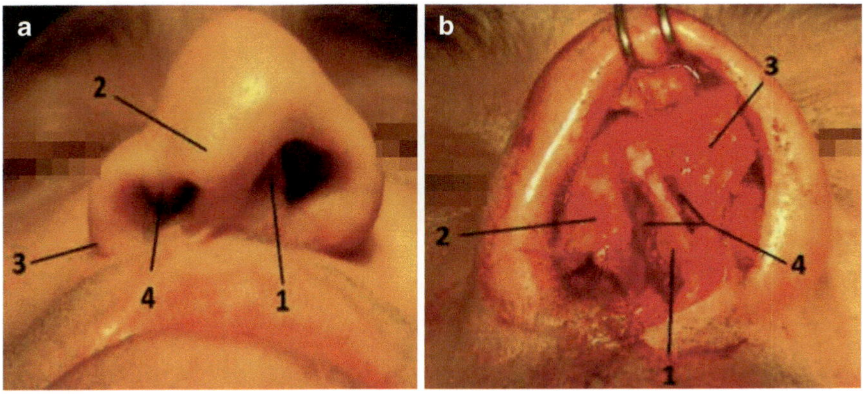

Fig. 6.6 Deviation of caudal septum observed before secondary cleft rhinoplasty. (**a**) 1: Caudal septum. 2. Nasal tip. 3. Alar base cleft side. 4. Nostril cleft side. (**b**) 1. Caudal septum. 2. Alar cartilage cleft side. 3. Alar cartilage noncleft side. 4. Septal mucosa

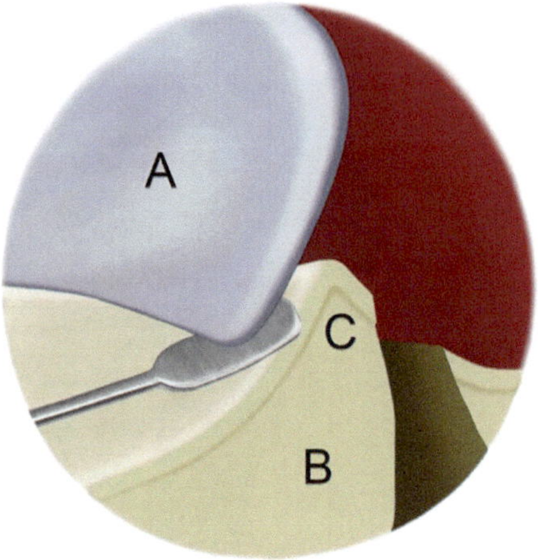

Fig. 6.7 Diagram of caudal septum dissection during Mc Comb modified technique. A. Caudal septum. B. Maxilla C. Anterior nasal spine

Fig. 6.8 Primary septoplasty during primary cleft rhinoplasty in a patient with unilateral cleft lip. 1. Caudal septum. 2. Septum mucosa. 3. Alae. 4. Columella. 5. Nasal tip. 6. Medial lip segment. 7. Lateral lip segment

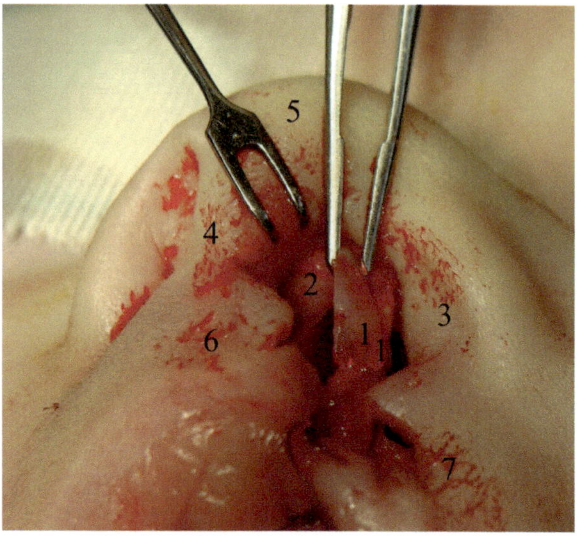

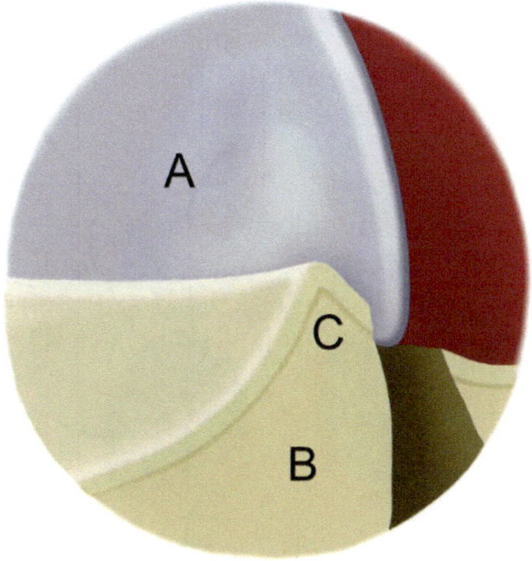

Fig. 6.9 Diagram of caudal septum reposition during Mc Comb modified cleft rhinoplasty. A. Caudal septum. B. Maxilla C. Anterior nasal spine

repair of the soft tissue platform which ignores the abnormal skeletal base. Skeletal base is finally repaired using the alveolar bone graft later during mixed dentition period (Figs. 6.11 and 6.12).

As I mentioned initially, these methods represent an alternative for conservative surgeons who may have a concern regarding the scar contracture of nasal vestibular incisions.

Cases (Figs. 6.13, 6.14, 6.15, 6.16, 6.17, 6.18, 6.19, 6.20, and 6.21)

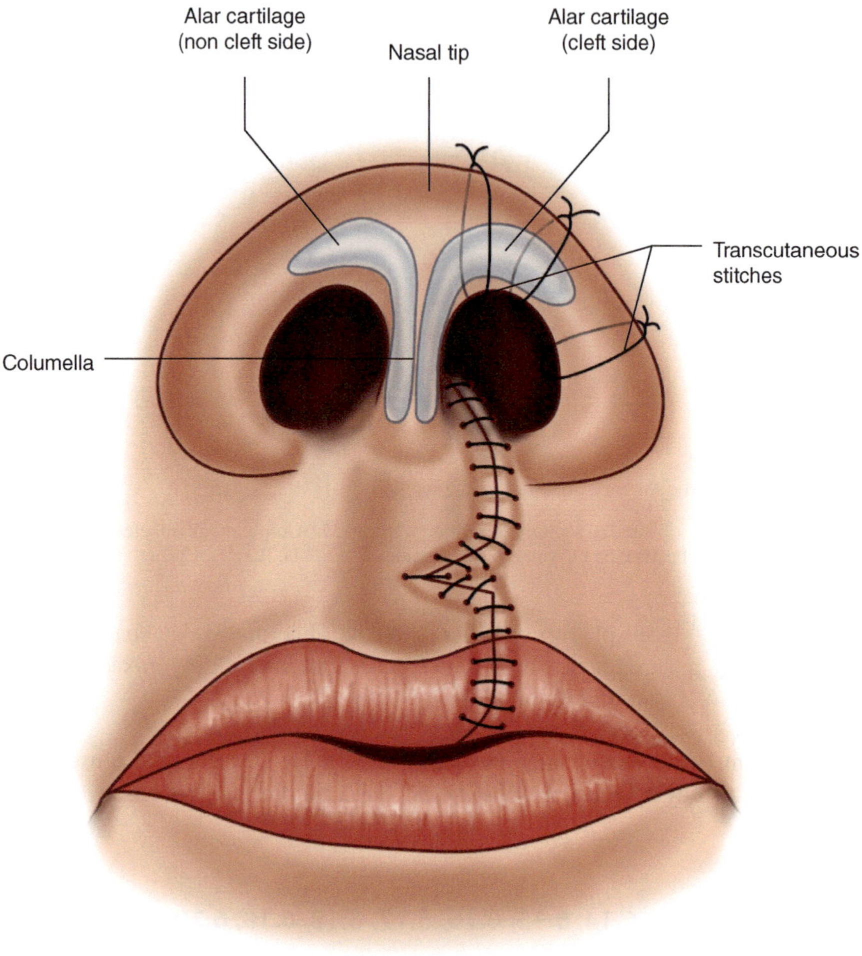

Fig. 6.10 Diagram of nasal tip reconstruction during Mc Comb modified cleft rhinoplasty

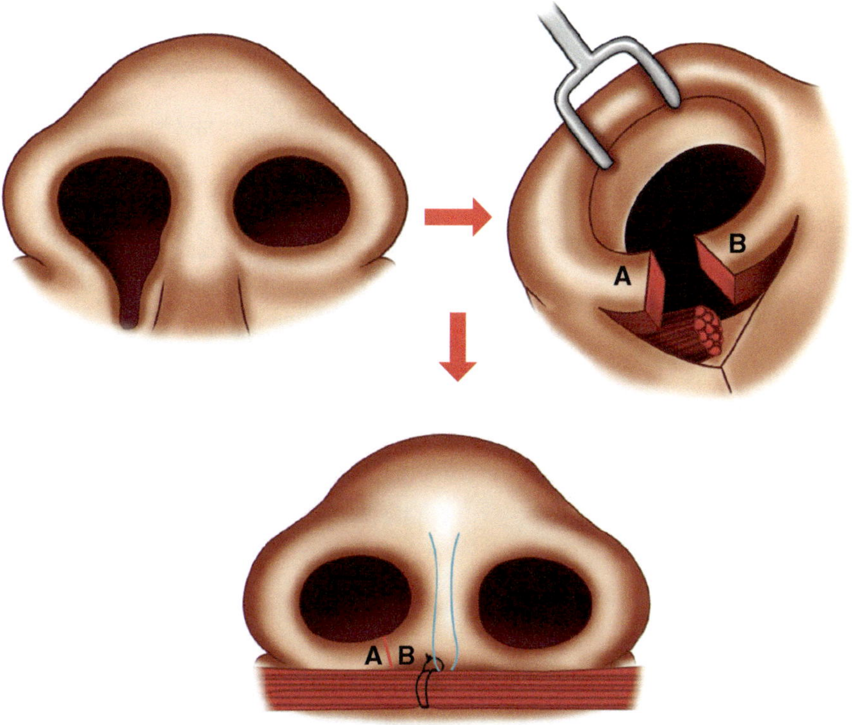

Fig. 6.11 Vestibular nasal floor reconstruction during Mc Comb modified technique. A: Alar flap. B: Columellar base flap

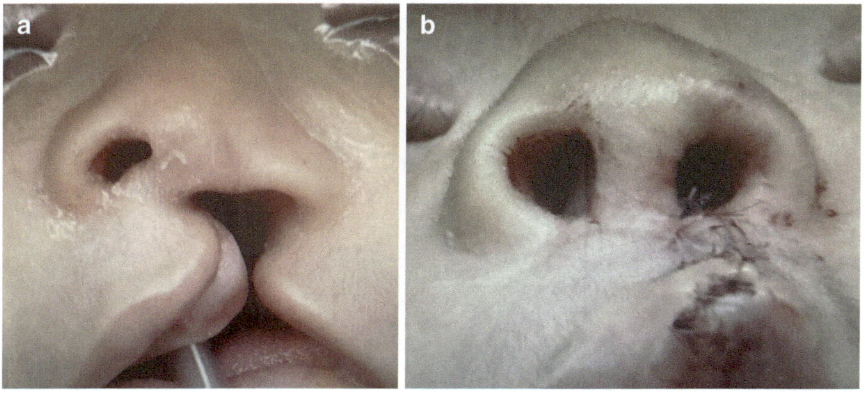

Fig. 6.12 Vestibular nasal floor reconstruction during Mc Comb modified technique. Vestibular segment of the nasal floor is repaired in a patient with unilateral cleft lip and palate. (**a**) Preoperative view. (**b**) Postoperative view

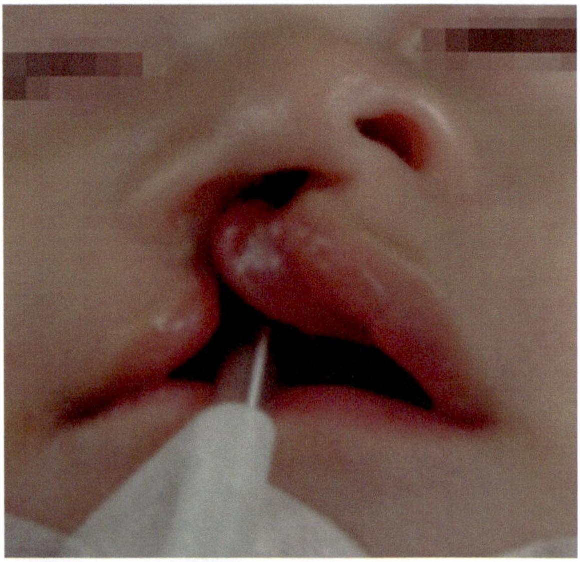

Fig. 6.13 Case 1. Preoperative view of a 3-month-old infant with complete unilateral cleft lip

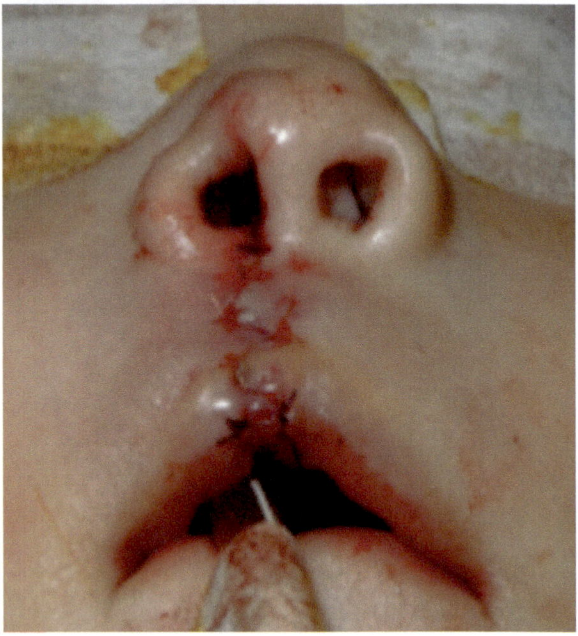

Fig. 6.14 Case 1. Immediate postoperative view of the infant shown in Fig. 6.13 after undergoing nasal repair using the Mc Comb modified technique

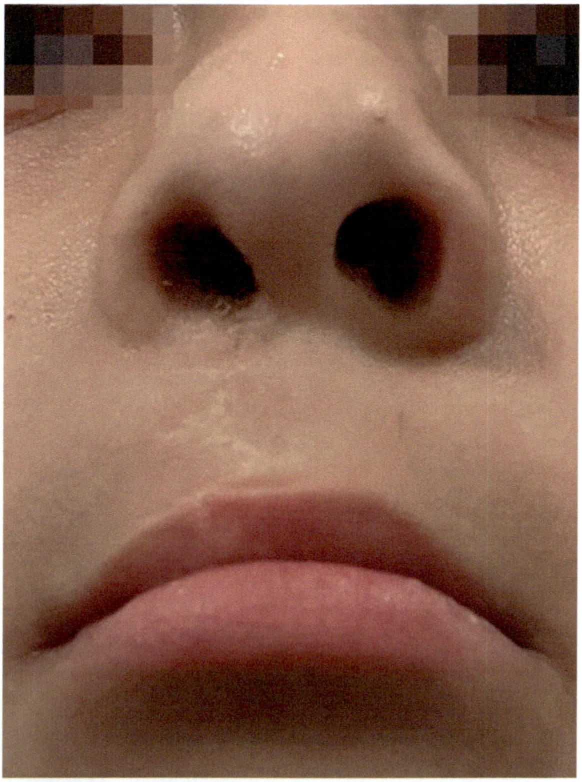

Fig. 6.15 Case 1. Long-term (10 years) postoperative view of the infant shown in Fig. 6.13 after undergoing nasal repair using the Mc Comb modified technique

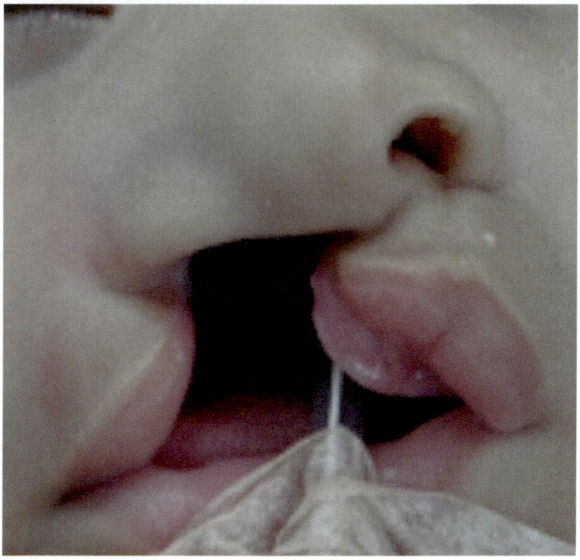

Fig. 6.16 Case 2. Preoperative view of a 3-month-old infant with complete unilateral cleft lip

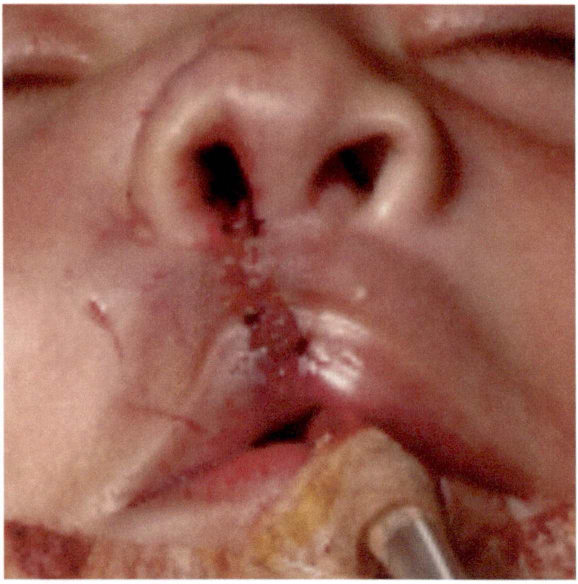

Fig. 6.17 Case 2. Immediate postoperative view of the infant shown in Fig. 6.16 after undergoing nasal repair using the Mc Comb modified technique

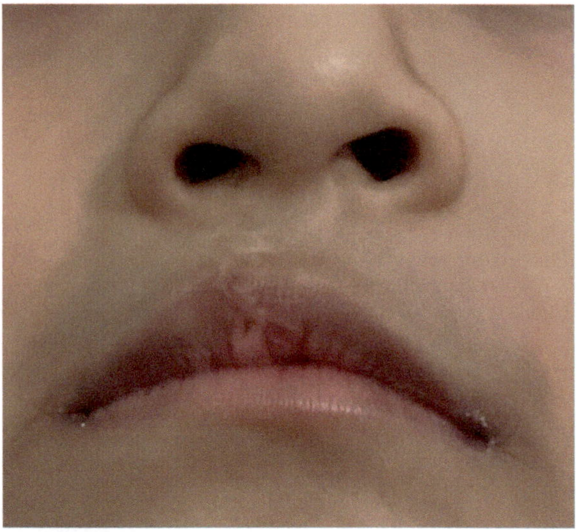

Fig. 6.18 Case 2. Long-term (9 years) postoperative view of the infant shown in Fig. 6.16 after undergoing nasal repair using the Mc Comb modified technique

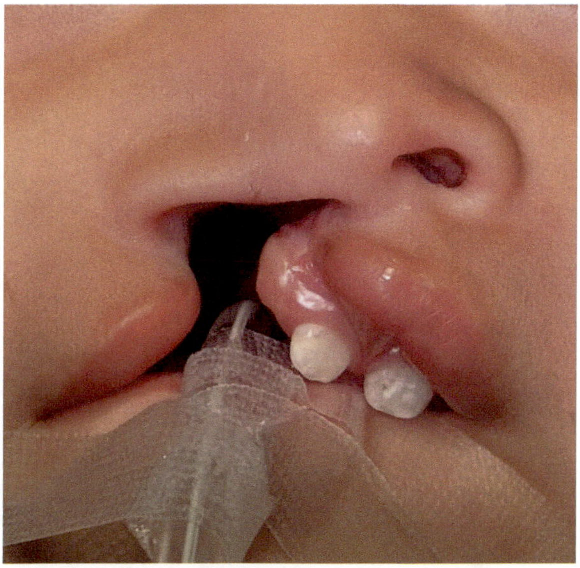

Fig. 6.19 Case 3. Preoperative view of a 3-month-old infant with complete unilateral cleft lip

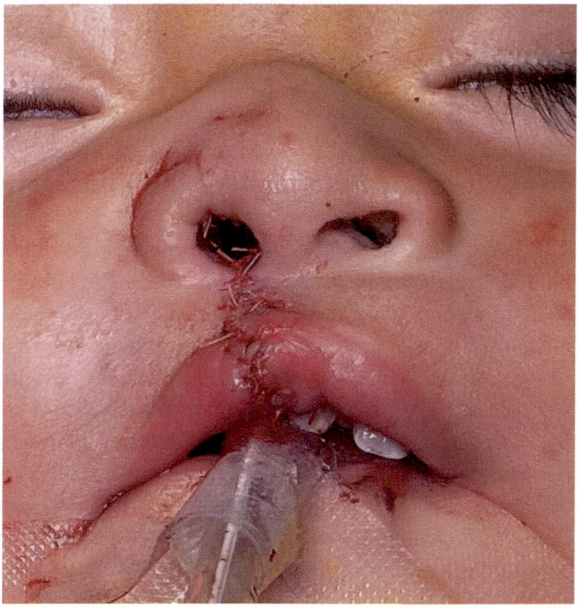

Fig. 6.20 Case 3. Immediate postoperative view of the infant shown in Fig. 6.19 after undergoing nasal repair using the Mc Comb modified technique

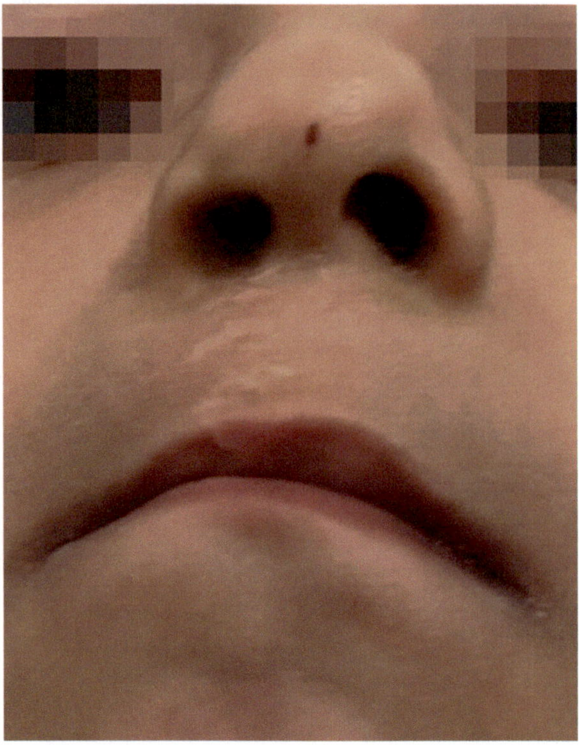

Fig. 6.21 Case 3. Long-term (10 years) postoperative view of the infant shown in Fig. 6.19 after undergoing nasal repair using the Mc Comb modified technique

The Composite Rotational Flap Rhinoplasty

This is a limited incision method for primary cleft rhinoplasty designed to be used in mild unilateral cleft lip nose forms (microform and incomplete forms). The method has been developed by the author and uses a composite flap (vestibular skin and cartilage) medially displaced in a rotational form; it is indicated for mild forms because they allow us preserve the lateral wall of the nasal vestibule preventing the development of lateral webs since the vestibular incision is not connected with lip incisions [11] (Figs. 6.22 and 6.23). In complete unilateral cleft lips, the release of the ala from its attachment to the pyriform aperture is mandatory; therefore, the lip and nose incisions are continuous, and the development of lateral web and intranasal scar contractures is more common in these cases. Its indication for microforms may be debatable because some associated nasal deformities are very mild and require only nasal base shortening.

Surgical Technique

Markings

The nose surgery starts performing the vestibular markings. The rotational composite flap design is composed by two lines: the marginal one which follows the lower border of the alar cartilage of the nose and a short intercartilaginous line

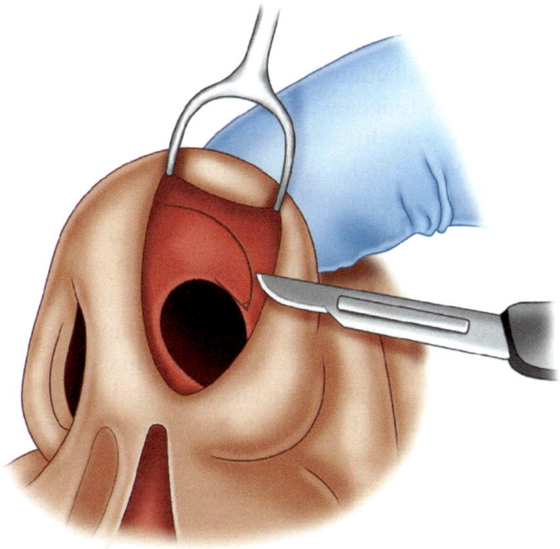

Fig. 6.22 Preoperative marking diagram for rotational composite flap cleft rhinoplasty in a patient with unilateral incomplete cleft lip

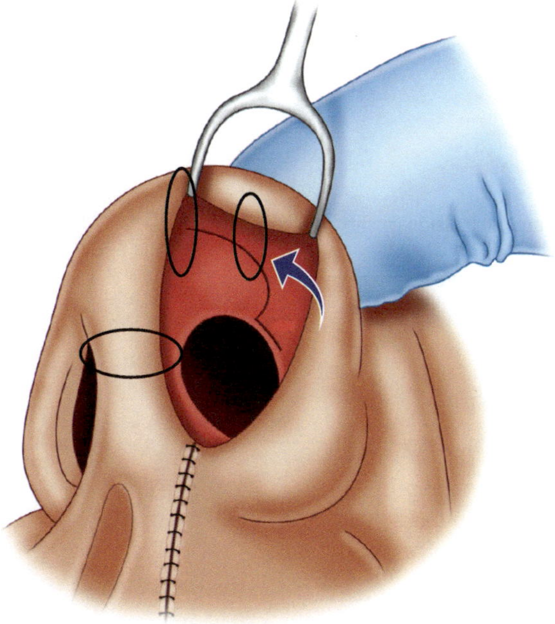

Fig. 6.23 Postoperative view for rotational composite flap cleft rhinoplasty in a patient with incomplete cleft lip

placed at the level of the limen nassi (intercartilaginous border) between the upper and lower lateral cartilages of the nose. The marginal line is an inferior curve which can be easily identified pushing the nasal tip from outside using the finger-tip, and then the border is more relevant. Another parameter to identify location of this line is the change of color of the vestibular skin; below the marginal border, the color of the skin is the same as the nasal skin, but above that line, there is a transitional epithelium (from skin to the nasal mucosa) and the color is red; therefore it is easy to locate the border of the alar cartilage following the line between these areas with different colors (Fig. 1.21). This line starts from the intercartilaginous border and finishes before the medial wall of the nasal vestibule at the level of cleft side nasal dome (Figs. 6.24 and 6.25). The intercartilaginous line is designed in continuity with the lateral end of the marginal marking and follows the intercartilaginous border (limen nassi) which is clearly identified. The extent of this marking is about 3–5 mm in order to release the lateral border of the alar cartilage and allow the rotation of the composite flap (Figs. 6.26, 6.27, and 6.28). Both lines are surrounding the alar cartilage to create the composite flap (composed by the vestibular skin and alar cartilage). The lateral wall of the nasal vestibule is preserved and prevents the development of lateral webs or scar contractures. The use of postoperative nasal conformers is optional using this technique because of the used limited incision.

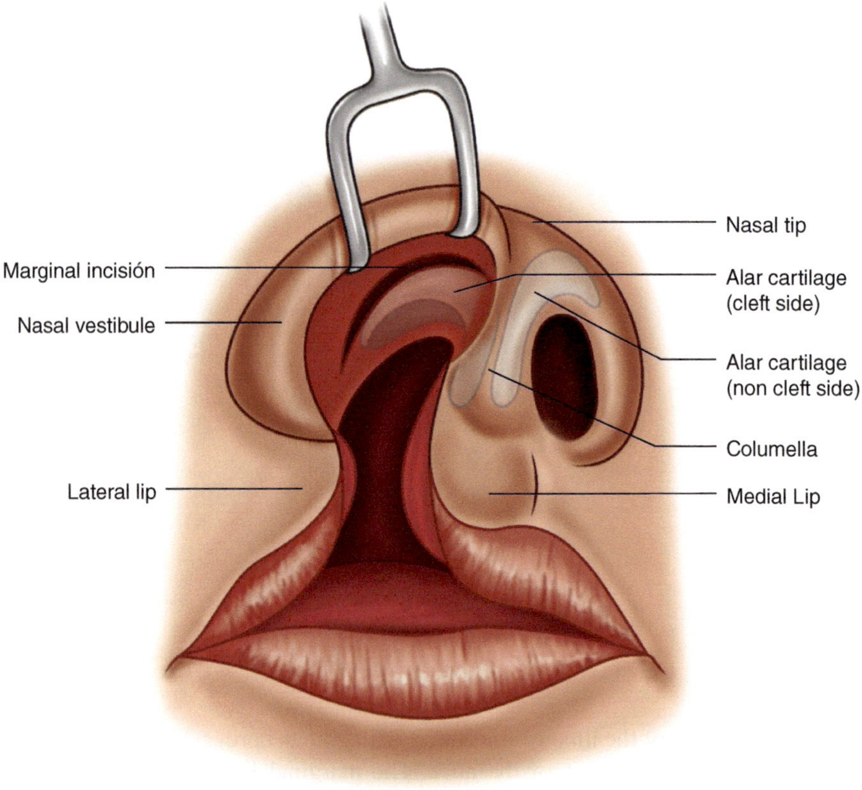

Fig. 6.24 Diagram of marginal incision during rotational composite flap cleft rhinoplasty

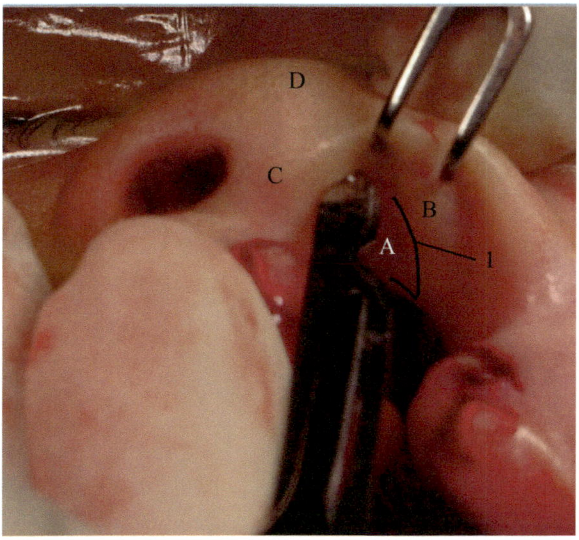

Fig. 6.25 1. Vestibular marginal border of the nasal vestibule (black line). A: Alar cartilage covered by transitional epithelium (red color area) B: Nasal vestibule. C: Columella. D. Nasal tip

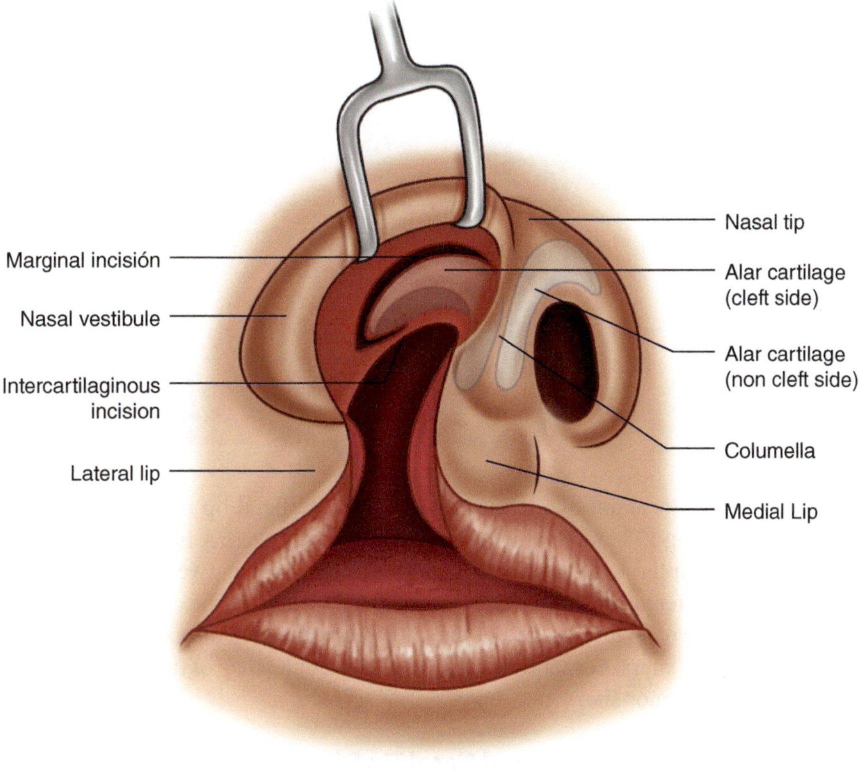

Fig. 6.26 Diagram of intercartilaginous incision during rotational composite flap cleft rhinoplasty

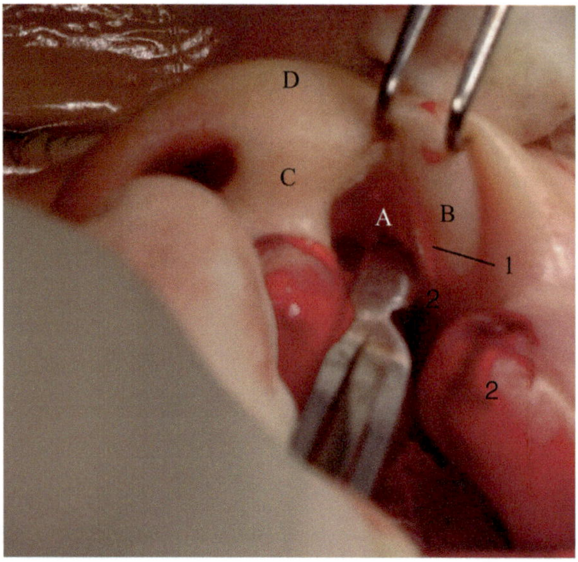

Fig. 6.27 Rotational composite flap incisions used for incomplete cleft lip nose repair. A: Rotational composite flap. B: Nasal vestibule. C: Nasal tip. D: Columella. 1: Marginal incision. 2: Intercartilaginous incision (Bisturí incision)

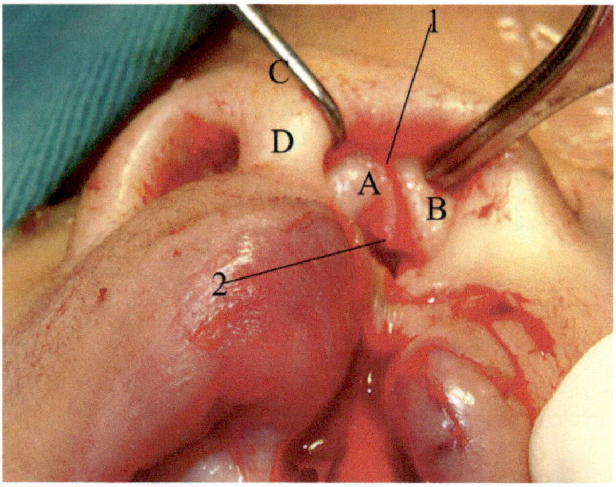

Fig. 6.28 Rotational composite flap after marginal and intercartilaginous incisions in a patient with unilateral incomplete cleft lip.
1. Marginal incision.
2. Intercartilaginous incision. A. Rotational composite flap. B. Nasal vestibule. C. Nasal tip. D. Columella

Incisions After local anesthetic infiltration and superficial lip incisions following lip markings using 11 blade scalpel, the nasal repair is started. A full-thickness nasal incisions through the vestibular skin are performed following vestibular markings (marginal and intercartilaginous) around the alar cartilage of the cleft side using 15 blade scalpel to create the composite flap. It is recommended the excision of a small triangle from the lateral corner of the flap to avoid redundancy of tissue after closure (ear dog) of the donor site.

Rotational Composite Flap and Nasal Tip Dissection

After identification of the alar cartilage through the marginal incision and using fine scissors, the composite flap (vestibular skin and alar cartilage) is dissected and elevated from lateral to medial side including alar cartilage and vestibular skin. Then, the nose dissection continues with the nasal tip including both sides through the vestibular incision and on the supracartilaginous plane separating the nasal skin from the cartilaginous structure of the nose (alar cartilages, domes, and lower dorsum). Both alar domes should be separated from the overlaying skin in order to facilitate the reposition of the structures from the cleft side (Figs. 6.29, 6.30, and 6.31). Some bleeding appears during this dissection; however, because of the closed approach of the nose, it is not possible to observe any important vessel to be cauterized. The bleeding uses to stop after application of the nasal transcutaneous stitches. In addition, the use of postoperative nasal packing (recommended after using the VYZ cleft rhinoplasty) is also optional in these cases.

Nasal Septum

The septal deviation associated with the incomplete cleft lips may vary in a wide spectrum, and some incomplete cleft lips have an important deviation; therefore in more severe nasal deformities associated with the incomplete cleft lips, the reposition of the nasal septum may be performed (Figs. 6.7, 6.8, and 6.9). This is achieved after dissection of the anterior nasal spine area through the medial lip incision in a similar form as I described before for the Mc Comb modified technique. After dissection and release of the noncleft nasal floor periosteum from the spine, the caudal septum is moved medially for suture fixation using 5/0 PDS (Fig. 6.9). I actually consider this maneuver as an alternative method since the columella can be perfectly repositioned only by muscular action. The caudal septoplasty is not correcting the whole septal deformity; therefore, a secondary correction is always necessary. In cases with nasal deformity associated with microform cleft lips, caudal septum treatment is not required.

Nasal Tip Reconstruction

Personally, I consider that the nose repair should be performed before the lip repair because the access to the nose through the nonrepaired cleft lip is easier than the access after lip repair. After elevating the rotational composite flap, it is displaced medially in a rotational form; this maneuver let us reposition the anterior portion of the nasal dome beside the dome at the noncleft side. This is a three-dimensional movement in three vectors: medial, posterior, and superior. I like to perform the fixation of the cartilage structures using the 5/0 PDS transcutaneous sutures. This material is monofilament being less reactive and producing less skin reaction and granulomas. These transcutaneous stitches are important to obliterate the space created after tip dissection and prevent the development of hematomas. Stitches are placed through the skin, starting from inside the nose and then exiting the skin at the level of the supraalar crease; the needle then returns through the same hole and finally enters the inside of the nose in front of the initial entrance, where the sutures are tied (Figs. 6.32, 6.33, 6.34, 6.35, and 6.36).

This is the recommended sequence (Fig. 6.36):

First stitch: After identification of the alar dome in the composite flap, this is medially displaced and fixed using a vertical transcutaneous stitch at the medial side of the supra alar crease. Then, the alar cartilage dome is in correct position.

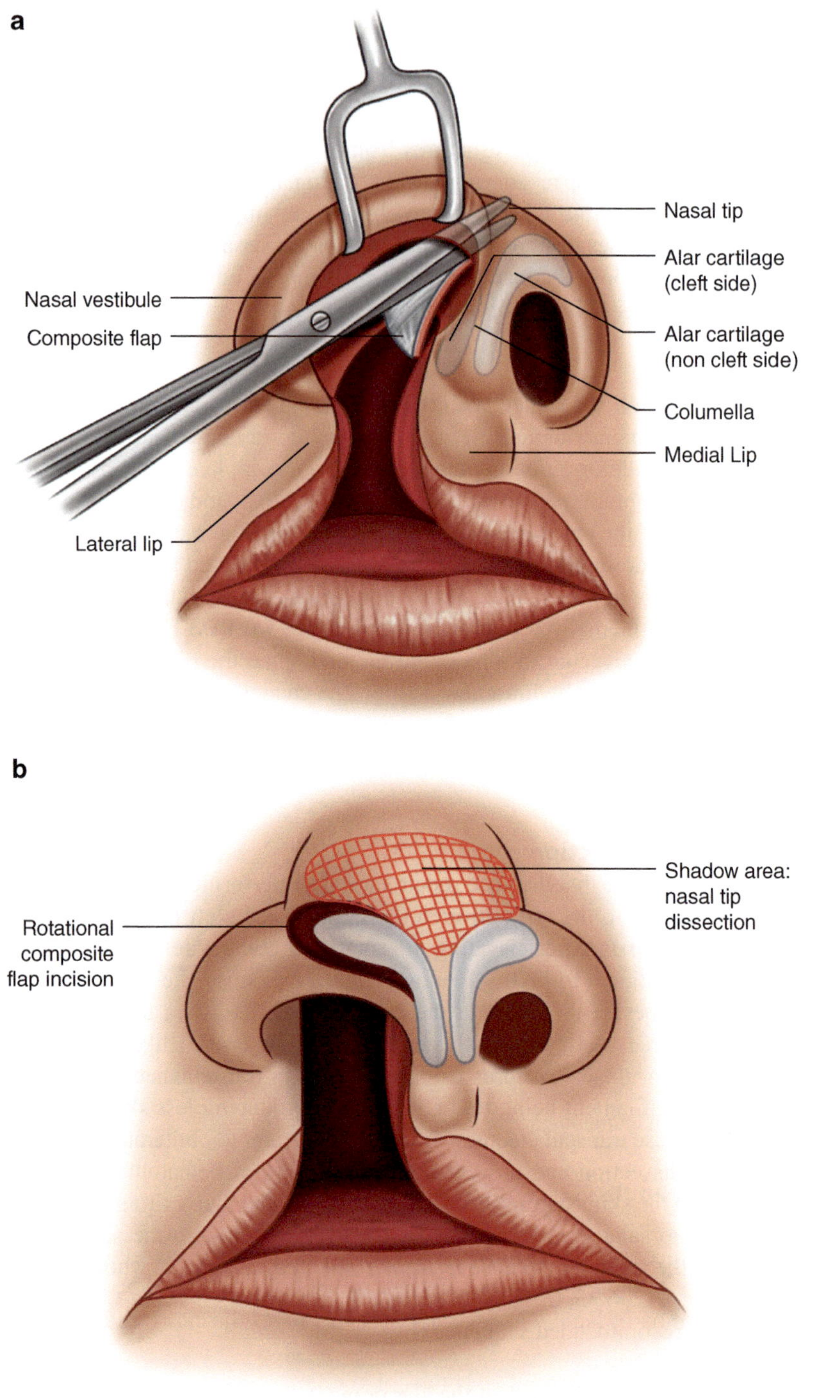

Fig. 6.29 Diagram of nasal tip dissection during unilateral rotational composite flap cleft rhinoplasty. A: Nasal tip dissection through the rotational composite flap incision. B: Shadow area: Extension of nasal tip dissection

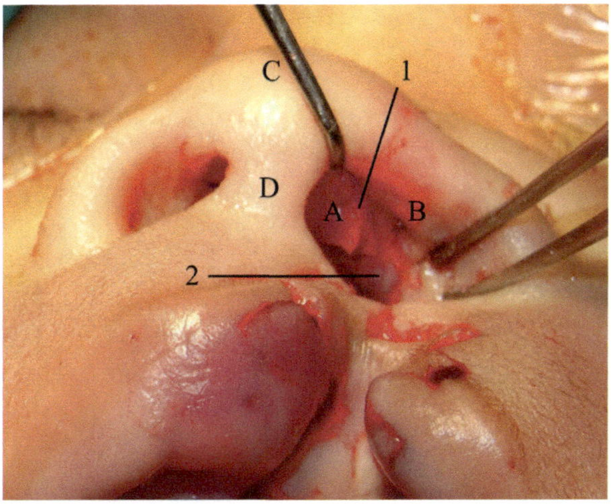

Fig. 6.30 Diagram of rotational composite flap elevation after nasal tip dissection.
1. Marginal incision.
2. Intercartilaginous incision. A. Rotational composite flap. B. Nasal vestibule. C. Nasal tip. D. Columella

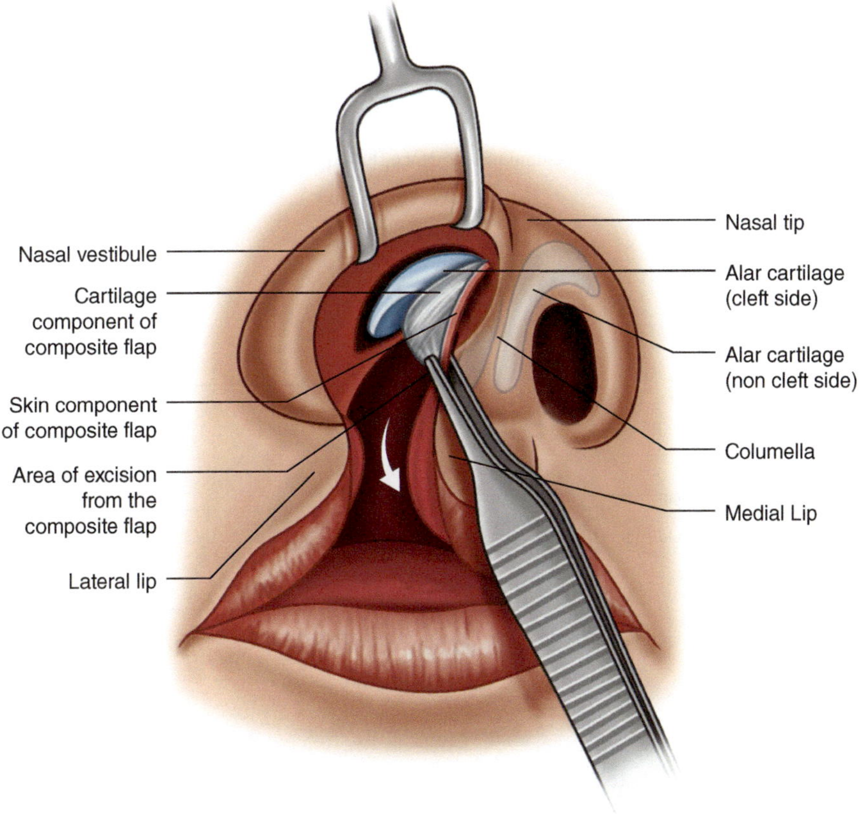

Fig. 6.31 Rotational composite flap elevation in a patient with unilateral incomplete cleft lip

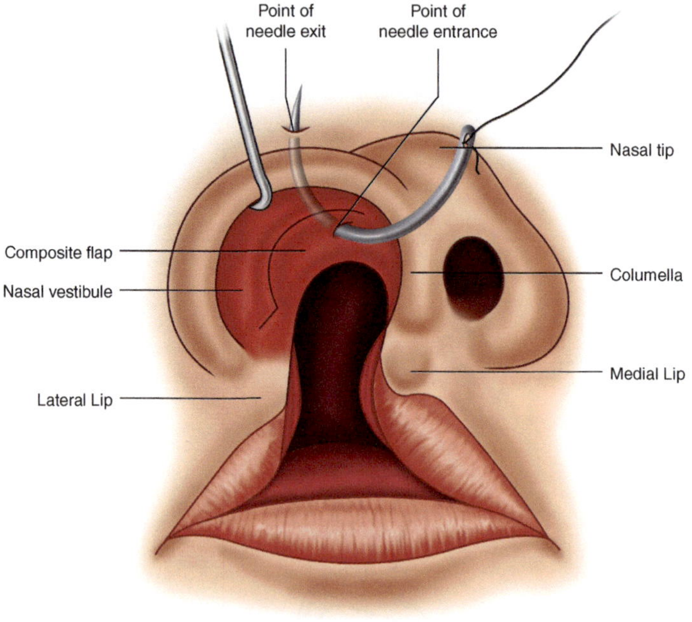

Fig. 6.32 Transcutaneous stitch technique sequence (initial step)

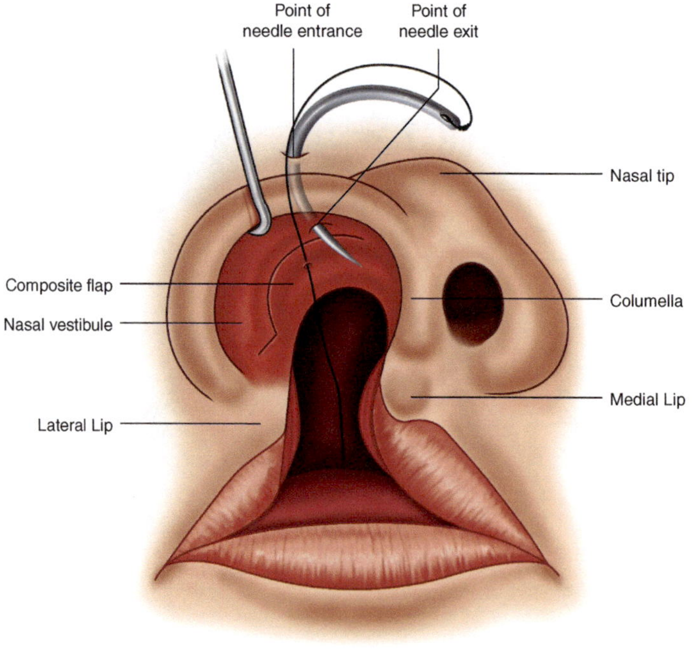

Fig. 6.33 Transcutaneous stitch technique sequence (second step)

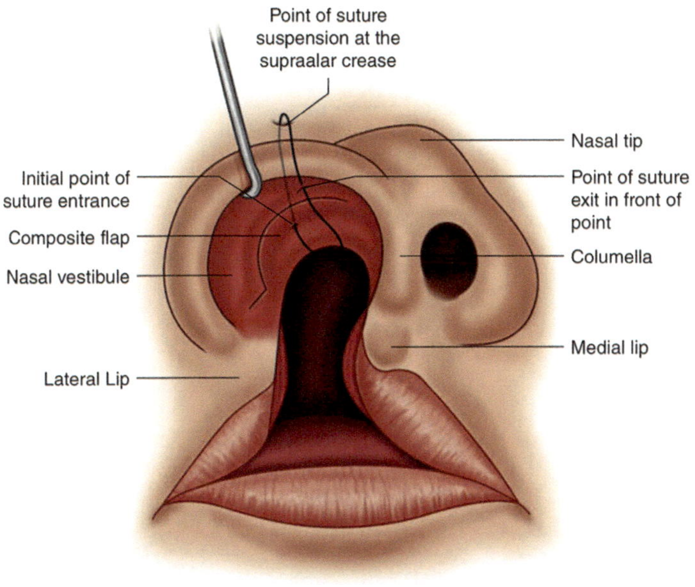

Fig. 6.34 Transcutaneous stitch technique sequence (third step)

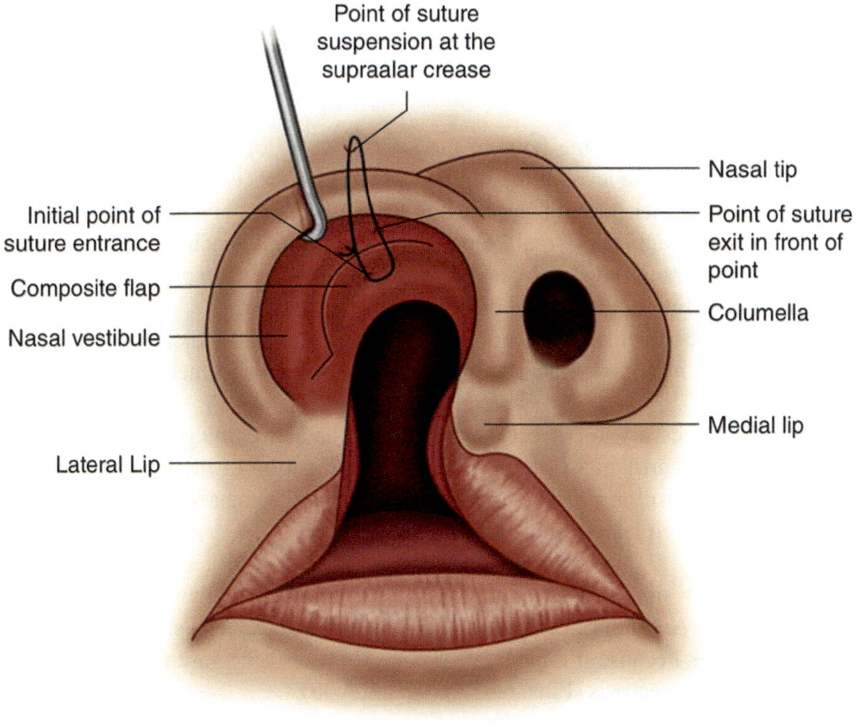

Fig. 6.35 Transcutaneous stitch technique sequence (final step)

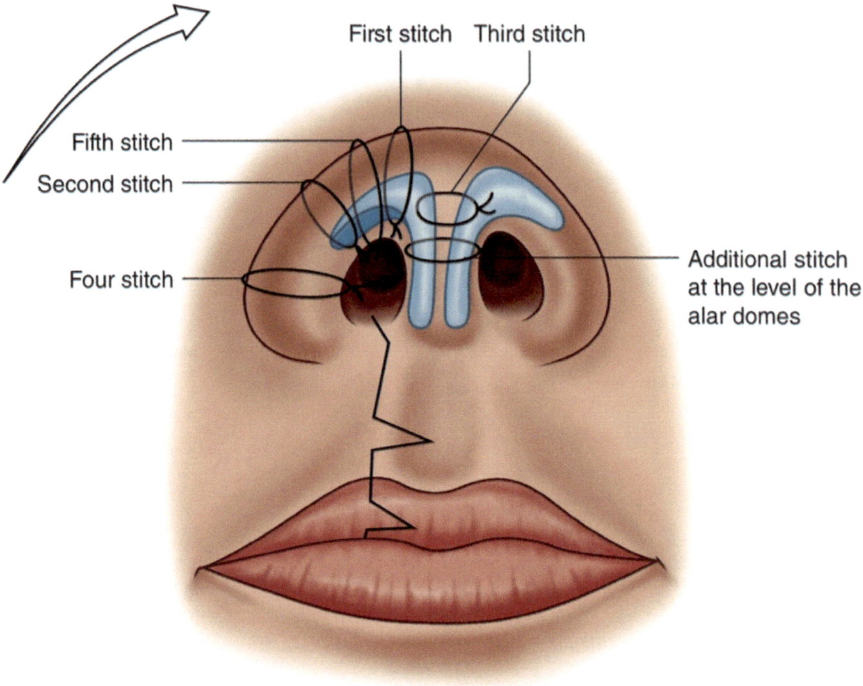

Fig. 6.36 Nasal tip reconstruction using transcutaneous stitches during rotational composite flap cleft rhinoplasty

Second stitch: Placed at the level of the lateral border of the flap using a similar vertical stitch at the level of the supra alar crease. These two sutures mobilize the flap medially after rotation and leaves a triangular donor site laterally.

Third stitch: Between the two alar domes using a transcutaneous stitch at the level of the midpoint of the alar domes. This suture creates the tip projection and definition according to the natural parameters of the patient.

Four stitch: Used to close the donor area of the flap. This is a lateral triangular raw surface which is closed using a simple stitch by advancement of the vestibular skin.

Fifth stitch: Necessary to correct the position of the alar cartilage in relation to the upper lateral cartilage of the nose. There is a luxation of the alar cartilage and requires a reposition over the upper lateral cartilage using a vertical transcutaneous stitch placed lateral to the internal nasal valve.

Finally a few simple stitches may be used to align correctly the borders of the composite flap. An important recommendation is not to exceed using these transcutaneous stitches because it may create a compromise of the vascular supply of the ala and develops necrosis (Figs. 6.37, 6.38, and 6.39).

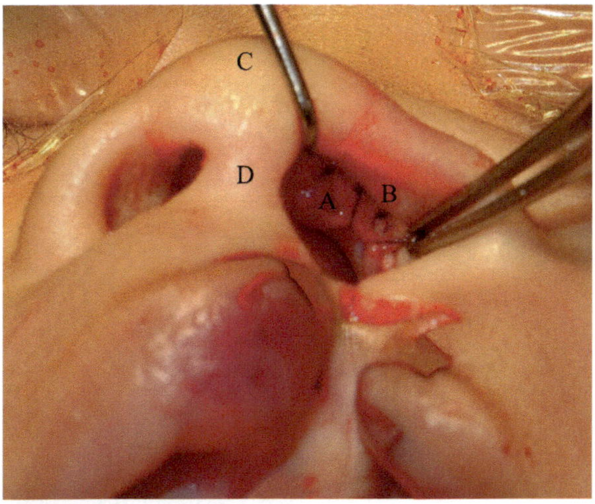

Fig. 6.37 Final closure of rotational composite flap cleft rhinoplasty in a patient with incomplete unilateral cleft lip. A: Rotational composite flap. B: Nasal vestibule. C: Nasal tip. D: Columella

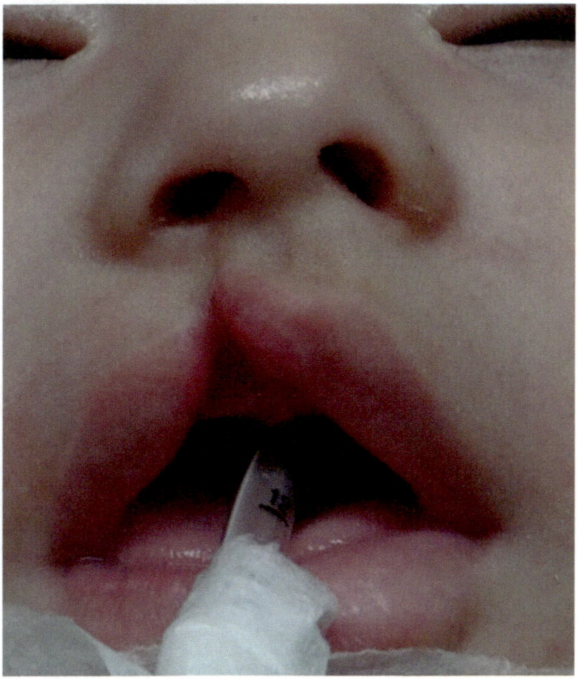

Fig. 6.38 A 3-month-old patient with unilateral incomplete cleft lip (preoperative view)

Nasal Floor

The repair of the nasal floor is the final step of cleft rhinoplasty and represents the correction of the most anterior portion of the nasal floor (vestibular segment). Based on our surgical protocol for cleft lip and palate repair, the other segments are closed in different times during primary and secondary palate

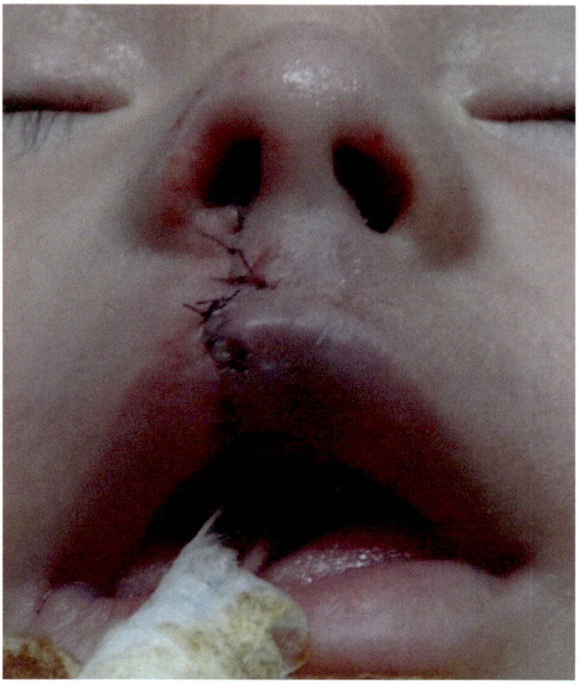

Fig. 6.39 Immediate postoperative view of the patient in Fig. 6.38 operated using the rotational composite flap technique

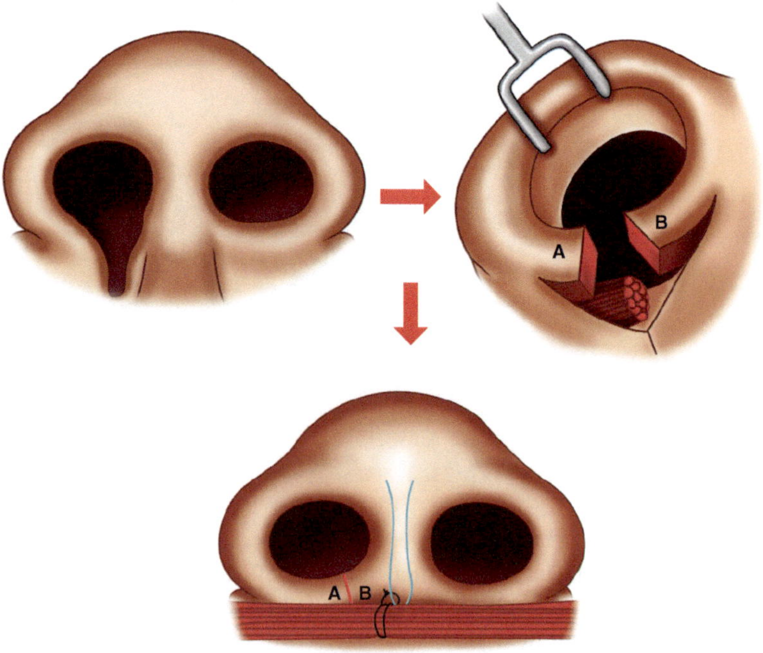

Fig. 6.40 Diagram of nasal floor repair during the rotational composite flap technique for unilateral cleft lip nose repair A. Alar base flap. B. Columellar base flap

repairs. The nasal floor reconstruction is performed during the cleft lip repair, and this is involving the use of two flaps: a medial cutaneous flap lateral to the base of the columella at the cleft border and a lateral flap, which is composed of the base of the ala (Fig. 6.40). These cutaneous flaps are supported by the muscular repair of the lip; the levator labii superioris alaeque nasi and orbicularis oris muscles are identified and repositioned allowing the final position of the nasal base (Figs. 6.41 and 6.42). This muscular reconstruction is providing support to the base of the nose but also acts over the caudal septum of the nose moving it medially and correcting the anterior septal deviation (membranous portion) and columella.

During cheiloplasty, the labial muscles are dissected and horizontally repositioned; their upper portion is sutured to the base of caudal septum. One muscle is relevant for nasal repair; this is the levator labii superioris alaeque nasi. This muscle also known as the quadratus labii is attached to the upper frontal process of the maxilla and inserts into the skin of the nostril and upper lip. The nasal fascicle of the levator labii superioris alaeque nasi muscle is identified during the muscular dissection and attached to the caudal septum previously exposed using PDS 5/0. This muscle pulls the membranous portion of the caudal septum to the midline addressing the position of the nasal columella and also brings support to the nose.

Cases (Figs. 6.43, 6.44, 6.45, 6.46, 6.47, 6.48, 6.49, 6.50, and 6.51)

Here I present long-term outcomes using the rotational composite flap rhinoplasty in patients with incomplete cleft lip and palate. None of them used presurgical nasal orthopedics or postoperative nasal conformers.

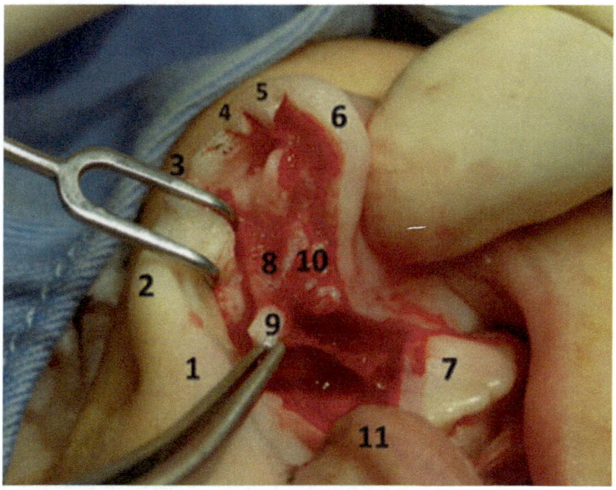

Fig. 6.41 Nasal fascicle of levator labii superioris alaeque nasi muscle is dissected to be repositioned allowing the final position of the nasal base. 1. Nasal tip. 2. Alae. 3. Cheek. 4. Lateral lip segment. 5. Triangular flap (Pool technique) 6. Vermillion 7. Maxilla 8. Levator labii superioris alaeque nasi muscle. 9. Fibrous tendon. 10. Orbicularis oris muscle.11. Medial lip segment

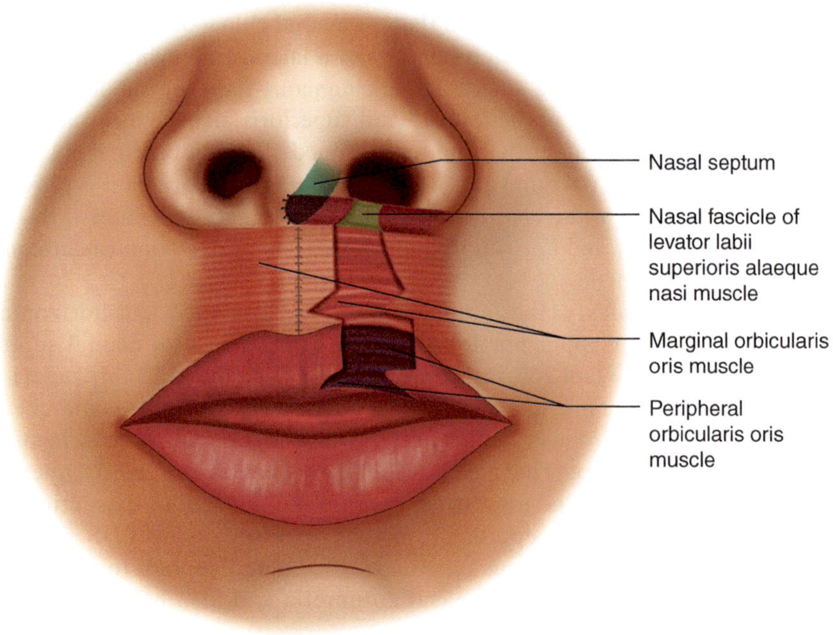

Fig. 6.42 Muscular reconstruction is providing support to the base of the nose acting over the membranous portion of caudal septum of the nose moving it medially and correcting the anterior septal deviation during rotational composite flap technique

Fig. 6.43 Case 1. Preoperative view of a 3-month-old infant with incomplete unilateral cleft lip

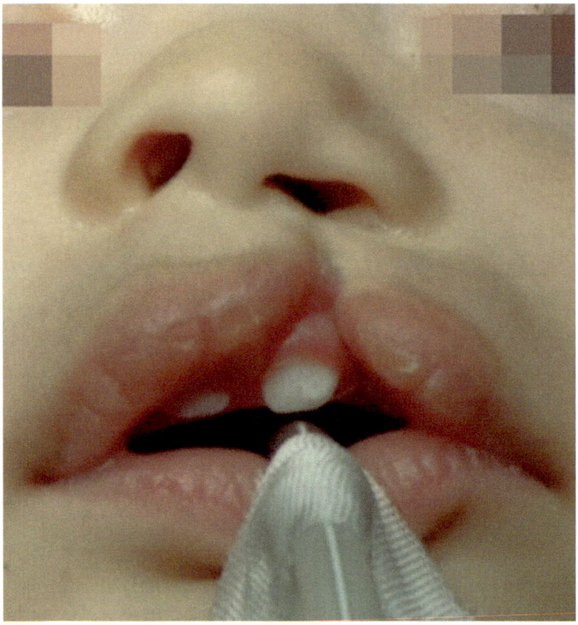

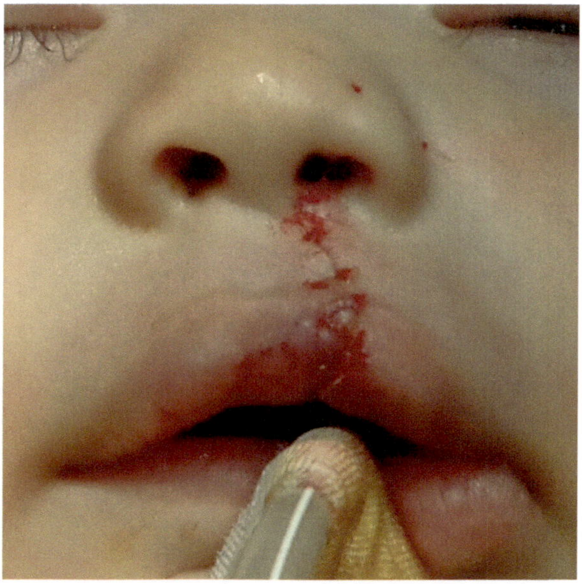

Fig. 6.44 Case 1. Immediate postoperative view of the infant shown in Fig. 6.43 after undergoing nasal repair using the rotational composite flap technique

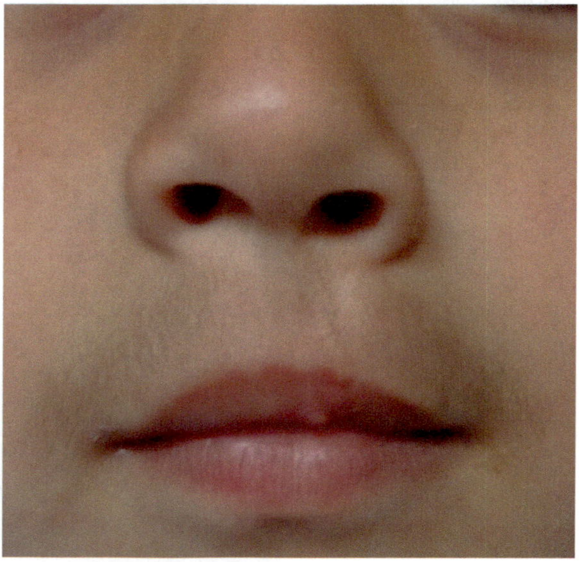

Fig. 6.45 Case 1. Postoperative view of the infant shown in Fig. 6.43 5 years after undergoing nasal repair using the rotational composite flap technique

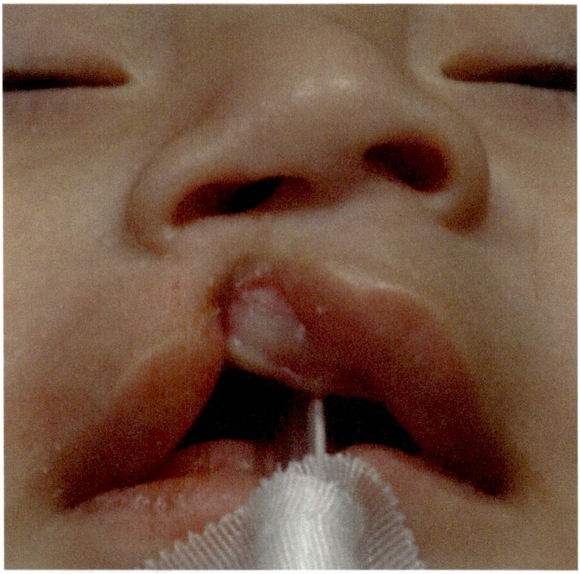

Fig. 6.46 Case 2. Preoperative view of a 3-month-old infant with incomplete unilateral cleft lip

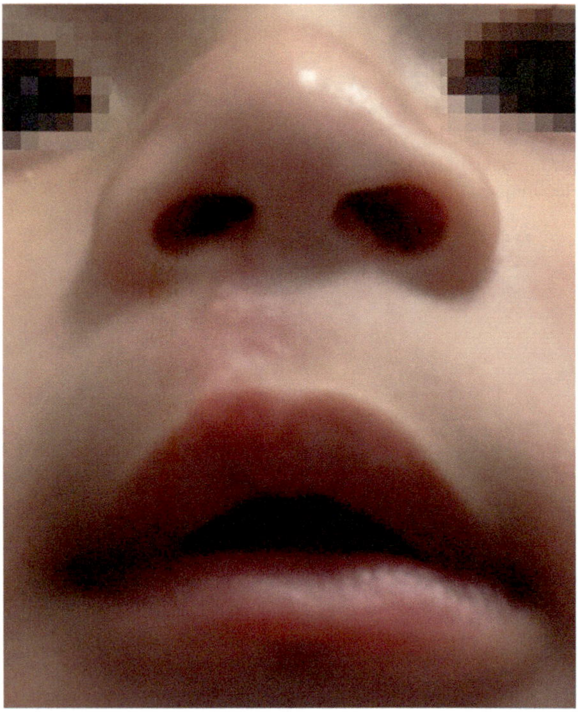

Fig. 6.47 Case 2. A 5-year postoperative view of the infant shown in Fig. 6.46 after undergoing nasal repair using the rotational composite flap technique

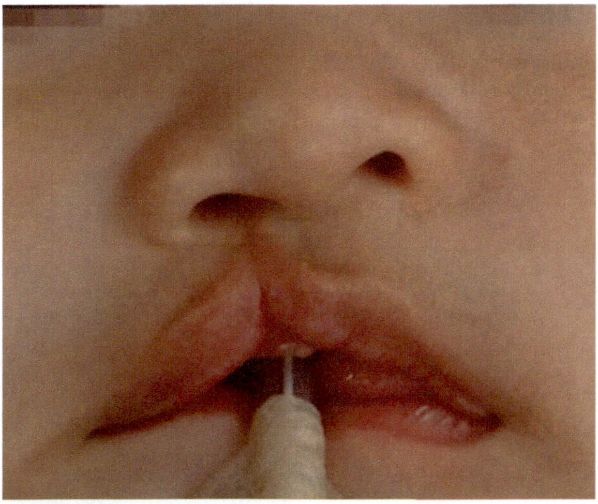

Fig. 6.48 Case 3. Preoperative view of a 3-month-old infant with incomplete unilateral cleft lip

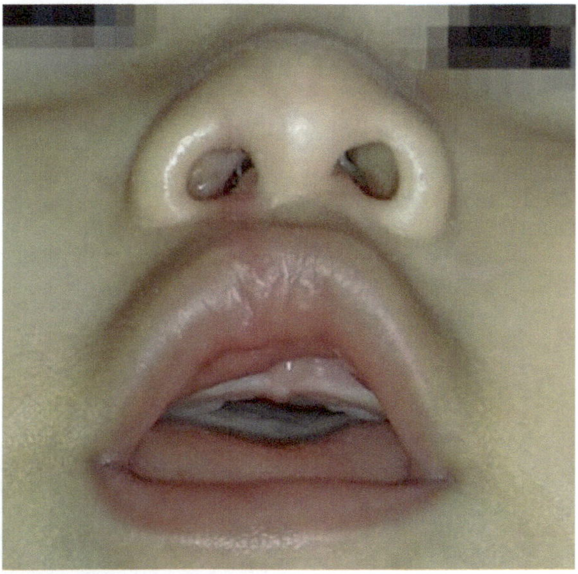

Fig. 6.49 Case 3. A 2-year postoperative view of the infant shown in Fig. 6.48 after undergoing nasal repair using the rotational composite flap technique

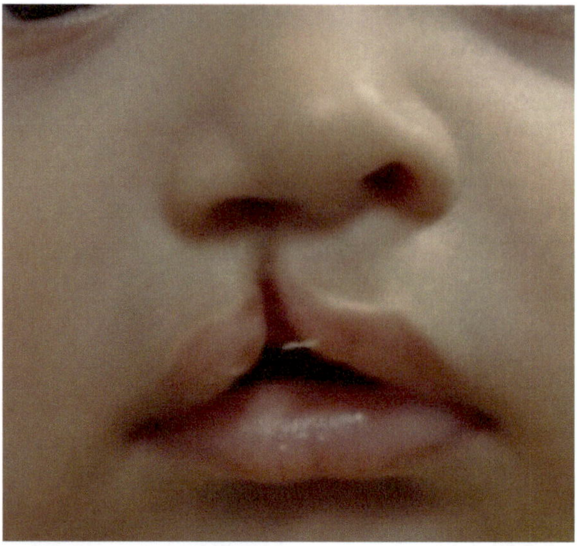

Fig. 6.50 Case 4. Preoperative view of a 3-month-old infant with incomplete unilateral cleft lip

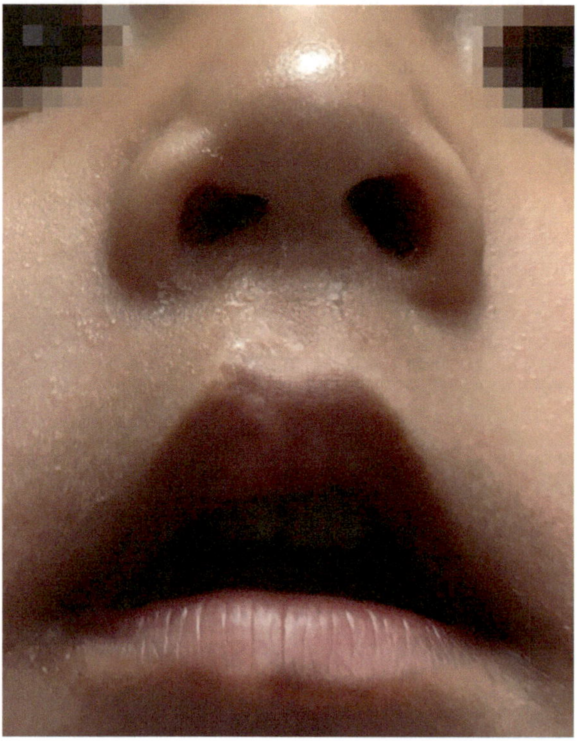

Fig. 6.51 Case 4. A 5-year postoperative view of the infant shown in Fig. 6.50 after undergoing nasal repair using the rotational composite flap technique

The V-Y-Z Cleft Rhinoplasty (Video 6.1)

Looking for answers after evaluation of the long-term outcomes using conservative methods, I decided to use a different technique to improve my work. Many of the primary cleft rhinoplasty techniques were used initially for secondary cases, and the V-Y advancement combined with lateral Z plasty was used with success in our secondary cases. Therefore, I decided to use this well-known method primarily expecting better outcomes even when the technique is more aggressive and the risk of complications is higher. It is clear now that this is not a true innovation since the technique has been currently used for secondary nose deformities and combines two previously described methods: Potter's and Berkeley's techniques [7, 8]. The technique was published in 2017, as the V-Y-Z cleft rhinoplasty for primary unilateral cleft lip nose repair observing good long-term outcomes after its initial use [20, 21]. The V-Y advanced composite flap was described by Potter in 1954 for secondary nasal deformities associated with unilateral cleft lip. The method is an effective form of nasal tip correction; however, it is not addressing the lateral vestibular web, and also the risk of lateral scar contracture is higher. This is the reason why the technique has been used in combination with lateral Z plasty (a technique previously described by Berkeley). The combination of these two techniques produces an expansion of the vestibule of the nose in a similar form as the presurgical orthopedic (NAM) is doing nonsurgically (however the effect of the orthopedics is temporary; that is why the surgery is always necessary); therefore the method was published by the author as the "surgical nasoalveolar molding" [10]. Its use by the author in primary cleft rhinoplasty is an innovative proposal that allows good outcomes after long-term follow-up [21]. The method is indicated for complete unilateral cleft lip nose cases because it is preventing the scar contracture developed by using a continuous incision from the nose to the lip in these cases. This lateral incision creates frequently a lateral web, and the lateral Z plasty prevents its development. We published a study comparing three methods, Mc Comb, Potter's, and V-Y-Z techniques, and observed increased risk of synechia using Potter and more nose deformity relapse and lateral web development after Mc Comb's method [9]. However, considering the extended incisions along the nasal vestibule, the use of postoperative nasal conformers is mandatory. If there is not option for their use, this method should not be used because of the risk of scar contracture and synechia. A total collapse of the nasal vestibule may be developed because of scar contracture if the patient does not follow the instructions and uses regularly the postoperative nasal conformer. The rotation composite flap method can be used as alternative if the use of nasal conformers cannot be guaranteed after surgery.

Surgical Technique

Markings

The nose surgery starts performing the vestibular markings. The advanced V-Y flap is designed following two lines: the marginal one which follows the lower border of the alar cartilage of the nose and the second an intercartilaginous line placed at the level of the limen nassi (intercartilaginous border) between the upper and lower lateral cartilages of the nose. Both markings are creating a V form composite flap (Figs. 6.52 and 6.53). The identification of the lower (marginal) and upper (intercartilaginous) lines can be done following the same parameters described for rotational composite flap markings. The skin area of the advancement V flap has a different color (red); therefore, it is easy to be identified during markings (Figs. 1.21 and 6.54). The lower line (marginal border) starts 2–3 mm before the level of the intercartilaginous border and finishes before the medial wall of the nasal vestibule at the level of cleft side nasal dome (Figs. 6.55, 6.56, and 6.57). The upper line (intercartilaginous border) starts from the lateral end of the lower line and then follows the intercartilaginous border finishing at the level of the medial wall of the nasal vestibule before the internal nasal valve (before it) (Figs. 6.55, 6.56, and 6.57). It is important to preserve the functional area of the nasal vestibule (nasal valves) preventing the development of scar contractures affecting function of these areas. Both lines are surrounding the alar cartilage to create the advancement composite flap (composed by the vestibular skin and alar cartilage). The lateral Z plasty is designed using two transpositional branches located at the lateral end of the V composite flap. This lateral design continues with the lip marking through the alar base (Figs. 6.58 and 6.59). This lateral Z plasty prevents the development of lateral webs or scar contractures. The use of postoperative nasal conformers is mandatory using this technique because of the used extended incisions.

Incisions After local anesthetic infiltration and superficial lip incisions following lip markings using 11 blade scalpel, the nasal repair is performed. Nasal incisions are performed following vestibular markings (marginal and intercartilaginous) around the alar cartilage of the cleft side using a 15-blade scalpel to create the

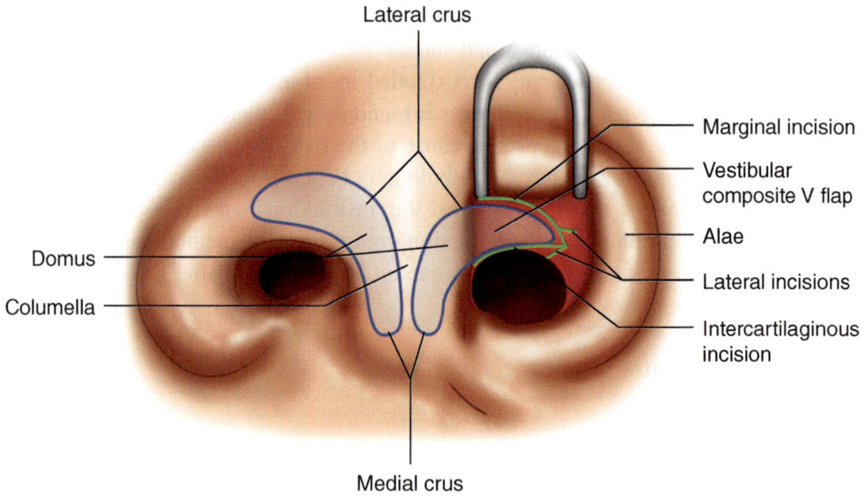

Fig. 6.52 Diagram of the VYZ surgical treatment for primary cleft rhinoplasty

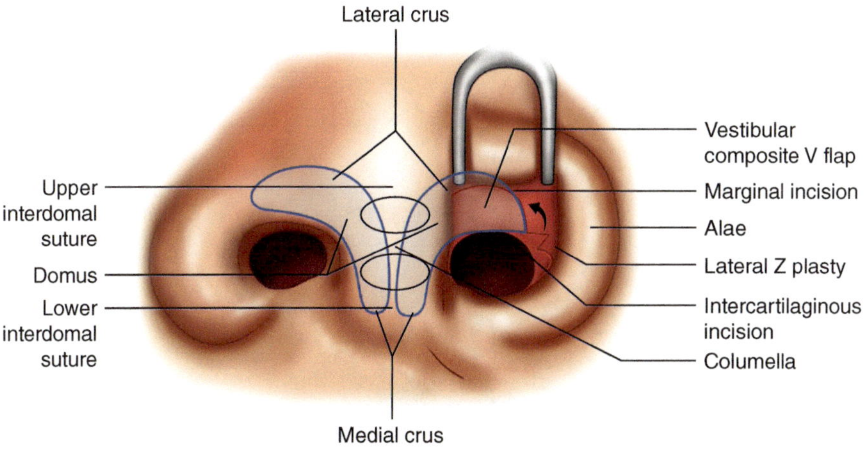

Fig. 6.53 Postoperative view of the vestibular lengthening achieved using the VYZ method for primary cleft rhinoplasty

Fig. 6.54 Vestibular marginal border of the nasal vestibule (black line). A: Alar cartilage covered by transitional epithelium (red color area) B: Nasal vestibule. C: Nasal tip. D. Columella

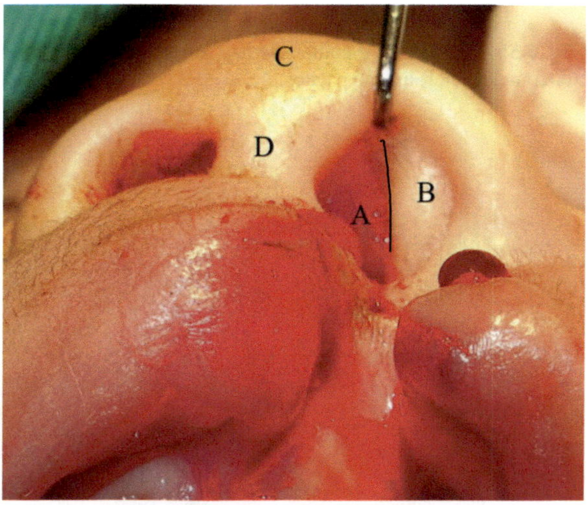

advanced V composite flap. Then the lateral Z plasty is incised following its markings and the incision continues with the lip through the alar base. All of them are full-thickness incisions preserving the alar cartilage and leaving included in the V advancement flap for its medial advancement.

V Composite Flap and Nasal Tip Dissection

After identification of the border of the alar cartilage through the marginal incision and using fine scissors, the V composite flap is dissected at the supra cartilaginous plane and elevated from lateral to medial sides. Then, the nose dissection continues with the nasal tip including both sides through the vestibular incision and on the supra cartilaginous plane separating the nasal skin from

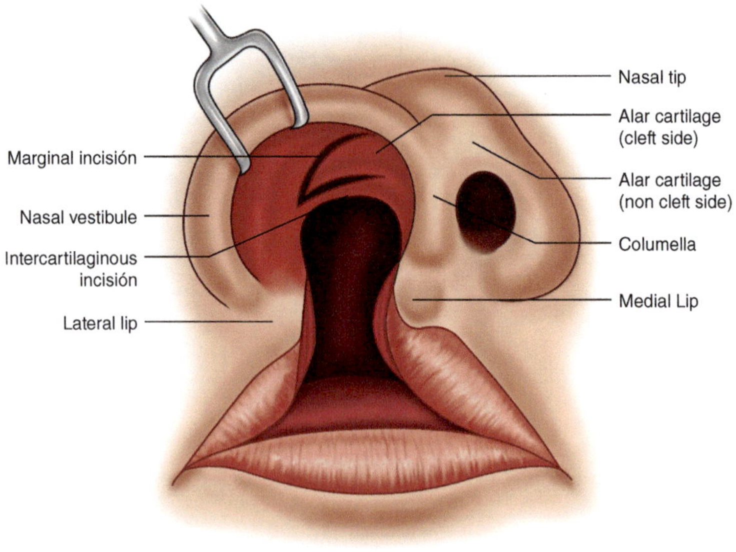

Fig. 6.55 Diagram of V composite flap surgical marking during unilateral VYZ cleft rhinoplasty for complete cleft lip and palate

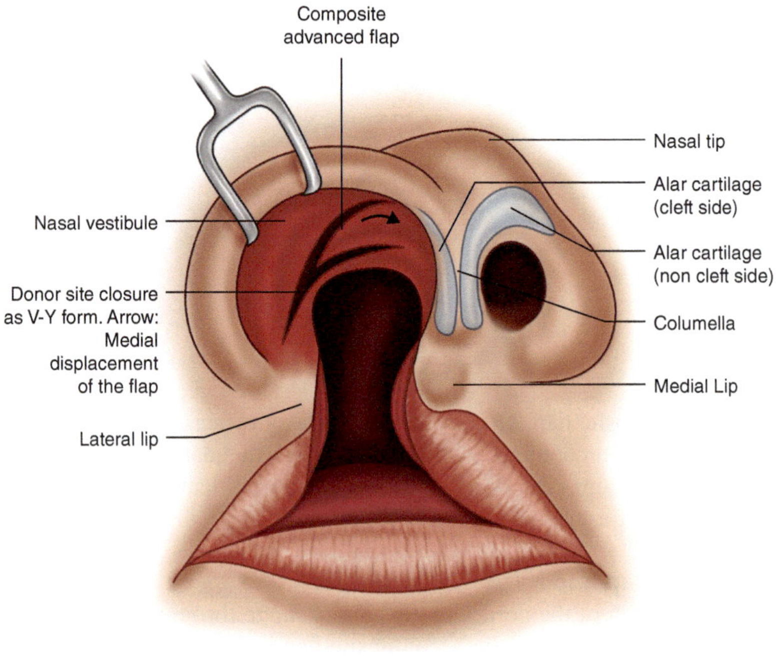

Fig. 6.56 Diagram of V-Y advancement of the composite flap during unilateral VYZ cleft rhinoplasty for complete cleft lip and palate

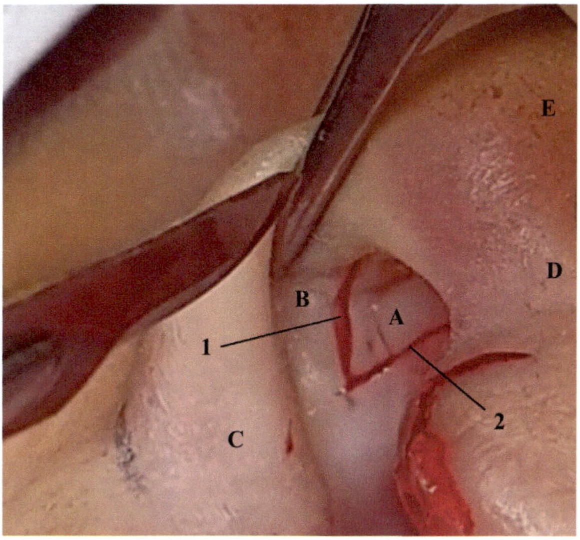

Fig. 6.57 VYZ cleft rhinoplasty for V composite flap incisions used for unilateral complete cleft lip nose repair. A: Rotational composite flap. B: Nasal vestibule. C: Alae. D: Columella. E: Nasal tip. 1: Marginal incision. 2: Intercartilaginous incision

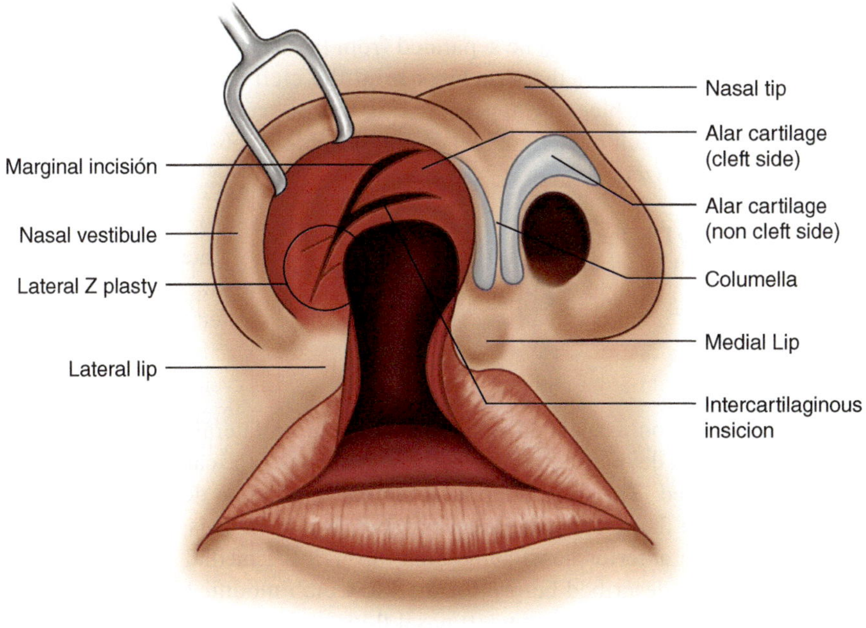

Fig. 6.58 Diagram of lateral Z plasty marking during VYZ technique

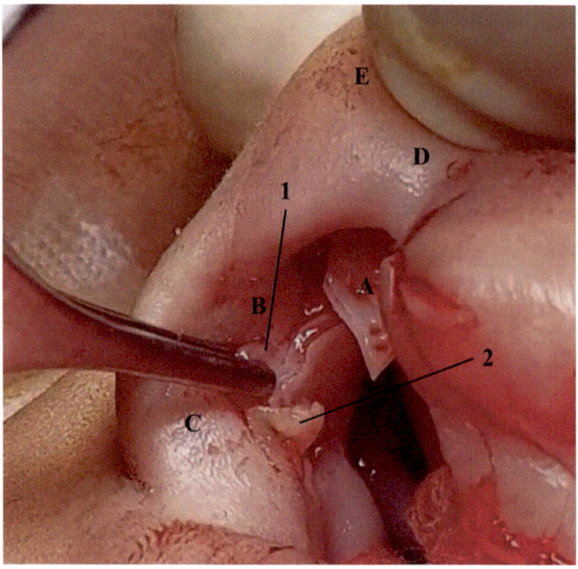

Fig. 6.59 Lateral Z plasty during VYZ cleft rhinoplasty used for unilateral cleft lip (Z plasty limbs are transposed). A: Rotational composite flap. B: Nasal vestibule. C: Alae. D: Columella. E: Nasal tip. 1: Medial branch of lateral Z plasty. 2: Lateral branch of lateral Z plasty

the cartilaginous structure of the nose (alar cartilages, domes, and lower dorsum). Both alar domes should be separated from the overlaying skin in order to facilitate the reposition of the structures from the cleft side (Figs. 6.60, 6.61, 6.62, and 6.63). Some bleeding appears during this dissection; however, because of the closed approach of the nose, it is not possible to observe any important vessel to be cauterized.

Lateral Z Plasty Dissection

Transpositional flaps are elevated at the subcutaneous level. Then the alar base is elevated using a supraperiosteal dissection from the pyriform aperture (Fig. 6.59).

Nasal Septum

The septal deviation associated with the complete unilateral cleft lips uses to have an important deviation; therefore, the reposition of the caudal nasal septum may be performed. The used method is similar to the one described for rotational composite flap technique (Figs. 6.7, 6.8, and 6.9). This is achieved after dissection of the anterior nasal spine area through the medial lip incision in a similar form as I described before for the Mc Comb modified technique. After dissection and release of the noncleft nasal floor periosteum from the spine, the caudal septum is moved medially for suture fixation using 5/0 PDS. The caudal septoplasty is not correcting the whole septal deformity; therefore a secondary correction is always necessary. I actually consider this maneuver as an alternative method for mild and moderate forms since the columella can be repositioned only by muscular action and recommended for severe cleft lip nasal deformities (see Cases).

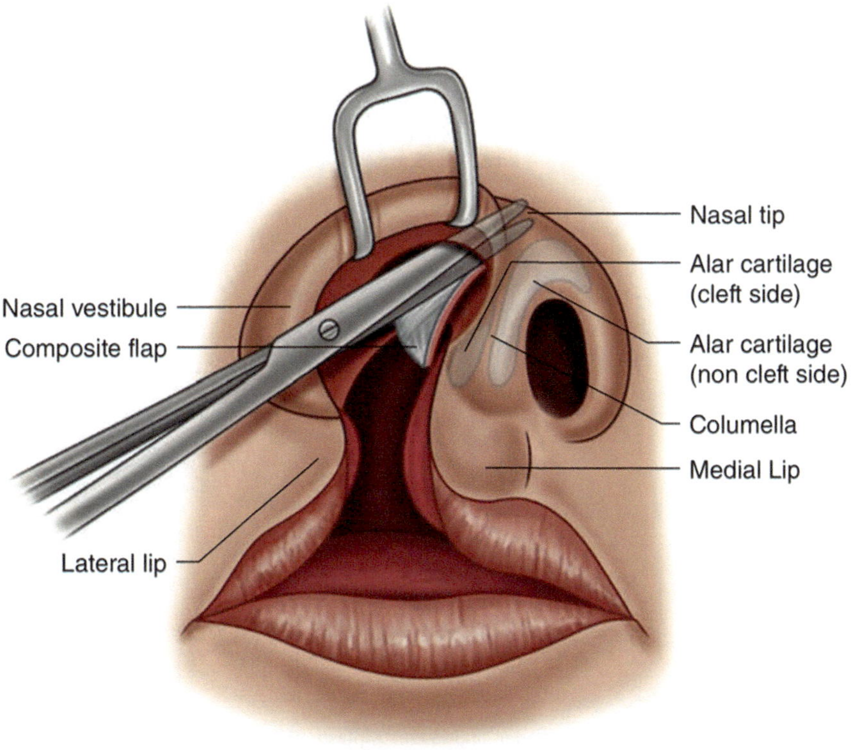

Fig. 6.60 Diagram of nasal tip dissection during VYZ technique for unilateral cleft lip and palate

Fig. 6.61 Nasal tip dissection during VYZ technique for primary unilateral cleft lip nose repair. A: V Composite flap. B: Nasal vestibule. C: Alae. D: Columella. E: Nasal tip. 1: V composite flap donor site

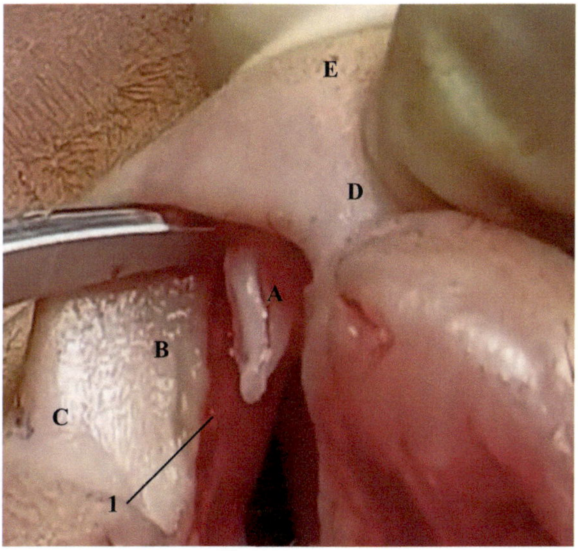

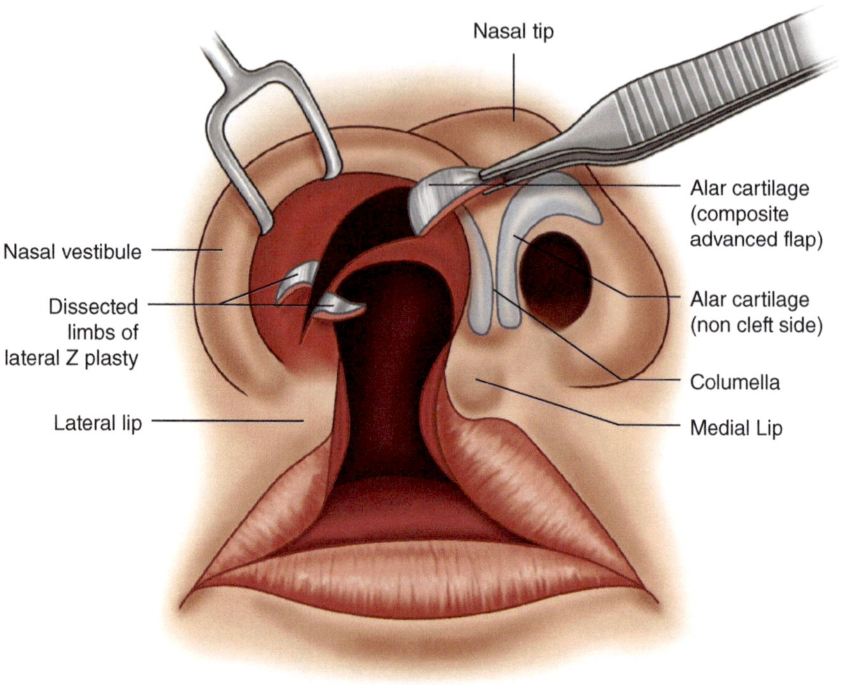

Fig. 6.62 Diagram of V composite flap and lateral Z plasty dissection during VYZ cleft rhinoplasty for complete unilateral cleft lip

Fig. 6.63 V composite flap elevation after nasal tip dissection during VYZ primary cleft rhinoplasty for complete unilateral cleft lip. A: V Composite flap. B: Alae. C: Columella. D: Nasal tip

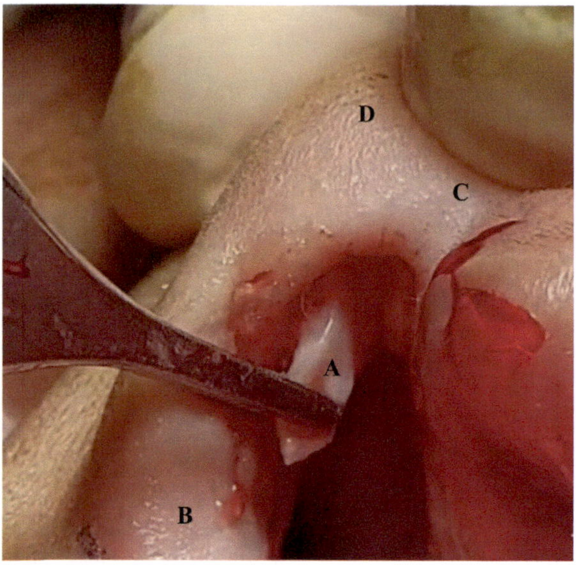

Nasal Tip Reconstruction

Nose repair should be performed before the lip repair because the access to the nose through the nonrepaired cleft lip is easier than the access after lip repair. After elevation, the composite flap is advanced medially and sutured using transcutaneous 5/0 PDS stitches. The medial advancement of the composite flap leaves a donor site which is closed using the vestibular skin and creates the Y form. Finally, the lateral Z plasty is transposed (Fig. 6.64). Similar to the rotational composite flap method, this is a three-dimensional movement in three vectors: medial, posterior, and superior.

The use of transcutaneous stitches allowed us to achieve the following two objectives: (1) repositioning the alar cartilage at the cleft side and (2) decreasing the space created by surgical dissection, which reduces the risks of postoperative bleeding and hematoma formation. These stitches are placed through the skin, starting from inside the nose and then exiting the skin at the level of the supra-alar crease; the needle then returns through the same hole and finally enters the inside of the nose in front of the initial entrance, where the sutures are tied (Figs. 6.32, 6.33, 6.34, and 6.35).

This is the recommended sequence (Fig. 6.65):

First stitch The alar cartilage dome of the composite flap is medially displaced and fixed using a vertical transcutaneous stitch. All these sutures leave and return the skin at the level of the supra alar crease. Special attention must be paid at the level of the soft triangle avoiding skin retraction due to the lack of cartilage in this area.

Second stitch: Placed at the level of the lateral corner of the triangular composite flap and using a similar vertical stitch at the level of the supraalar crease.

Third stitch: Between the two alar domes using a transcutaneous stitch at the level of the anterior border of the alar domes.

Fourth stitch: They are placed to transpose the branches of the lateral Z plasty closing the donor site of the V-Y advanced flap. The suture leaves and returns at the level of the alar crease (alar facial groove).

Fifth stitch: Used to correct the position of the alar cartilage in relation to the upper lateral cartilage. This is repositioned using a vertical transcutaneous stitch placed lateral to the internal nasal valve.

Finally, few simple stitches may be used to align correctly the borders of the V-Y and lateral Z plasty. A similar recommendation should be taken in consideration to prevent not to exceed the number of these transcutaneous stitches in order to prevent alar necrosis.

The combination of V-Y advancement and lateral Z plasty produces a vestibular lengthening which facilitates the medial displacement of the alar cartilage and prevention of lateral web, a common problem after primary cleft rhinoplasty. The outcome observed after using this method is similar to the change produced by the presurgical orthopedic nasal molding which expands the nasal vestibule but only temporarily. That is the reason why always the presurgical nasal molding should be

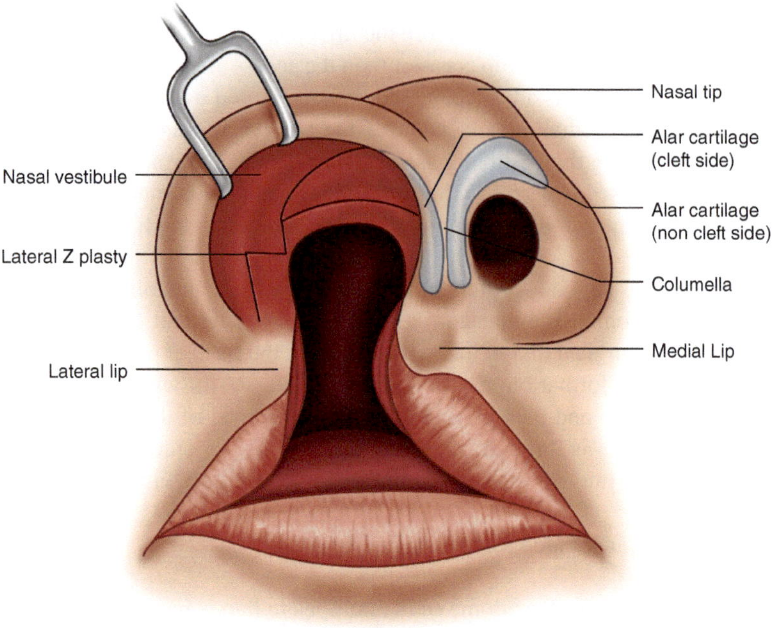

Fig. 6.64 Diagram of nasal tip repair after V-Y composite flap advancement plus lateral Z plasty transposition

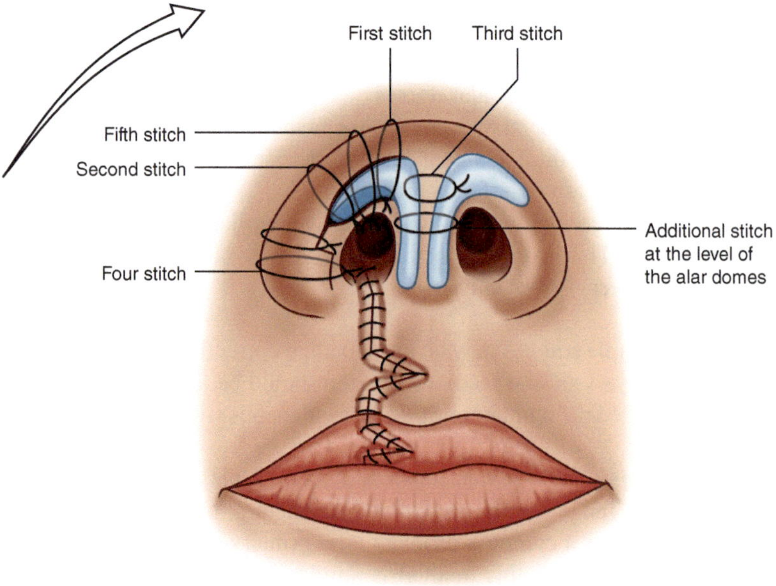

Fig. 6.65 Transcutaneous stitches during VYZ technique

combined with the primary cleft rhinoplasty. That is the reason why the technique developed by the author has been named as "the surgical nasoalveolar molding"; the nose and the maxillary arch can be effectively molded by surgical effect only [10] (Figs. 6.66, 6.67, and 6.68).

Nasal Floor

The repair of the nasal floor is the final step of cleft rhinoplasty and represents the correction of the most anterior portion of the nasal floor (vestibular segment). Based on our surgical protocol for cleft lip and palate repair, the other segments are closed in different times during primary and secondary palate repair. The anterior section of the nasal floor repair is performed in a similar form as described for the rotational composite flap technique (Fig. 6.40). The anterior section of the nasal floor is repaired using the medial cutaneous flap lateral to the base of the columella at the cleft border and the base of the ala. The alar is released by a lateral lip incision at the piriform margin in combination with an upper buccal sulcus incision performing a supraperiosteal dissection over the maxilla. The structural support of the anterior segment of the nasal floor is provided by the muscular repair of the upper lip; the levator labii superioris alaeque nasi and orbicularis oris muscles are identified and repositioned, allowing the final position of the nasal base (Figs. 6.41 and 6.69). This muscular reconstruction is providing support to the base of the nose but also acts over the caudal septum of the nose moving it medially and correcting the anterior septal deviation.

The nasal fascicle of the levator labii superioris alaeque nasi muscle is identified during the muscular dissection and attached to the caudal septum previously exposed using PDS 5/0. This muscle pulls the membranous portion of the caudal septum to

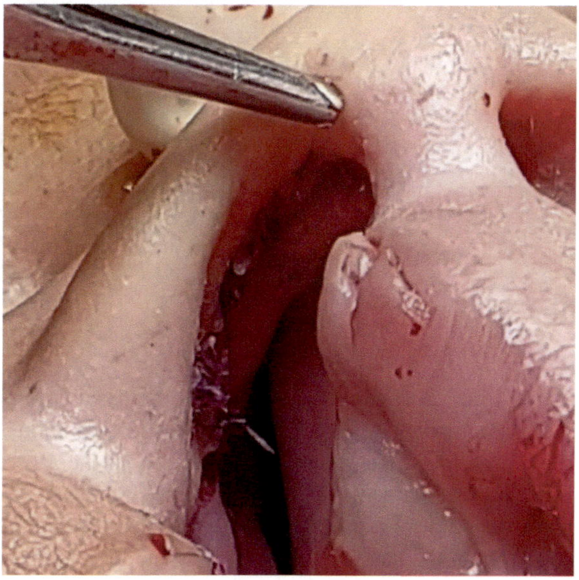

Fig. 6.66 The surgical nasal molding effect of the VYZ cleft rhinoplasty. The nasal vestibule has been expanded as a consequence of vestibular lengthening produced by VY advancement and lateral Z plasty

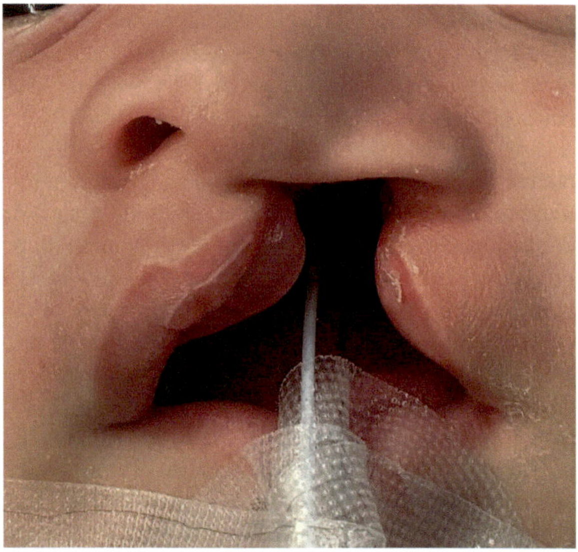

Fig. 6.67 A 3-month-old patient with unilateral complete cleft lip and palate (preoperative view)

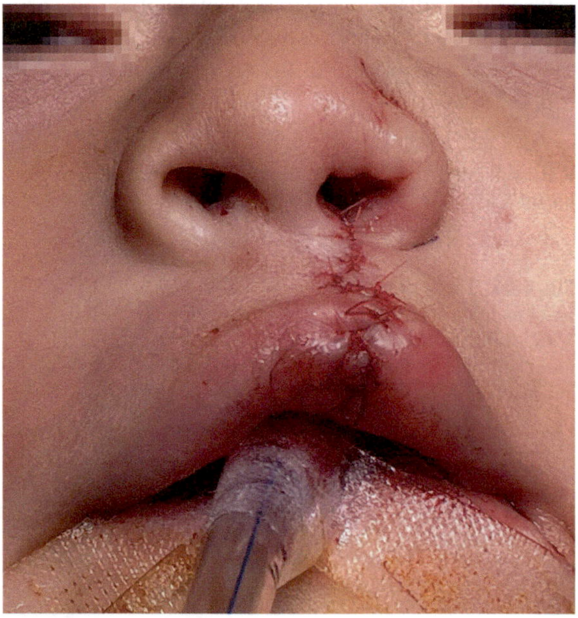

Fig. 6.68 Immediate postoperative view of the patient in Fig. 6.67 operated using the VYZ technique

the midline addressing the position of the nasal columella and bringing support to the base of the nose. A common misconception about the nasal floor repair is that the normal position cannot be achieved until the alveolar bone graft is performed; this theory explains why a lower position of the nasal base is expected after primary cleft lip and nose repair. The author has been studied the effect of muscular reconstruction on the base of the nose position, and this procedure is effective providing

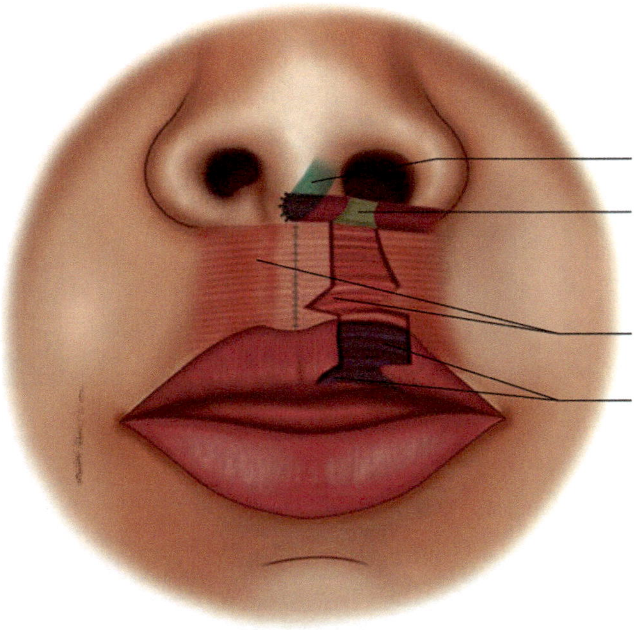

Fig. 6.69 Muscular reconstruction is providing support to the base of the nose acting over the membranous portion of the caudal septum of the nose moving it medially and correcting the anterior septal deviation during VYZ technique

nose asymmetry after long-term follow-up; therefore, alveolar bone graft is not necessary to achieve this outcome [10, 21].

In addition, muscular repair during cheiloplasty molds the maxillary arch in a more physiological form in comparison with molding plates. This is an author hypothesis. During his experience, adequate maxillary segment molding after cleft lip and palate repair was observed; however, comparative studies are required to obtain definitive conclusions regarding this topic (Fig. 6.70).

The effect of the proposed primary cleft cheilorhinoplasty produces a similar outcome as the presurgical orthopedic (nasoalveolar molding) using plates and nasal stents; therefore the author named the method as the "surgical nasoalveolar molding" [10].

Cases (Figs. 6.71, 6.72, 6.73, 6.74, 6.75, 6.76, 6.77, 6.78, 6.79, 6.80, 6.81, 6.82, 6.83, 6.84, 6.85, 6.86, 6.87, 6.88, 6.89, 6.90, 6.91, and 6.92)

Here I present long-term outcomes using the VYZ rhinoplasty in patients with complete cleft lip and palate. None of them used presurgical orthopedics and only one (case 4) used postoperative nasal conformers.

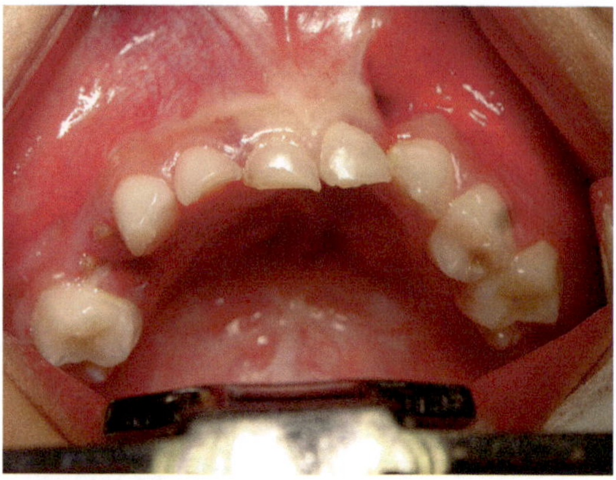

Fig. 6.70 Maxillary arch molding after cleft lip primary cheiloplasty

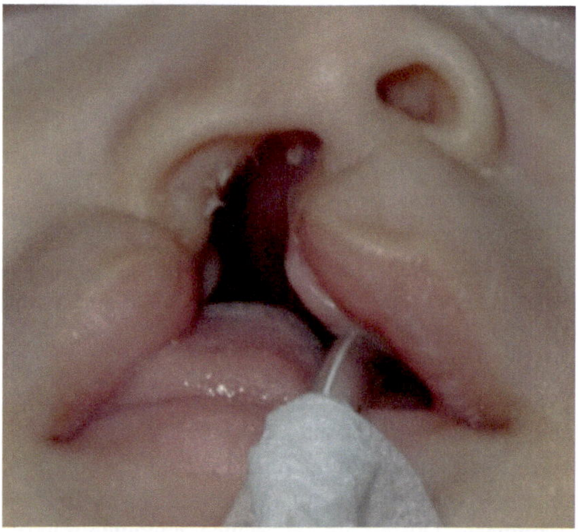

Fig. 6.71 Case 1. Preoperative view of a 3-month-old infant with complete unilateral cleft lip

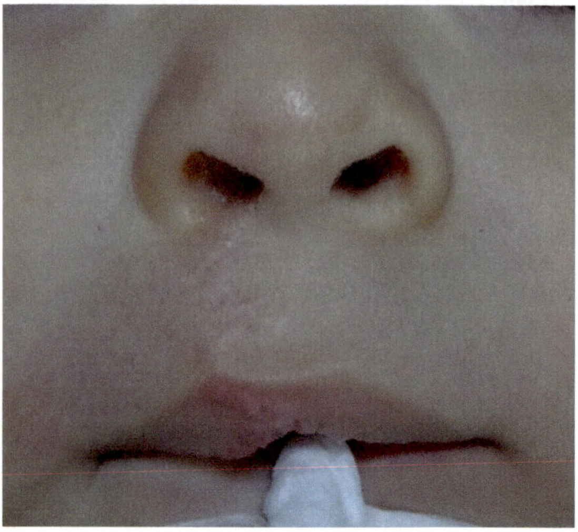

Fig. 6.72 Case 1. A 1-year postoperative view of the infant shown in Fig. 6.71 after undergoing nasal repair using the VYZ technique (frontal view)

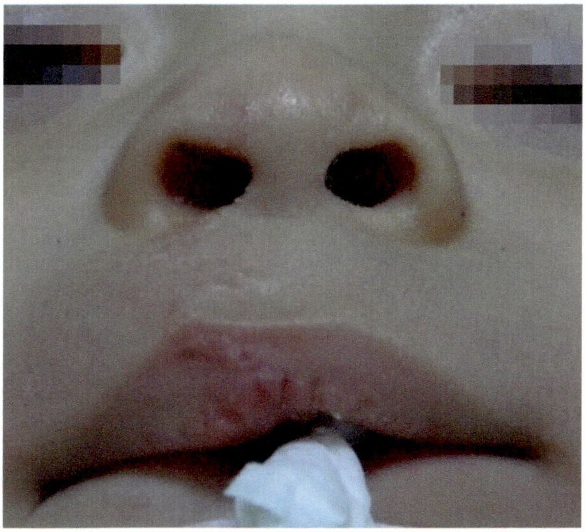

Fig. 6.73 Case 1. A 1-year postoperative view of the infant shown in Fig. 6.71 after undergoing nasal repair using the VYZ technique (worm eye view). No presurgical orthopedics and no postoperative nasal stents

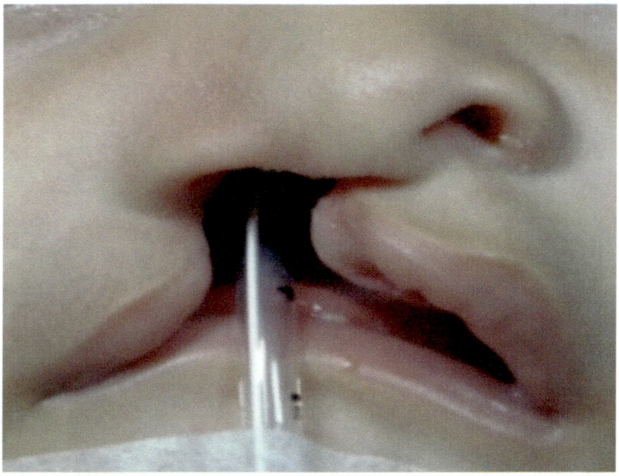

Fig. 6.74 Case 2. Preoperative view of a 3-month-old infant with complete unilateral cleft lip (frontal view)

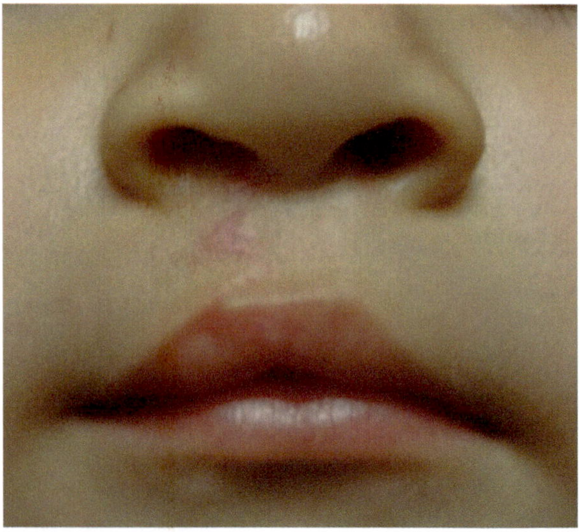

Fig. 6.75 Case 2. One-year postoperative view of the infant shown in Fig. 6.74 after undergoing nasal repair using the VYZ technique (frontal view). No presurgical orthopedics and no postoperative nasal stents

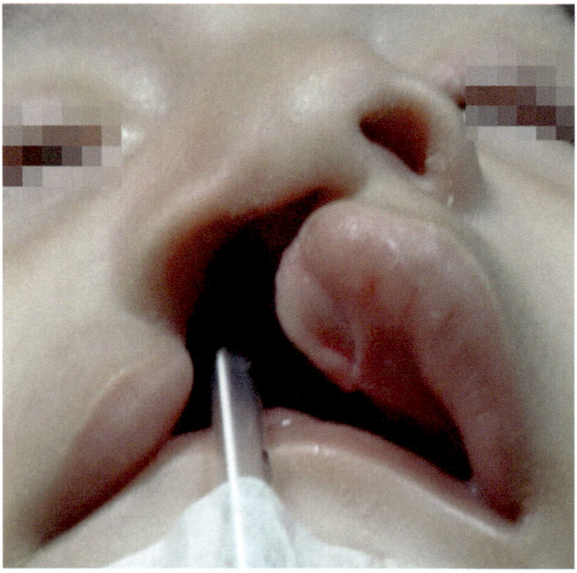

Fig. 6.76 Case 2. Preoperative view of a 3-month-old infant with complete unilateral cleft lip (worm eye view)

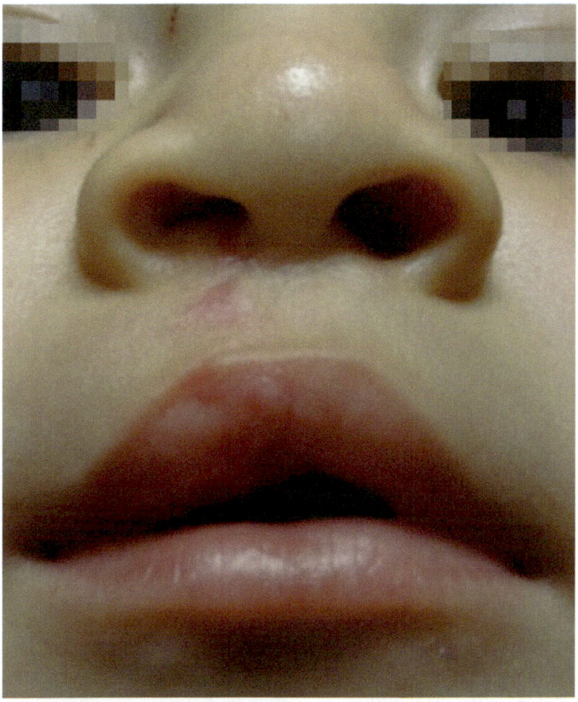

Fig. 6.77 Case 2. A 1-year postoperative view of the infant shown in Fig. 6.76 after undergoing nasal repair using the VYZ technique (worm eye view). No presurgical orthopedics and no postoperative nasal stents

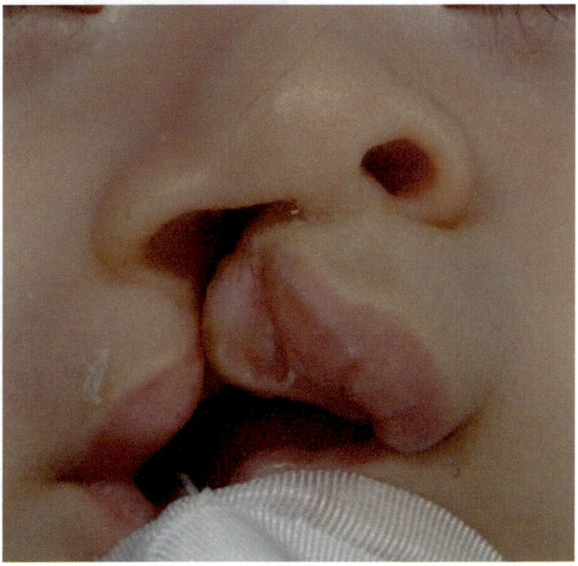

Fig. 6.78 Case 3. Preoperative view of a 3-month-old infant with complete unilateral cleft lip

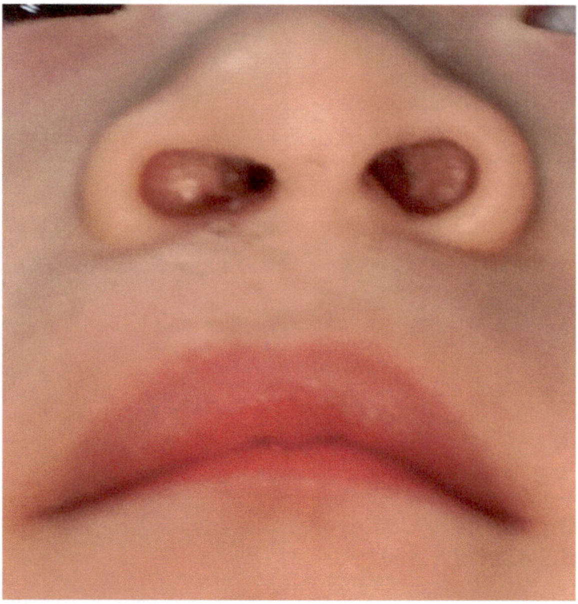

Fig. 6.79 Case 3. One-year postoperative view of the infant shown in Fig. 6.78 after undergoing nasal repair using the VYZ technique. No presurgical orthopedics and no postoperative nasal stents

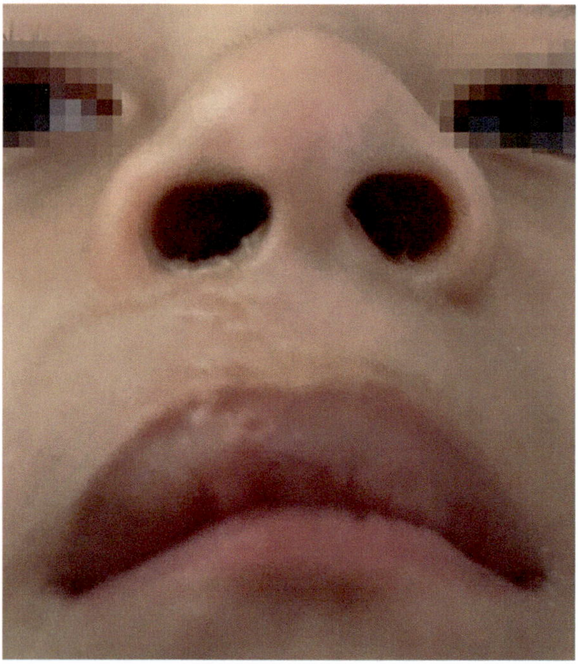

Fig. 6.80 Case 3. Long-term (10 years) postoperative view of the infant shown in Fig. 6.78 after undergoing nasal repair using the VYZ technique

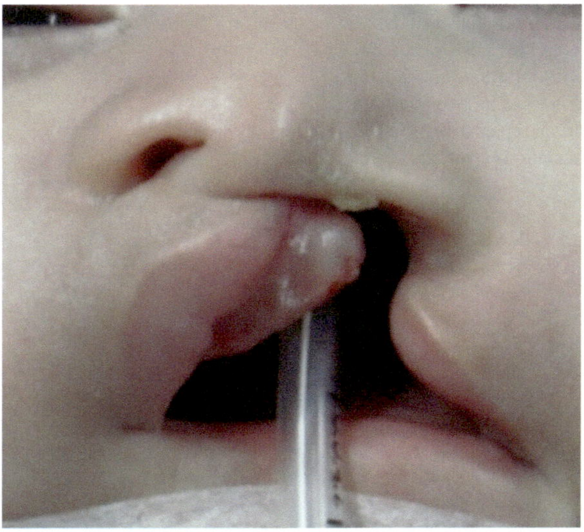

Fig. 6.81 Case 4. Preoperative view of a 3-month-old infant with complete unilateral cleft lip (frontal view)

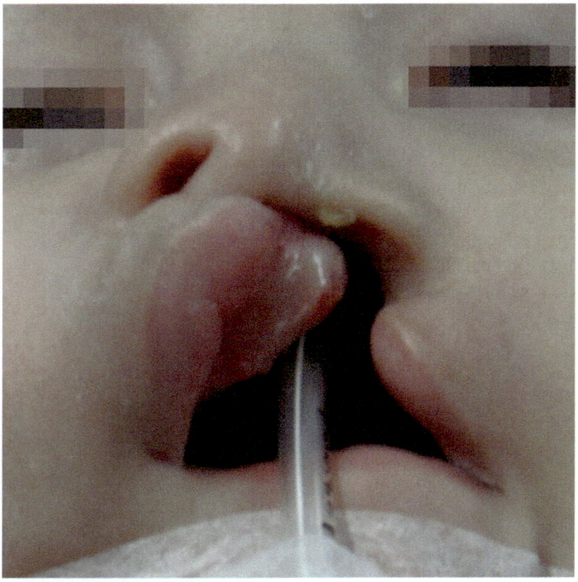

Fig. 6.82 Case 4. Preoperative view of a 3-month-old infant with complete unilateral cleft lip (worm eye view)

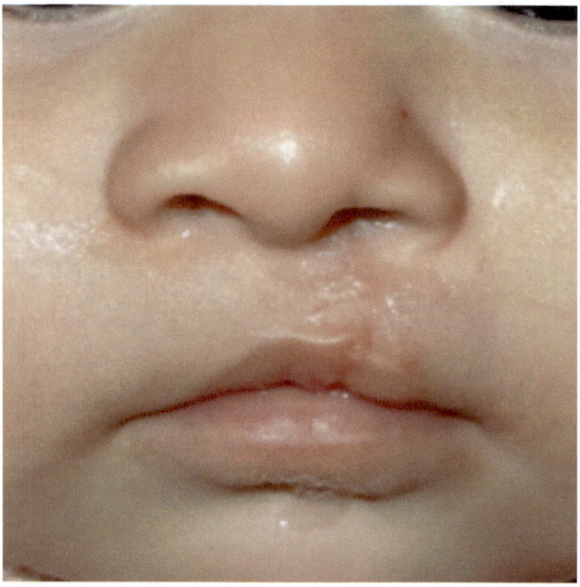

Fig. 6.83 Case 4. One-year postoperative view of the infant shown in Fig. 6.81 after undergoing nasal repair using the VYZ technique (frontal view)

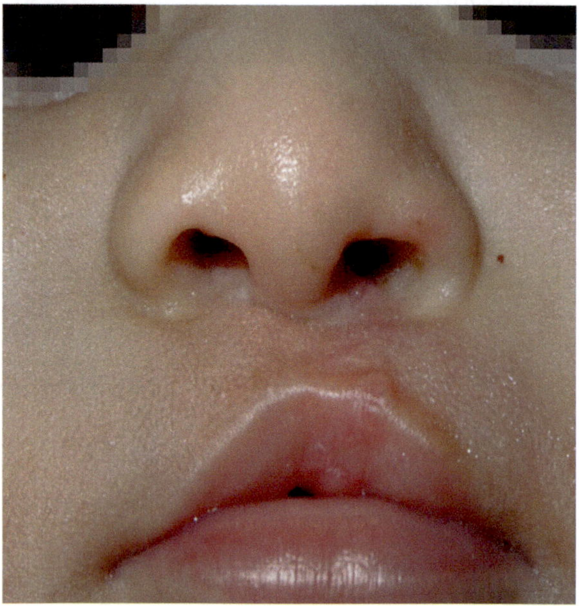

Fig. 6.84 Case 4. One-year postoperative view of the infant shown in Fig. 6.81 after undergoing nasal repair using the VYZ technique (worm eye view). No presurgical orthopedics. Nasal conformers used during 6 months

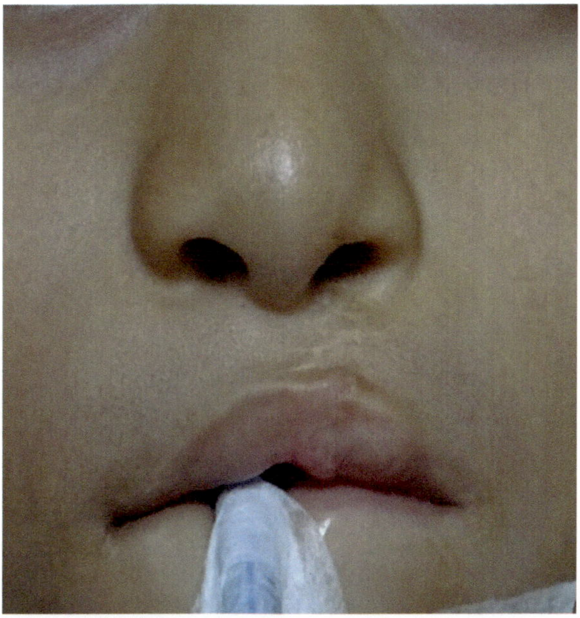

Fig. 6.85 Case 4. Long-term (10 years) postoperative view of the infant shown in Fig. 6.81 after undergoing nasal repair using the VYZ technique (frontal view)

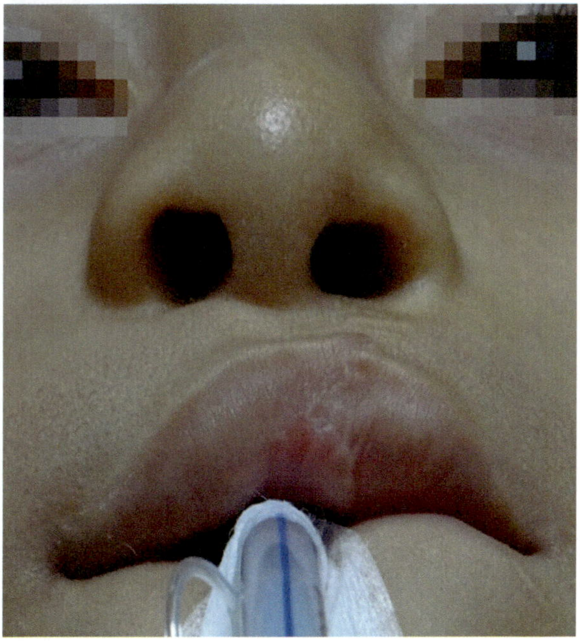

Fig. 6.86 Case 4. Long-term (10 years) postoperative view of the infant shown in Fig. 6.81 after undergoing nasal repair using the VYZ technique (worm eye view)

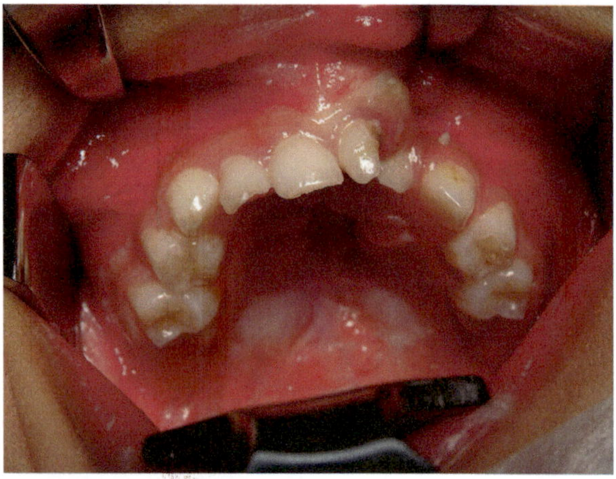

Fig. 6.87 Case 4. Long-term (8 years) postoperative view of the maxillary arch of the patient shown in Fig. 6.81 after alveolar molding effect of cleft lip repair using modified Pool technique

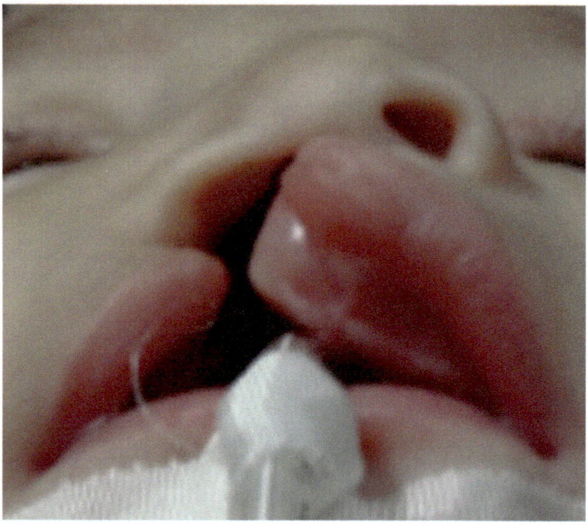

Fig. 6.88 Case 5. Preoperative view of a 3-month-old infant with complete unilateral cleft lip

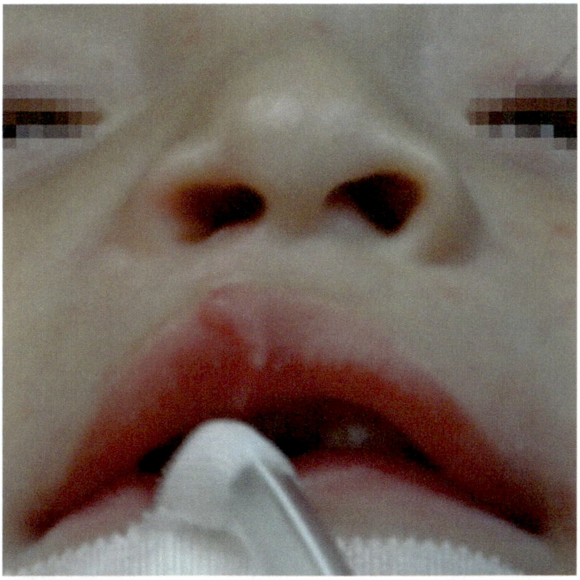

Fig. 6.89 Case 5. A 1-year postoperative view of the infant shown in Fig. 6.88 after undergoing nasal repair using the VYZ technique (frontal view). No presurgical orthopedics and no postoperative nasal stents

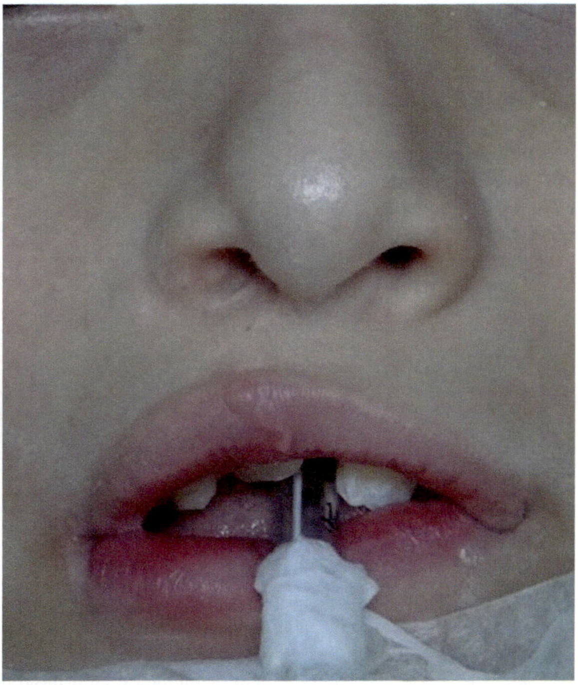

Fig. 6.90 Case 5. Long-term (10 years) postoperative view of the infant shown in Fig. 6.86 after undergoing nasal repair using the VYZ technique (frontal view)

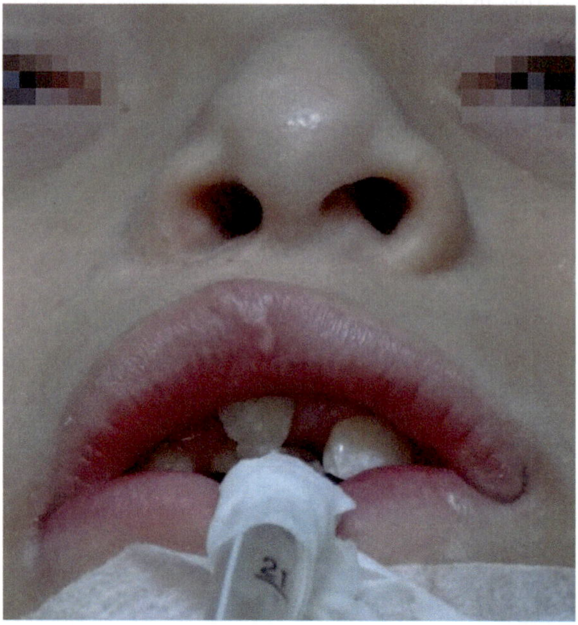

Fig. 6.91 Case 5. Long-term (10 years) postoperative view of the infant shown in Fig. 6.88 after undergoing nasal repair using the VYZ technique (worm eye view)

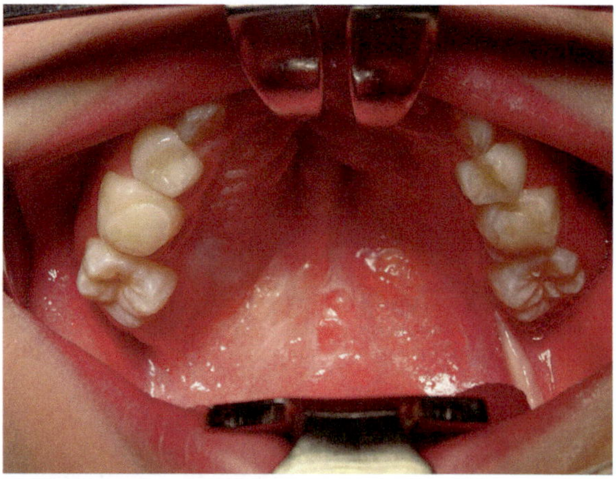

Fig. 6.92 Case 5. Long-term (9 years) postoperative view of the maxillary arch of the patient shown in Fig. 6.88 after alveolar molding effect of cleft lip repair using modified Pool technique

References

1. Haddock N, McRae M, Cutting C. Long-term effect of primary cleft rhinoplasty on secondary cleft rhinoplasty in patients with unilateral cleft lip–cleft palate. Plast Reconstr Surg. 2012;129(3):740–8.
2. Salyer K. Early and late treatment of unilateral cleft nasal deformity. Cleft Palate Craniofac J. 1992;29:556–69.
3. Salyer K, Genecov E, Genecov D. Unilateral cleft lip-nose repair: a 33-year experience. J Craniofac Surg. 2003;14:549–58.
4. Mc Comb H. Treatment of the unilateral cleft lip. Plas Reconstr Surg. 1975;55(5):596–601.

5. Garland K, McNeely B, Dubois L, Matic D. Systematic review of the long-term effects of pre-surgical orthopedic devices on patient outcomes. Cleft Palate Craniofac J. 2022;59(2):156–65.
6. Uzel A, Alparslan ZN. Long-term effects of presurgical infant orthopedics in patients with cleft lip and palate: a systematic review. Cleft Palate Craniofac J. 2011;48(5):587–95.
7. Potter J. Some nasal tip deformities due to alar cartilage abnormalities. Plas Reconstr Surg. 1954;13(5):359–66.
8. Berkeley W. The cleft lip nose. Plast Reconstr Surg. 1959;23:567.
9. Rossell-Perry P. Primary cleft rhinoplasty: surgical outcomes and complications using three techniques for unilateral cleft lip nose repair. J Craniofac Surg. 2020;31(6):1521–5.
10. Rossell-Perry P. The surgical nasoalveolar molding: a rational treatment for unilateral cleft lip nose deformity and literature review. Plast Reconstr Surg Glob Open. 2020;8(8):e3044.
11. Rossell-Perry P. Rotational composite flap technique for primary incomplete cleft nose deformity. Plast Reconstr Surg Glob Open. 2020;8(6):e2870.
12. Doyle DJ, Hendrix JM, Garmon EH. American Society of Anesthesiologists classification. [Updated 2023 Aug 17]. In: StatPearls [Internet]. Treasure Island: StatPearls Publishing; 2023. Available from: https://www.ncbi.nlm.nih.gov/books/NBK441940
13. Schalet G, Langlie J, Kim M, Thaller S. The rule of 10s for cleft repair: a historical review of the literature. J Craniofac Surg. 2023;34(3):884–7.
14. Chow I, Purnell CA, Hanwright PJ, Gosain AK. Evaluating the rule of 10s in cleft lip repair: do data support dogma? Plast Reconstr Surg. 2016;138(3):670–9.
15. Raghavan U, Vijayadev V, Rao D, Ullas G. Postoperative management of cleft lip and palate surgery. Facial Plast Surg. 2018;34(06):605–11.
16. Bösenberg AT, Kimble FW. Infraorbital nerve block in neonates for cleft lip repair: anatomical study and clinical application. Br J Anaesth. 1995;74(5):506–8.
17. Feriani G, Hatanaka E, Torloni MR, da Silva EM. Infraorbital nerve block for postoperative pain following cleft lip repair in children. Cochrane Database Syst Rev 2016;4(4):CD011131.
18. Rossell-Perry P. Modification of Reichert's technique based on natural landmarks and individual designs for unilateral repair of cleft lip. Scand J Plast Reconstr Surg Hand Surg. 2008;42(3):113–21.
19. Raymond WT, Mercan E, Fisher DM, Hopper RA, Birgfeld CB, Gruss JS. Unilateral cleft lip nasal deformity: foundation-based approach to primary rhinoplasty. Plast Reconstr Surg. 2019;144(5):1138–49.
20. Rossell-Perry P. Primary unilateral cleft lip nasal deformity repair using VYZ plasty: an anthropometric study. Indian J Plast Surg. 2017;50(02):180–6.
21. Rossell-Perry P, Gavino-Gutierrez A. Mixed dentition period follow-up of primary unilateral cleft nose deformity repair. Plast Reconstr Surg Glob Open. 2023;11(10):e5313.

The Bilateral Cleft Lip Nose Deformity

7

Percy Rossell-Perry

Contents

Introduction

Nasal deformity in bilateral cleft lip is complex and varies from minor to severe (Figs. 7.1, 7.2, and 7.3); James Barrett Brown mentioned "Bilateral cleft lip is twice as difficult to repair as unilateral, and the results are only half as good" also Ralph Millard Jr. said "the presence of the projecting premaxilla and how it is to be handled has always been and continues to be a difficult variable and at the core of some of the controversies" [1].

The nasal tip is commonly flattened, the columella is absent, and the alar base is very wide in combination with muscular distortion and severe dentoskeletal disturbance (Figs. 7.4, 7.5, and 7.6).

Skeletal deformity is characterized by prominent premaxilla (to different degrees) and hypoplastic maxillary segments. The existing discrepancy between the central and lateral segments creates a complex scenario for lip and nose reconstruction.

As Harold Gillies mentioned in relation to complex deformities, "the skeleton is first" [1]; the basic treatment of these problems should consider first consider

P. Rossell-Perry (✉)
Health of Science Faculty, School of Human Medicine, Peruvian University Union (UpeU), Lima, Peru
e-mail: percy.rossell@upeu.edu.pe

P. Rossell-Perry (ed.), *Atlas of Primary Cleft Rhinoplasty*,
https://doi.org/10.1007/978-3-031-68012-0_7

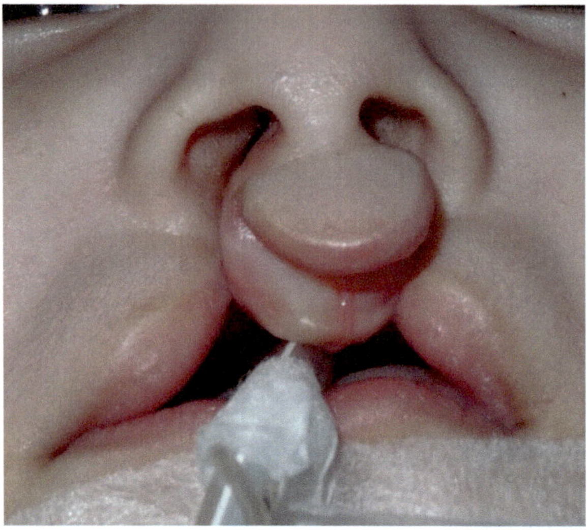

Fig. 7.1 Mild bilateral cleft lip nasal deformity

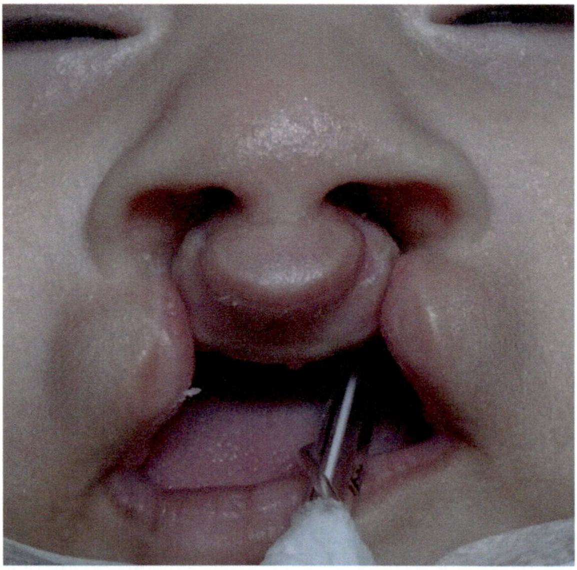

Fig. 7.2 Moderate bilateral cleft lip nasal deformity

skeletal repair; however this is not possible to be done because of the growth disturbance of the bones produced by its early correction.

The different types of presurgical orthopedics help us to improve skeletal proportions in order to facilitate the lip and nose repair in bilateral cleft lip forms. The surgical type (represented by the lip adhesion) and nonsurgical type (represented by lip taping, elastic bandage, nasoalveolar molding, and others) help us to improve skeletal proportions to prevent bad outcomes and complications after primary bilateral cleft lip and nose repair. The nasal septum does not have an important role in

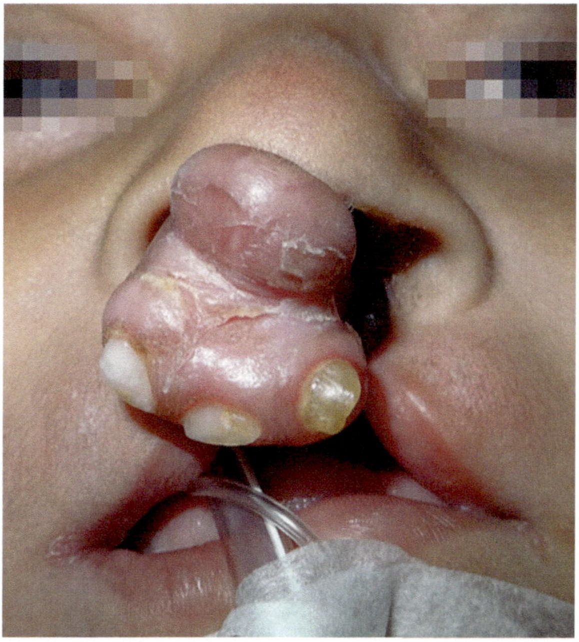

Fig. 7.3 Severe bilateral cleft lip nasal deformity

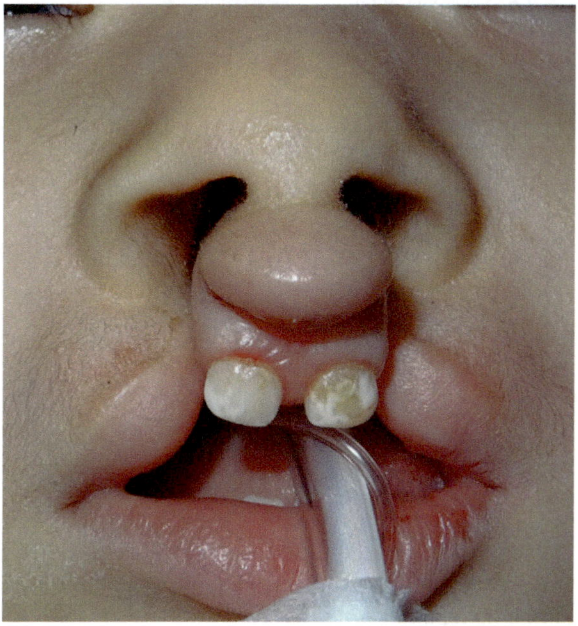

Fig. 7.4 Mild nasal tip and columella deformity in the bilateral cleft lip

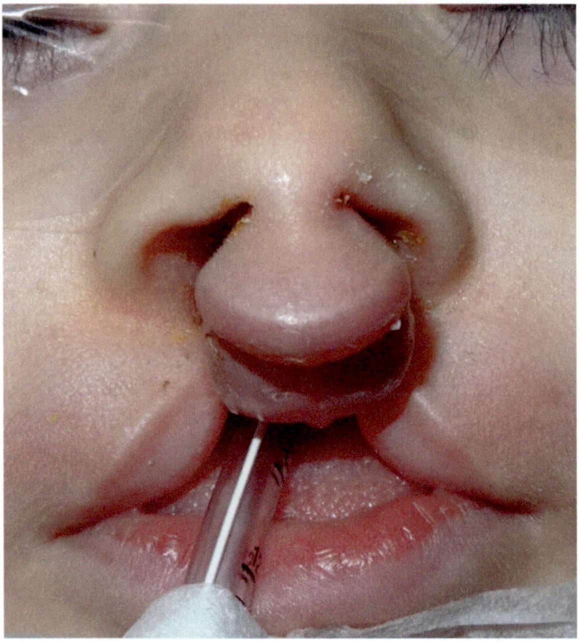

Fig. 7.5 Moderate nasal tip and columella deformity in the bilateral cleft lip

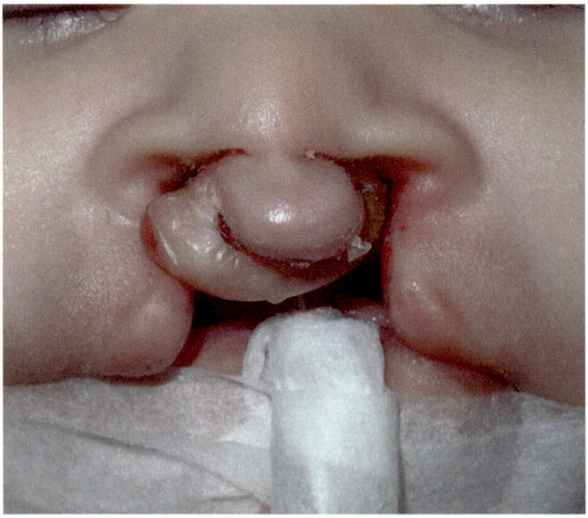

Fig. 7.6 Severe nasal tip and columella deformity in the bilateral cleft lip

the nose deformity associated with the bilateral cleft lip in comparison with unilateral forms. The nasal floor is usually wider than normal and requires shortening during lip repair.

The alar cartilages are affected bilaterally, appearing dislodged from their natural position and wider and rotated outwardly in a flare.

The vestibule of the nose seems to be stretched bilaterally, and this finding supports the use of vestibular lengthening techniques as the bilateral VYZ is used to normalize the position of the cartilages of the tip of the nose [2].

The effects of these methods reproduce the temporal effects of the nasal molding using presurgical orthopedics; therefore, the author named this technique as the "surgical nasoalveolar molding."

Two basic types of bilateral cleft lip have been described, as follows: complete and incomplete forms. But these types may be presented in combination with mild forms.

Nasal deformity associated with the bilateral cleft lip correlates well according to these different types.

Microforms are associated with incomplete or complete forms and should be identified to develop an adequate surgical plan for the treatment of bilateral cleft lip nose.

The Incomplete Bilateral Cleft Lip Nose Deformity (Figs. 7.7, 7.8, and 7.9)

The spectrum of incomplete cleft lips may vary from microforms to extended incomplete clefts on one or both sides of the bilateral cleft lip. Nose deformity usually correlates with the severity of these forms.

Based on nose components, we may describe the characteristics of the incomplete bilateral cleft lips and their applications to the surgical treatment.

Nasal floor The nasal floor has four sections as follows: nostril sill, primary palate (alveolus), secondary palate (hard palate), and soft palate. The nostril sill and

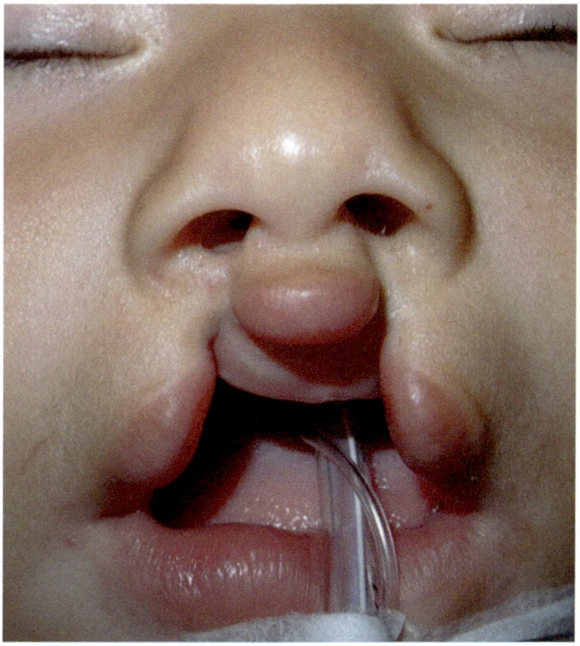

Fig. 7.7 Incomplete bilateral cleft lip nose deformity

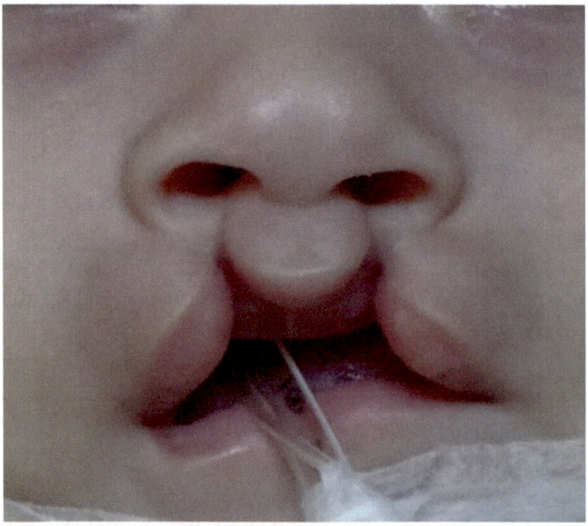

Fig. 7.8 Incomplete bilateral cleft lip nose deformity

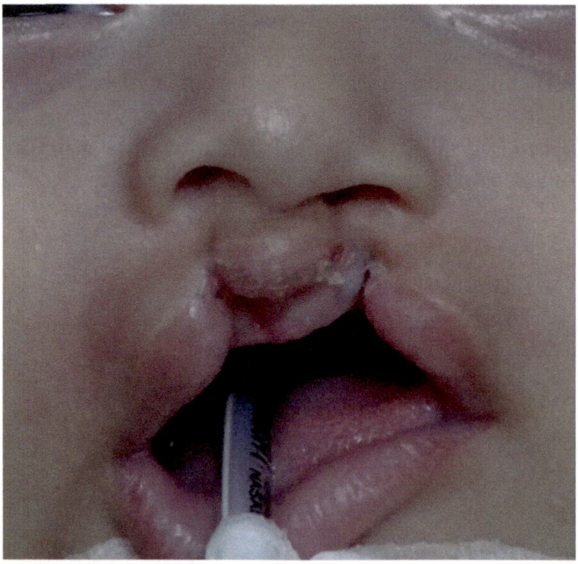

Fig. 7.9 Incomplete bilateral cleft lip nose deformity

primary palate may be partially affected by incomplete forms. This is why the nasal deformity associated with these types of clefts is mild.

Columella The columella in incomplete bilateral cleft lip nose forms is short but longer that those in complete forms requiring both types of lengthening.

Alar base The alar base in incomplete cleft lips is wider than that in the normal population and requires bilateral shortening. The requirement for alar base shortening depends on the severity of the nose deformity on each side.

Nasal tip Flattening of the nasal tip is common and depends on the degree of the alar cartilage distortion. The lack of the tip projection in bilateral cleft lip requires improvement even in incomplete forms.

Nasal septum The nasal septum is not affected as it is in its complete form. However, there may be partial deviation in combined forms when a complete form is combined with minor forms (incomplete).

Alar cartilage Inward buckling and retrodisplacement of the alar dome are observed on both sides, affecting the form and extension of the vestibule.

Nostril These components are more symmetric than unilateral clefts; however, asymmetry may exist between the two sides. Wide nostrils were also observed on both sides.

Maxilla The existence of a cleft may vary among patients with incomplete cleft lips. Sometimes there is a simple notch or absence of any cleft or combination of both. Commonly, all of these variants have an aligned maxillary arch in the bilateral cleft lips.

Complete Bilateral Cleft Lip Nose Deformity (Figs. 7.10, 7.11, and 7.12)

This is the most complex nasal deformity of the cleft lip and palate involving distortion of the skeleton and soft tissues.

The most important factor associated with the severity of the nasal deformity in complete bilateral cleft lips is the position of the premaxilla. Severely protruding premaxilla is related to severe nasal deformities characterized by short or absent columella, underprojected nasal tips, laterally displaced alar bases, and flared alae [3].

Therefore, it is essential in complete bilateral cleft lip nose repair and early premaxilla management (using different strategies such as Naso Alveolar Molding or bilateral lip adhesion before primary cleft rhinoplasty.

Based on the nose components, we may describe the characteristics of the complete bilateral cleft lips and their application in surgical treatment.

Nasal floor The nasal floor has four sections as follows: nostril sill, primary palate (alveolus), secondary palate (hard palate), and soft palate. All these elements in the bilateral complete cleft lip and palates are absent. The nostril sill is repaired primarily using the lateral and medial elements of the cleft and is supported by the muscular reconstruction. The alar bases (lateral elements of the cleft) are attached to the skeletal structure (the pyriform aperture of the maxilla). They should be released for proper alignment of both sides during primary repair.

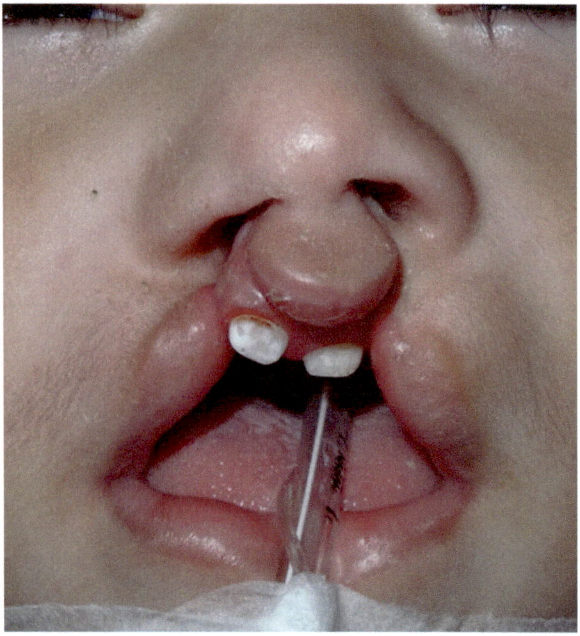

Fig. 7.10 Complete bilateral cleft lip nose deformity

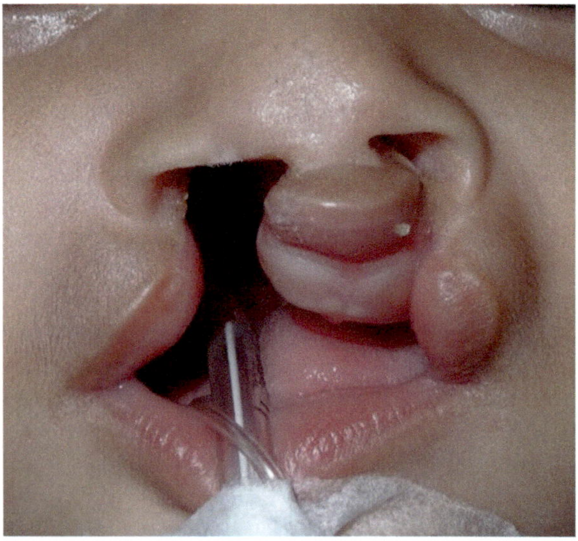

Fig. 7.11 Complete bilateral cleft lip nose deformity

This segment is usually wider and shortening is necessary during nasal floor repair.

Muscular repair is also important for providing support for the nasal sills. The presence of the Simonart's band is not relevant for reconstructive purposes, and it is usually resected during primary lip and nose repair.

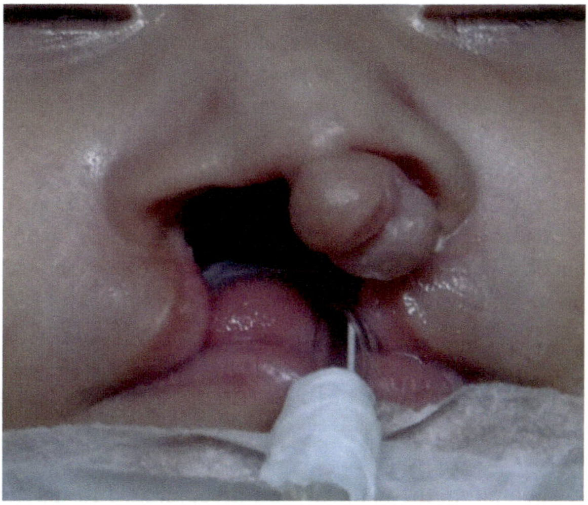

Fig. 7.12 Complete bilateral cleft lip nose deformity

Columella Repair of the shortening or absence of the columella is the key point in bilateral cleft lip nose deformity. Initially, it was repaired by columellar lengthening using lip tissues (Millard banked forked flap method); however, the outcome appears to be unnatural. Later, Mulliken proposed columellar repair using nasal tissues considering that "the columella is in the nose." Actually, based on this concept, the columella is repaired by bilateral alar cartilage and dome repositioning [4].

Nasal tip This structure is commonly affected and characterized by flattening because of the inwards buckling and retrodisplacement of the alar domes on both sides. Corrections of the alar cartilage structures allow us to improve the columellar length and nasal tip projection.

Nasal septum This structure may be affected in asymmetric forms of bilateral cleft lips and may require correction. However, this approach is limited to the caudal portion during primary lip repair.

Alar cartilage Bilateral malpositioning of these structures is associated with columellar and nasal tip deformities in bilateral cleft lips. These findings also explain the vestibular shortening observed in these patients. The use of presurgical orthopedics such as NAM (nasoalveolar molding) expands the nasal vestibule; however, this effect is temporary; primary rhinoplasty is always necessary for long-term outcomes. The most important effect of the presurgical treatments for bilateral cleft lip nose repair is on the prominent premaxilla. The author described the "surgical nasal molding" to surgical extension of the vestibule without presurgical treatment [2].

Premaxilla The skeletal structure of the complete bilateral cleft lip plays an important role in the nose deformity. Early management is essential to provide an adequate scenario for primary lip and nose correction in bilateral cleft lips. The premaxilla projection depends mainly on the degree of the maxillary hypoplasia, and the role of the presurgical orthopedic or lip adhesion treatment is extremely important and should be provided at an early age (the first week of life) to guarantee adequate correction of this segment.

Late treatment of this segment may result in poor lip and nasal outcomes, and setback osteotomy may be required for its correction.

The goal of primary bilateral cleft rhinoplasty is to normalize the nasal appearance through columellar lengthening, narrowing and increasing the projection of the nasal tip, and decreasing the alar base width.

The Bilateral Cleft Lip Combined Forms (Figs. 7.13, 7.14, and 7.15)

By definition, the bilateral cleft lip combined forms include combinations of complete, incomplete, and microforms with their associated nasal deformities. Nasal deformities are asymmetric and require different treatments for each side. Even when the cleft is complete or incomplete on both sides, there are always minor or major differences. Some publications reported symmetrically forms as the most common type I consider asymmetrical forms to be more common [5]. Asymmetrical bilateral cleft lip is either complete or incomplete with an incomplete or microform deformity on the other side. The presence of minor forms is often underestimated and produces unnatural outcomes after correction of one side only. Both sides should be repaired according to the type of cleft lip and nose deformity. The characteristics of the nasal deformity on each side are presented according to the

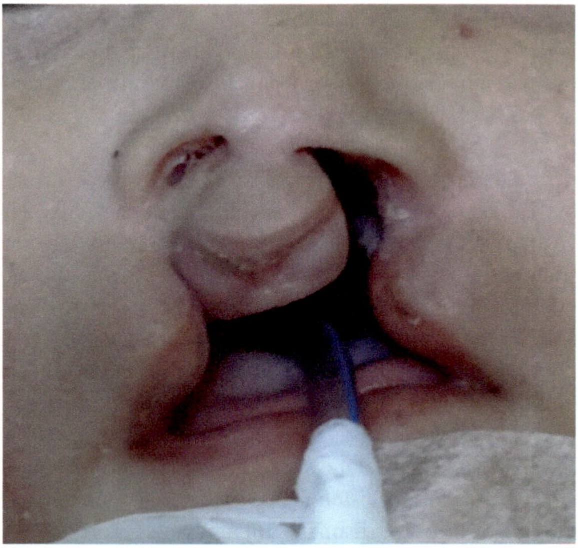

Fig. 7.13 Combined forms of bilateral cleft lip nose deformity

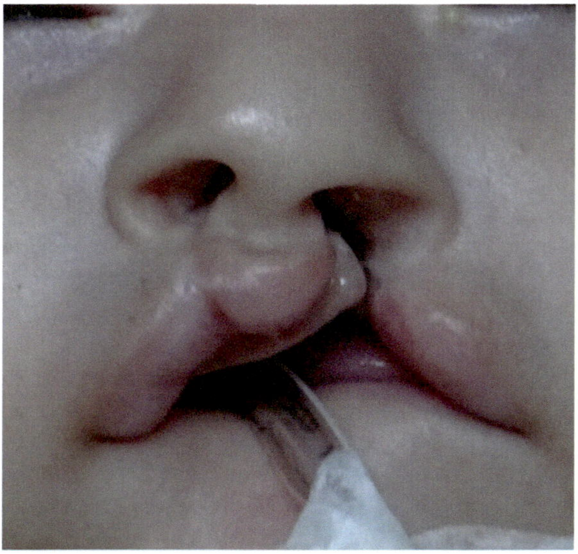

Fig. 7.14 Combined forms of bilateral cleft lip nose deformity

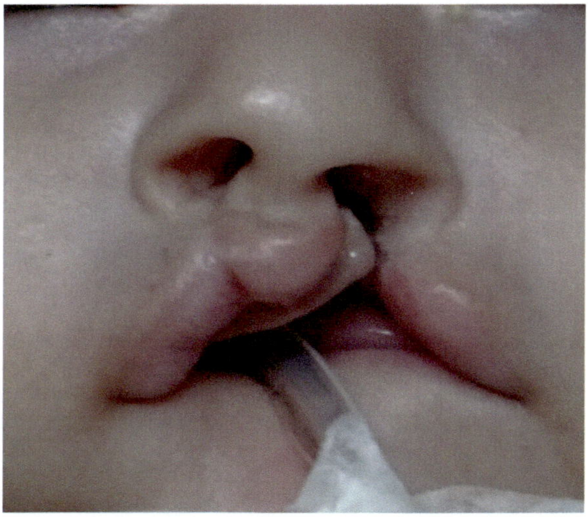

Fig. 7.15 Combined forms of bilateral cleft lip nose deformity

description for each type of unilateral cleft lip described in Chap. 5; with this type of cleft lip, it is more difficult to achieve nose symmetry after surgical repair.

Surgical Protocol

Bilateral cleft rhinoplasty is a well-accepted treatment for primary lip repair actually. The synchronous correction of the nasal deformity at the time of lip repair is considered actually as a major advance in bilateral cleft lip nose management [4, 6].

Table 7.1 Bilateral cleft lip nasal repair surgical protocol

Age	Degree of severity	Surgery
0–3 months	Severe complete	Presurgical orthopedics/lip adhesion
3–6 months	Incomplete	Rotational composite flap technique
	Complete	VYZ technique
5 years	All complete	Alveolar cleft closure
		Intermediate rhinoplasty or revision
>5 years	Persistent severe	Premaxilla setback
7–9 years	All complete	Alveolar bone graft
16–18 years		Secondary rhinoplasty

Repair of the nasal deformity associated with the bilateral cleft lip is challenging owing to complex characteristics requiring more surgeon's experience and skills. Since neonatal presurgical management uses orthopedics or lip adhesion to the secondary rhinoplasty refinement during the adulthood, the nose deformity associated with cleft lip requires different interventions from those of the interdisciplinary cleft team to achieve good functional and aesthetic outcomes. The time and management during the patient's life are presented in Table 7.1.

References

1. Millard DR. A rhinoplasty tetralogy: corrective, secondary, congenital, reconstructive. Boston: Little Brown & Company; 1996.
2. Rossell-Perry P, Olivencia-Flores C, Delgado-Jimenez MP, Ormeño-Aquino R. Surgical naso-alveolar molding: a rational treatment for bilateral cleft lip nose and systematic review. Plast Reconstr Surg Glob Open. 2020;8(9):e3082.
3. Byrd HS, Ha RY, Khosla RK, Gosman AA. Bilateral cleft lip and nasal repair. Plast Reconstr Surg. 2008;122(4):1181–90.
4. Mulliken JB. Primary repair of bilateral cleft lip and nasal deformity. Plast Reconstr Surg. 2001;108(1):181–94.
5. Yuzuriha S, Oh A, Mulliken J. Asymmetrical bilateral cleft lip: complete or incomplete and contralateral lesser defect. Plast Reconstr Surg J. 2008;122(5):1494–504.
6. Trott JA, Mohan N. A preliminary report on one stage open tip rhinoplasty at the time of lip repair in bilateral cleft lip and palate: the Alor Setar experience. Br J Plast Surg. 1993;46(3):215–22.

Surgical Techniques for Bilateral Cleft Lip Nose Repair

8

Percy Rossell-Perry

Contents

Introduction

Complex nature of the bilateral cleft lip and palate deformity involves soft tissue and skeletal components. According to the basic principles in plastic reconstructive surgery, the skeleton should be addressed first in order to facilitate the

P. Rossell-Perry (✉)
Health of Science Faculty, School of Human Medicine, Peruvian University Union (UpeU), Lima, Peru
e-mail: percy.rossell@upeu.edu.pe

P. Rossell-Perry (ed.), *Atlas of Primary Cleft Rhinoplasty*,
https://doi.org/10.1007/978-3-031-68012-0_8

soft tissue repair later and improve surgical outcomes. However, it is not recommended to be done primarily because of the long-term impact over the facial growth. In addition, hypoplasia of the soft tissues, affecting mainly the prolabium, makes nasal repair more difficult. Role of presurgical treatments in this scenario is relevant, and different methods have been described for this purpose. The presurgical orthopedics like naso alveolar molding (NAM) and the surgical lip adhesion are probably the most important methods used to improve skeletal deformity to facilitate lip and nose repair. This is the key point in primary bilateral cleft rhinoplasty since it is very difficult to achieve good nasal outcomes with skeletal deformity. Bilateral cleft rhinoplasty is a well-accepted treatment during primary lip repair actually. The synchronous correction of the nasal deformity at the time of lip repair is considered actually as a major advance in bilateral cleft lip nose management, and scientific evidence accumulated during the last years has been supported its utility and safety [1, 2]. During the last 30 years, I avoided the primary rhinoplasty initially, and then I used more conservative methods for nose repair during bilateral cleft lip surgery, specifically the Mc Comb method, but the main issue during this time was the high rate of relapse; later I used the Mulliken's technique improving rates of relapse. However, I observed increased number of complications related to the non-preservative nature of this method. Soft tissue resection creates scar related problems; therefore, I decided to change the strategy to more preservative methods through closed approach. During the appearance of the nasoalveolar molding (NAM), the method was included in our protocol but during short time because of lack of improvement in nasal outcomes. Previous experience addressing unilateral cleft lip nose let me introduce the following techniques in bilateral cleft lip nose management. A combination of Potter's concept (the V-Y advancement) and Berkeley's method (lateral Z plasty) has been used efficiently during my experience operating bilateral cleft lip nose. The efficacy of this technique for primary bilateral cleft rhinoplasty was published and included in our protocol for bilateral primary nose management [3]. Considering the extended incisions along the nasal vestibule, the use of postoperative nasal conformers is mandatory.

The rotation composite flap method can be used as alternative; however, this method may be limited to correct severe forms of bilateral cleft lip noses [4]. Because of the observed differences of the nose deformity between the incomplete and complete cleft lips, a more conservative method, the rotational composite flap, was used for nasal repair in incomplete bilateral cleft lips with good outcomes. A combination of these techniques is recommended for nasal treatment of the combined forms of bilateral cleft lips. If there is no option for their use, this surgical technique should not be used because of the risk of scar contraction and synechia. Finally, it is important to highlight that no surgical technique is effective in complete bilateral cleft lip and palate without prior positioning of the premaxilla through presurgical treatments. In this chapter, I describe these methods for bilateral primary cleft rhinoplasty in detail and present well-illustrated outcomes.

Presurgical Considerations

Age for primary lip cheilorhinoplasty in bilateral patients should be performed around 3–6 months; however, there could be a delay in comparison with unilateral cleft lip because of the required presurgical treatments. It is important to note that the efficacy of the presurgical treatments is observed at early age during the first weeks of age.

Preoperative Evaluation

Like unilateral forms, pediatric evaluation is essential to determine nutritional and acute or chronic diseases, and patients qualified for primary surgery must have physical status of class 1 or 2 based on parameters from the American Society of Anesthesiology (ASA) [5]. Greater attention must be paid to syndromic cases which are more associated with bilateral cleft lip and palate. Increased rate of perioperative complications is observed in this group of patients. The "rule of ten" (10 pounds of weight, 10 grams of hemoglobin per deciliter, and 10 weeks of life) is also valid for bilateral cleft lip and palate; however, the most important parameter seems to be the weight of the child [6]. Presurgical evaluation should be completed with the following tests: full blood count, hemostasis, urine test, ECG, and cardiologic evaluation. The preoperative anesthesia evaluation should be performed the night before the surgery or even better the same day by pediatric anesthesiologist to identify if any active disease is present. In case of urinary or respiratory infection, the surgery should be delayed 2–4 weeks until the health status is improved. Presurgical instructions should include nothing per oral guidelines, and the recommended fasting time is this: breast milk (4 h) and solids (6 h) and the surgical team should confirm this information from the parents [7]. Signed informed consent should be always obtained after enough information has been provided to the parents. The surgical center must have a well-implemented postanesthetic care unit (PACU) and guaranteed access to pediatric intensive care unit (ICU).

Instruments

Surgical markings in cleft lip surgery are done in millimeters; therefore, we have to consider that this surgery by definition is a microsurgery since we are working in a very small area and adequate surgical instruments are recommended to perform it. Surgical loupes are mandatory, and I like the 3.5× magnification to be more precise during markings and surgical performance. The surgical instrumental set for bilateral primary cleft rhinoplasty is the same as the set used for unilateral cases and used in combination with proper illumination during the procedure (*see* Chap. 6).

The use of temperature monitors and warming devices is recommended during pediatric anesthesia, and the use of pediatric head positioning cushion is essential to limit any movement of the head during the surgery guaranteeing surgical precision and preventing neck injuries. Surgical asepsis is performed using diluted iodine or chlorhexidine solutions, and fenestrated surgical drapes are commonly used in these surgeries. Throat packs are used to prevent aspiration of blood during cleft rhinoplasty surgery.

Anesthesia

The primary cleft rhinoplasty in a child should be performed under general anesthesia provided by a pediatric anesthesiologist. Patient is intubated in supine position, and the endotracheal tube is centrally fixed using adhesive tapes. The use of local anesthetic is recommended to reduce the dose of general anesthesia and surgical bleeding during the procedure (because of the addition of vasoconstrictor). I personally like to perform lip markings before asepsis and anesthetic infiltration. Considering the maximum dose of xylocaine as 5 mg/kg, I recommend the 1% concentration because of the increased amount of solution required for both sides in bilateral cleft lips. If the baby weighs 6 kg, we may use 6 cc of xylocaine 1% distributed in 2 cc for each lateral segments and 2 cc for prolabium and nose for nerve block and local infiltration. A 0.2 ml of epinephrine (1:200,000) is added to the solution. Other local anesthetics like bupivacaine is not used because of the increased risk of side effects including cardiac arrest.

A combination of nerve block and local infiltration is used for nose anesthesia as follows:

Step 1. Infraorbital Nerve Block (Fig. 8.1)

The infiltration for bilateral infraorbital nerve block can be done through two different approaches using a fine needle (30-gauge needle), the external and internal approaches. I like to use the internal approach; this is closer to the infraorbital nerve which is located 1 cm from the base of the alae nasi or the border of the pyriform aperture [8]. After location of the nerve position, using a syringe and fine needle, 1 of xylocaine 1% is infiltrated in both sides.

Step 2. External Nasal Nerve Block (Fig. 8.2)

External branches of anterior ethmoidal nerve are blocked bilaterally. This nerve arises from the nasociliary and exits between the border of the nasal bone and the upper lateral cartilage. It provides sensation to the nasal tip and medial aspect of the alae. The nerve approaches to the supraperichondral level from the notch conformed by the nasal bones (medially) and upper maxilla, more precise at the lowest point of the nasomaxillary suture. This point can be easily identified by palpation following the lower border of the nasal skeleton. The nerve block is done during local infiltration of the nasal vestibule, and I recommend this option. After location of the nerve position, using a syringe and fine needle 1 cc of xylocaine, 1% is infiltrated in the area to proceed with the nerve block.

Step 3. Central Segment and Nasal Vestibule Infiltration

The central segment of the bilateral cleft lip is composed by the prolabium and nose, and it is infiltrated using 2 cc distributed as follows: 0.5 cc for prolabium, 0.5 cc to the tip of the nose, and 0.5 cc for each side of the nose (vestibules). A small amount may be used for caudal septum additionally. Even when the

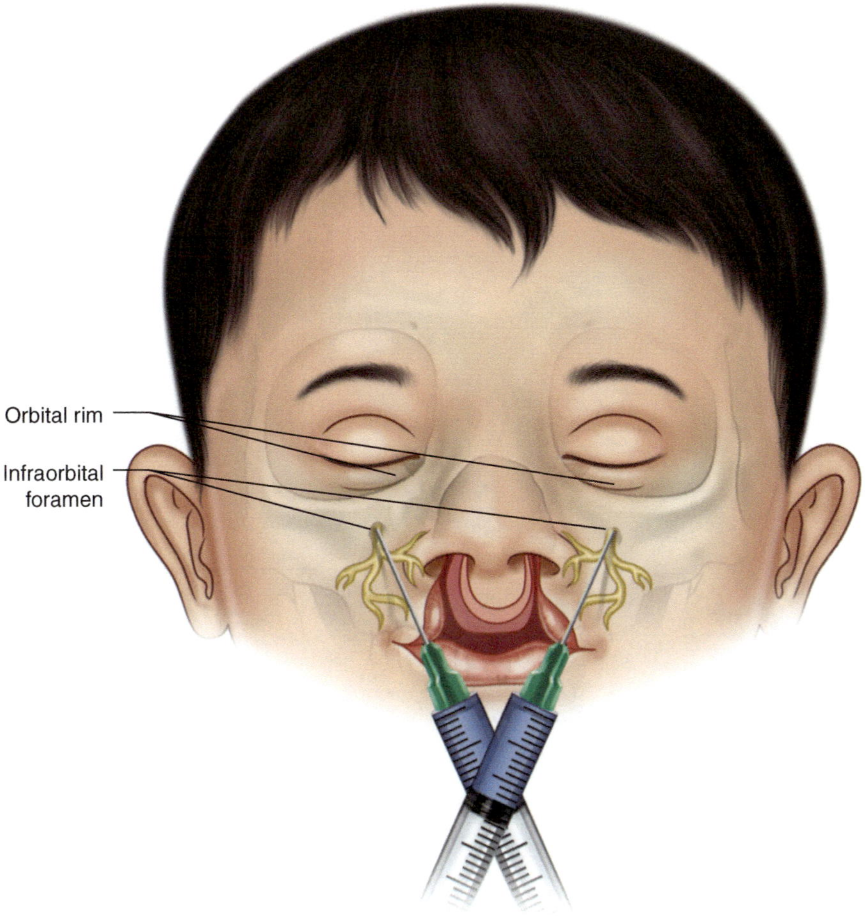

Fig. 8.1 Bilateral infraorbital nerve block internal approach before bilateral cleft lip nose repair

external nasal nerve blocks are enough to produce local anesthesia for the central segment in bilateral cleft lips, additional local infiltration is necessary for internal structures and the tip of the nose and to reduce bleeding during surgery. The solution is infiltrated over the supra perichondral level of the nasal tip and vestibules of the nose. A fine needle is introduced through the nasal vestibule, specifically over the marginal border (lower border of alar cartilage). Infiltration of the nasal vestibules helps to the surgeon with the alar and dome cartilages of the nose, developing a dissection of these structures. This maneuver makes easier the dissection of the nasal cartilages. In addition, the internal nasal valve (angle of medial intersection between the marginal and inter cartilaginous borders) infiltration let the surgeon block the nasal tip branches of the external nasal nerve.

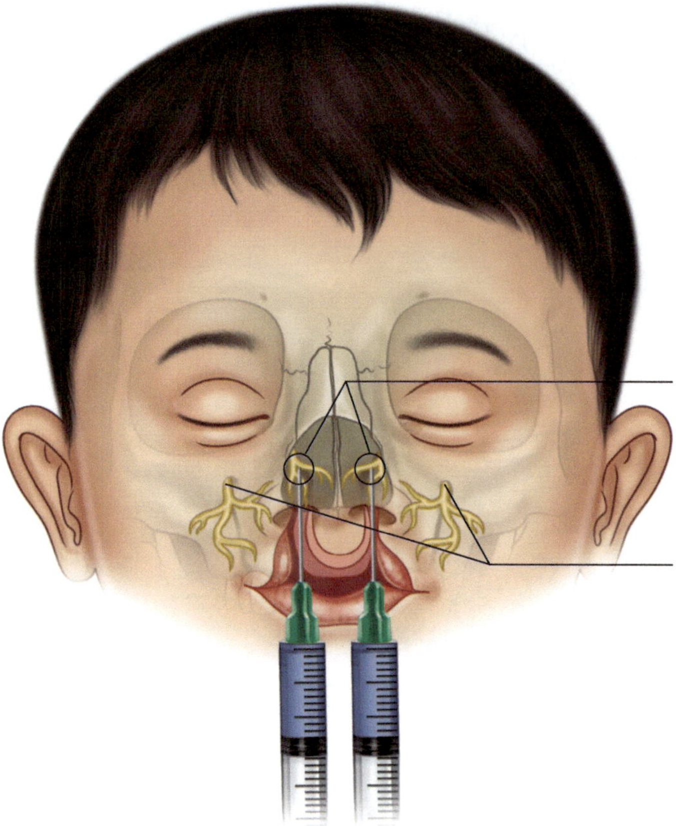

Fig. 8.2 Bilateral external nasal nerve block procedure before bilateral cleft lip nose repair

Step 4. Lateral Segment Infiltration

The lateral segments of the bilateral cleft lip are effectively anesthetized using the bilateral infraorbital nerve block. In a 6 Kg of weight patient, 2 cc of local anesthetic is used for each lateral segment. One cc is used for infraorbital nerve block and 1 cc is used for local infiltration of the lateral segment in both sides. The infiltration is applied around the cleft borders of the lateral lip segments on each side. Even when the infraorbital nerves blocks are enough to produce local anesthesia for the lateral segments in bilateral cleft lips, additional local infiltration is necessary to reduce bleeding during surgery.

Step 5. Postoperative Bilateral Infraorbital Nerve Block

Multimodal anesthesia is actually used for pain control and includes nerve blocks, analgesics, and short-acting opioids. The main objective is the reduction of opioid use preventing its nondesirable side effects. The infraorbitary nerve block is commonly used in combination with other analgesics (NSAID) for postoperative pain control in cleft lip and nose repair [9].

Mc Comb Modified Technique

The Mc Comb technique for nasal correction in cleft lip deformity has been described as a conservative method and represents an alternative to address the nose when the surgeon does not have enough skill or expertise. Applying the principle "primun non nocere," it makes sense to be conservative in order to prevent complications after surgery; therefore this method could be considered as alternative especially for beginners. This technique may prevent the development of postoperative synechia because of the limited nasal incisions but not the development of lateral web which is created due to scar contracture and lateral incisions used for release of the alae from the lateral segment [10]. The main issue observed using this method is the high rate of nose deformity relapse.

Surgical Technique

The technique I performed initially uses an approach through extension of the lateral lip incision into the nose and partial degloving of alar cartilage bilaterally to finally reposition them using transcutaneous stitches.

Nasal Tip Dissection Nose surgery starts after lip incisions, and the intranasal alar base incision (an extension of the lateral lip incision) is used to dissect the alar cartilages bilaterally. Through this maneuver, we have access to the lower lateral cartilages to dissect them from the overlying skin, and then the dissection is completed over the alar domes bilaterally to allow reposition of the displaced cartilages (Fig. 8.3). This is a degloving maneuver to release the cartilage structure from its abnormal position allowing its repositioning medially.

Caudal Septum Dissection Nasal septum is not affected in more symmetrical forms of bilateral cleft lips; however, dissection of the caudal septum may be necessary in symmetrical forms of the bilateral cleft lip and palate. The procedure is similar to that described for unilateral forms.

Nasal Structure Reposition The reposition of the dissected structures is done by placement of transcutaneous stitches from vestibular lining to skin across the cartilages into desired position bilaterally. The alar domes are shifted at the genu providing optimal projection of the nasal tip. Several sutures are necessary to achieve optimal position and nasal shape (Fig. 8.4).

Nasal Floor Repair Finally, the anterior nasal floor is repaired. The floor of the nasal vestibule is done by reposition of the alar base into proper position in both sides. The role of muscular repair in bilateral forms supporting the anterior nasal floor is less relevant because of the muscular hypoplasia observed in lateral cleft sides. Skeletal base is finally repaired using the alveolar bone graft later during mixed dentition period.

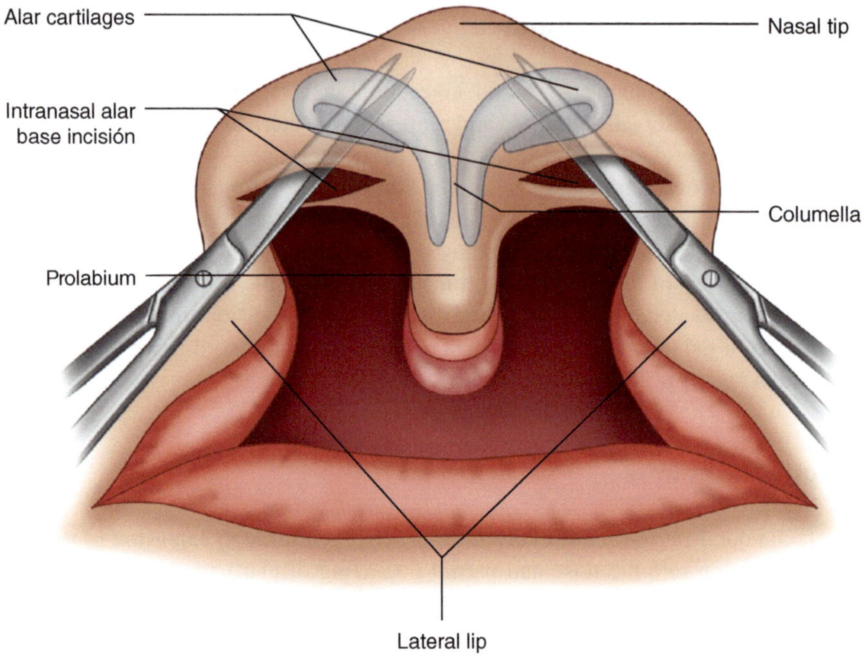

Fig. 8.3 Nasal tip dissection during bilateral Mc Comb cleft rhinoplasty

Fig. 8.4 Nasal structure reposition during Mc Comb modified technique

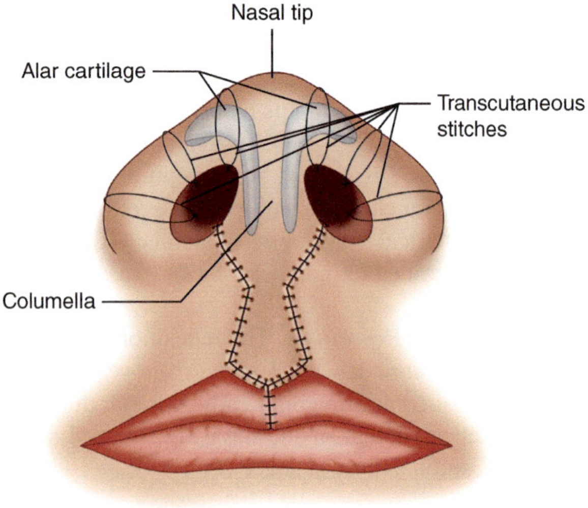

Cases (Figs. 8.5, 8.6, 8.7, 8.8, 8.9 and 8.10)

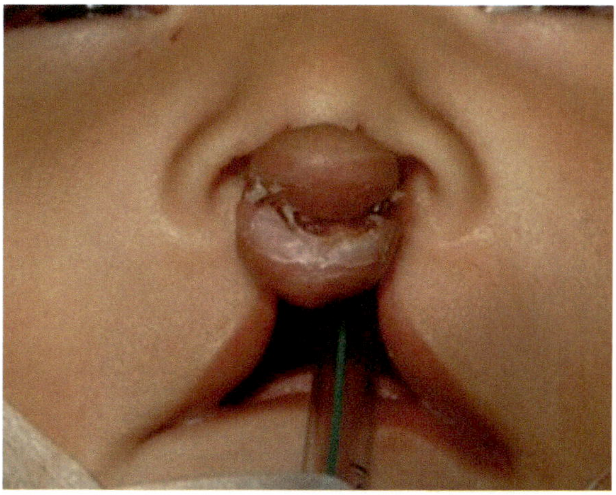

Fig. 8.5 Case 1. Preoperative view of a 3-month-old infant with complete bilateral cleft lip

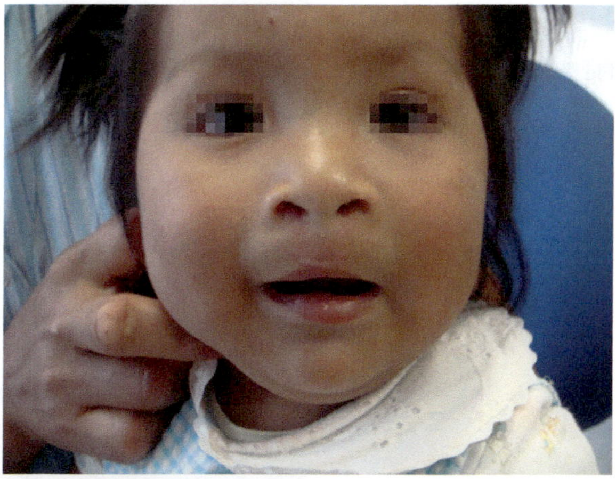

Fig. 8.6 Case 1. A 3-year-old postoperative view of the infant shown in Fig. 8.5 after undergoing nasal repair using the Mc Comb modified technique

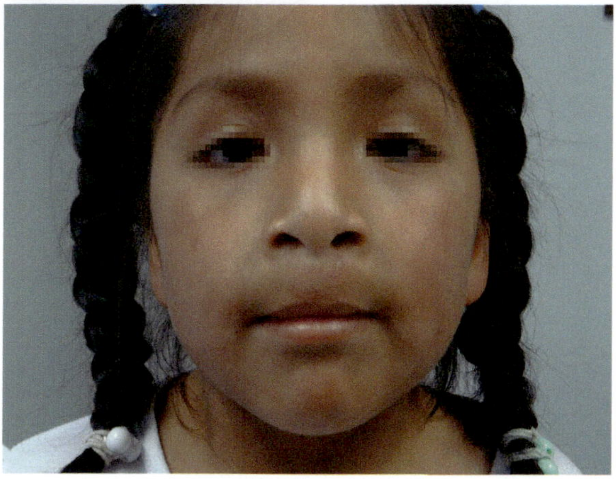

Fig. 8.7 Case 1. A 7-year postoperative view of the infant shown in Fig. 8.5 after undergoing nasal repair using the Mc Comb modified technique

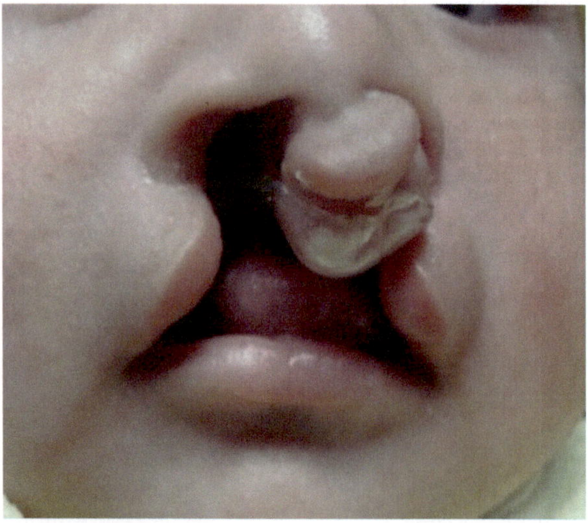

Fig. 8.8 Case 2. Preoperative view of a 3-month-old infant with severe complete bilateral cleft lip

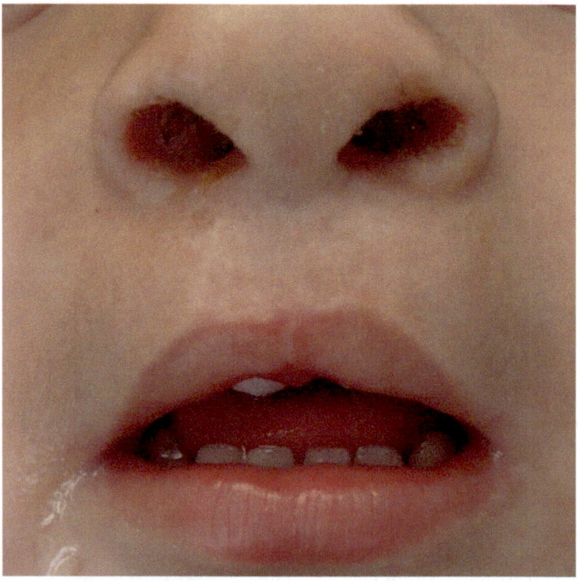

Fig. 8.9 Case 2. A 3-year-old postoperative view of the infant shown in Fig. 8.5 after undergoing nasal repair using the Mc Comb modified technique

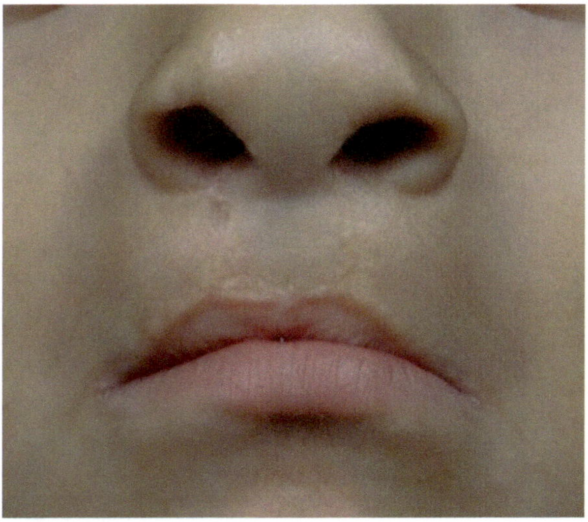

Fig. 8.10 Case 2. A 8-year-old postoperative view of the infant shown in Fig. 8.8 after undergoing nasal repair using the Mc Comb modified technique

The Composite Rotational Flap Rhinoplasty for Microforms and Incomplete Bilateral Cleft Lip Nose

This surgical technique developed by the author is a limited incision method for primary cleft rhinoplasty and designed initially to be used in mild unilateral cleft lip nose forms (microform and incomplete forms). The advantage of this method is that it allows us preserve the lateral wall of the nasal vestibule preventing the development of lateral webs since the vestibular incision is not connected with lip incisions. A composite flap (vestibular skin and cartilage) is designed and medially displaced in a rotational form (Figs. 8.11 and 8.12). It is indicated for bilateral incomplete cleft lips or incomplete side in combined forms of bilateral cleft lips.

Surgical Technique

Markings

Surgery starts performing markings. They are composed by two lines, the inferior curved line following all the lower border of the alar cartilage (marginal incision) and the upper one at the level of the intercartilaginous border. The marginal border (produced by the lower border of the alar cartilage) represents a change in the epithelium of the vestibule of the nose. This line can be easily identified because of the change of the color; above the line is red and below is the same color as the nasal skin. The nasal lining of the vestibule consists of squamous epithelium and changes to a different one, the pseudostratified ciliated columnar respiratory epithelium. The marginal line starts from the intercartilaginous border laterally and finishes before the medial wall of the nasal vestibule medially (Figs. 8.13 and 8.14). The second marking is performed in continuity with the lateral side of the marginal marking and

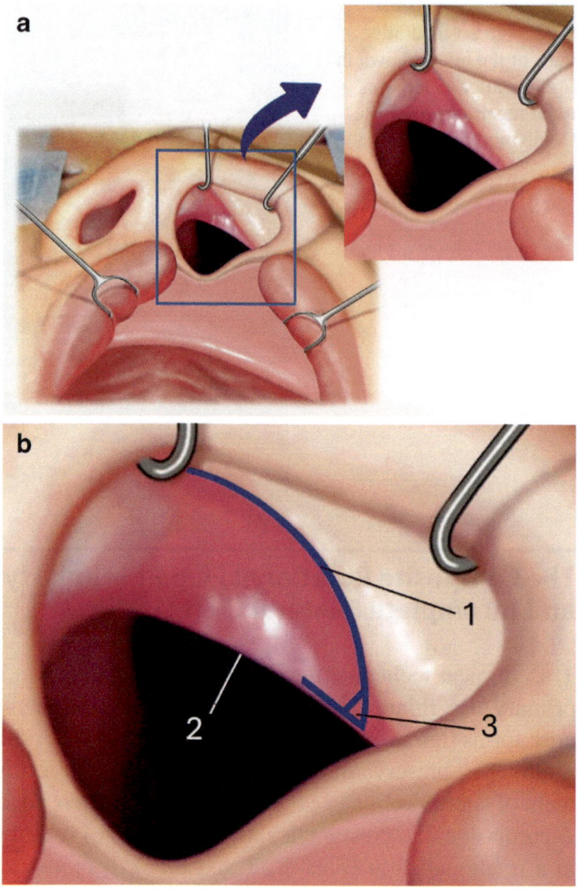

Fig. 8.11 The rotational composite flap cleft rhinoplasty. Surgical marking diagram. 1. Composite flap. 2. Marginal incision. 3. Intercartilaginous incision (small triangular area for resection)

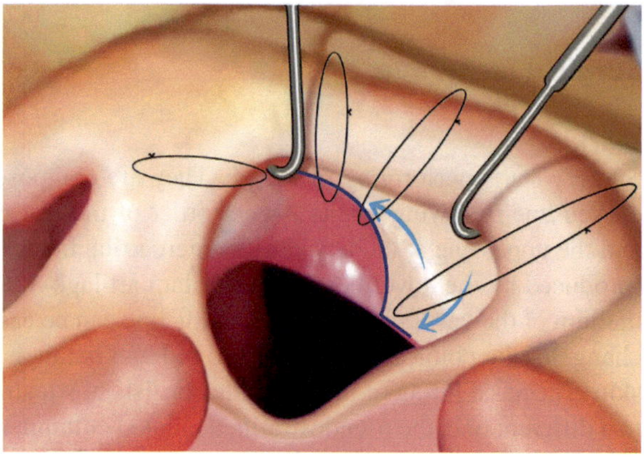

Fig. 8.12 The rotational composite flap cleft rhinoplasty. Medial rotation and lateral advancement donor site closure using transcutaneous stitches. 1. Composite flap. 2. Marginal incision. 3. Intercartilaginous incision. 4. Columella. 5. Alae. 6. Lateral crus. 7. Domes. 8. Medial crus. Green arrow: rotational medial displacement

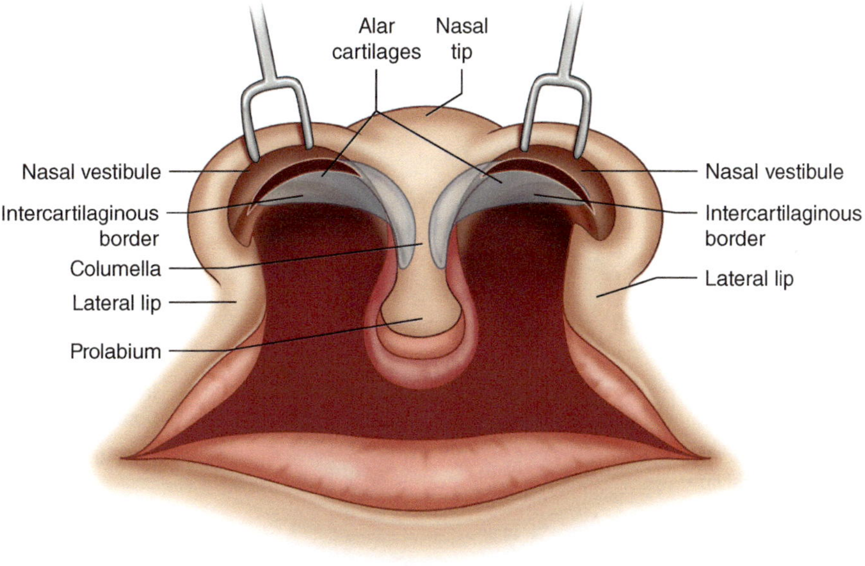

Fig. 8.13 Diagram of marginal marking during rotational composite flap technique for bilateral cleft lip nose repair

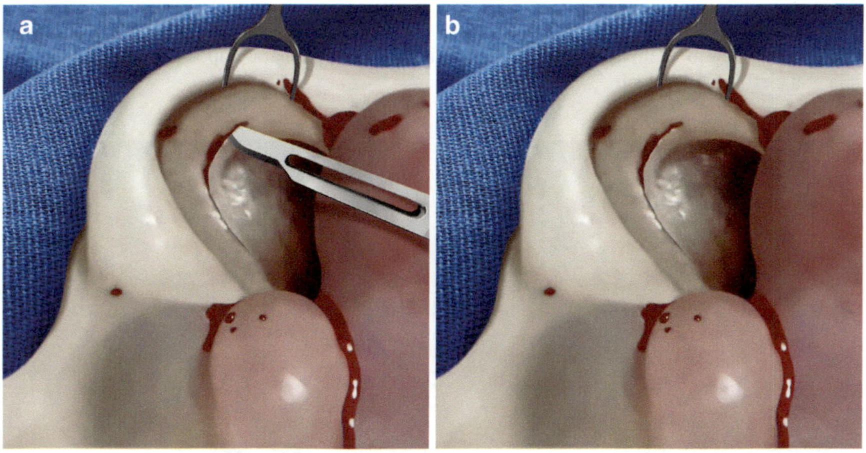

Fig. 8.14 Right marginal incision during rotational composite flap technique for bilateral cleft lip nose repair. (**a**) and (**b**) Right marginal incision

follows the intercartilaginous border (limit between the upper and lower lateral cartilages of the nose) (Figs. 8.15 and 8.16). The upper line is designed in continuity with the lateral end of the marginal marking and follows the intercartilaginous border (limen nassi), and its extension is around 3–5 mm. This short marking let the surgeon to release the lateral border of the alar cartilage and allow the rotation of the

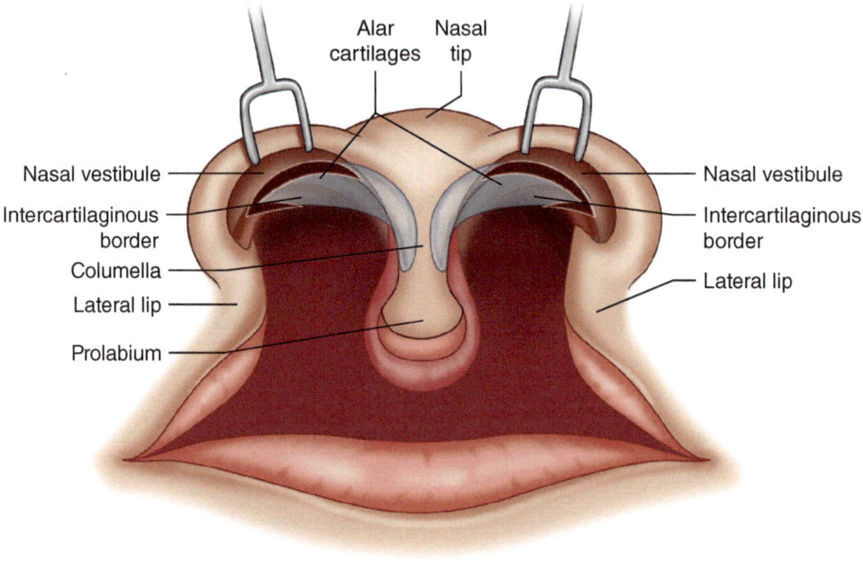

Fig. 8.15 Diagram of intercartilaginous marking during rotational composite flap technique for bilateral cleft lip nose repair

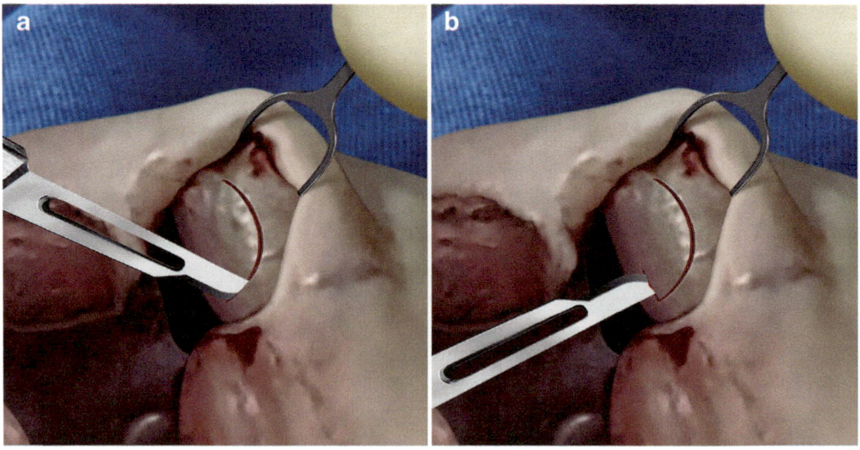

Fig. 8.16 Left marginal and intercartilaginous incision during rotational composite flap technique for bilateral cleft lip nose repair. (**a**) Left marginal incision (**b**) Left intercartilaginous incision

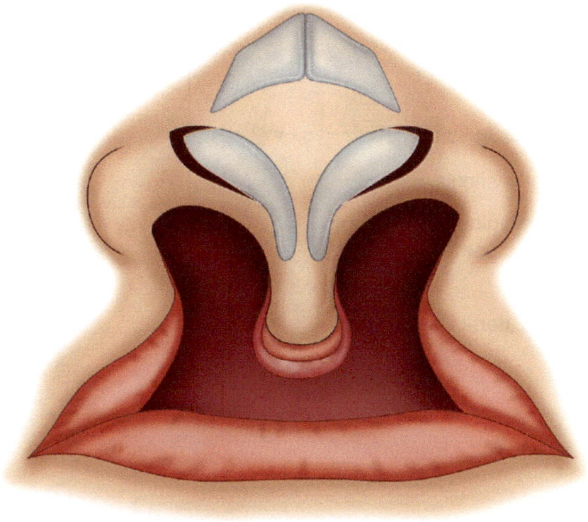

Fig. 8.17 Position incisions of the rotational composite flap cleft rhinoplasty for bilateral cleft lip

composite flap. Both lines are surrounding the alar cartilage to create the composite flap (composed by the vestibular skin and alar cartilage). Main benefit of this method is the preservation of the lateral wall of the nasal vestibule which prevents the development of scar contractures inside the nose. These markings are performed in both sides in bilateral incomplete cleft lips (Fig. 8.17).

Incisions After local anesthetic infiltration and superficial lip incisions following lip markings using 11 blade scalpel, the nasal repair is performed. Nasal incisions are performed following vestibular markings (marginal and intercartilaginous) around the alar cartilage of the cleft side using a 15-blade scalpel to create the composite flap (Figure). It is recommended the excision of a small triangle from the lateral corner of the flap to avoid redundancy of tissue after closure. These incisions are performed in both sides in incomplete bilateral cleft lips.

Rotational Composite Flap and Nasal Tip Dissection

After identification of the alar cartilage and using a semiopen approach through the marginal incision and using fine scissors, the composite flap (vestibular skin and alar cartilage) is dissected on the supracartilaginous plane and elevated from lateral to medial side including alar cartilage and vestibular skin in both sides. A small triangle is resected at the lateral end of the composite flap to facilitate its closure after medial rotation. Interdomal fatty tissue is preserved and the dissection continues over the upper lateral cartilages. Then, the nose dissection continues with the nasal tip including both sides through the vestibular incision and on the supracartilaginous plane separating the nasal skin from the cartilaginous structure of the nose (alar cartilages, domes, and lower dorsum). Both alar domes should be separated from the overlaying skin in order to facilitate the reposition of the structures from the cleft side (Figs. 8.18 and 8.19).

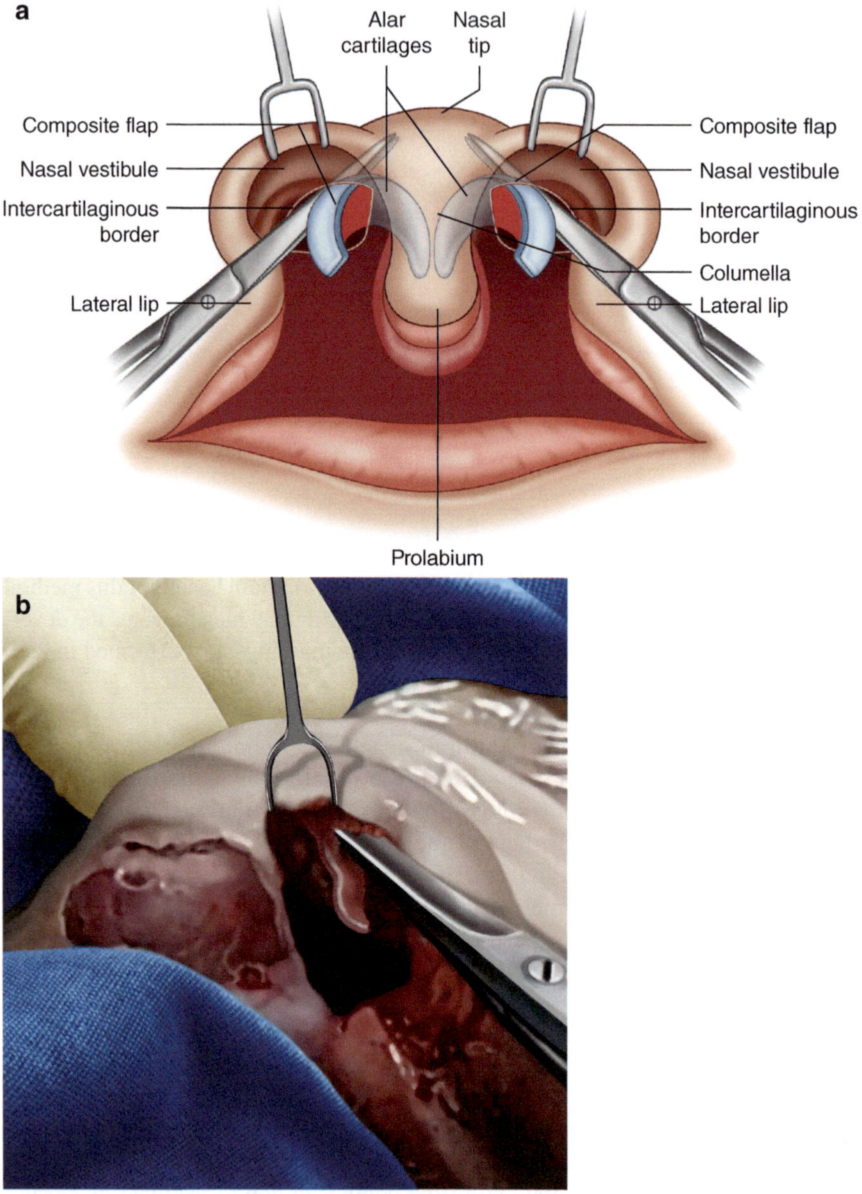

Fig. 8.18 (**a**) Diagram of nasal tip dissection during rotational composite flap technique for bilateral cleft lip nose repair. (**b**) Nasal tip dissection during rotational composite flap technique for bilateral cleft lip nose repair

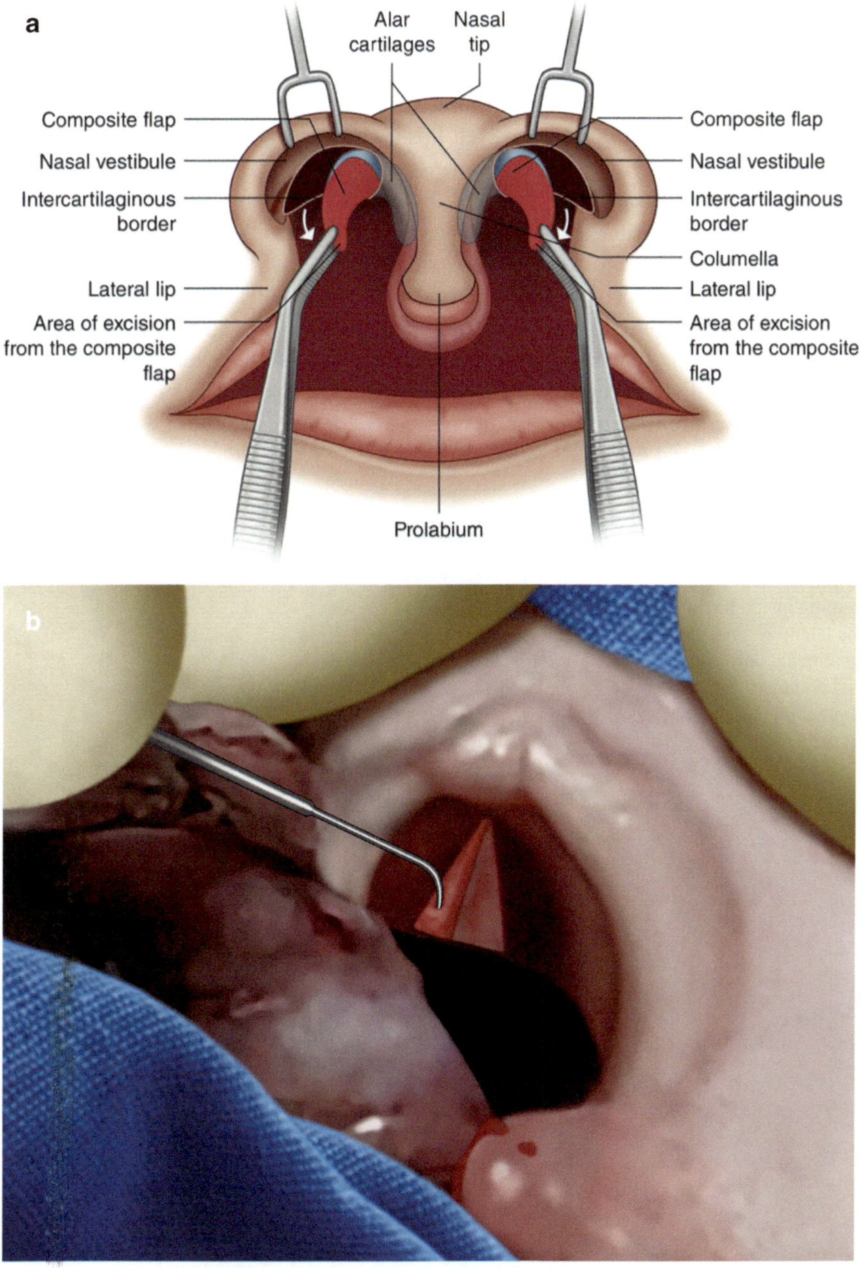

Fig. 8.19 (**a**) Diagram of bilateral composite flap elevation after nasal tip dissection. (**b**) Rotational composite flap elevation left side

Nasal Septum

The septal deviation associated with the bilateral cleft lips is less frequently observed in comparison with unilateral forms; therefore its early correction is not necessary. However, it may be considered in asymmetrical forms. In these cases, the caudal septum is corrected as in unilateral cleft lips (*see* Chap. 6).

Nasal Tip Reconstruction

After elevating the rotational composite flap in both sides, they are displaced medially in a rotational form and fixed using five 5/0 PDS transcutaneous sutures. These sutures are important to obliterate the space created after tip dissection and prevent the development of hematomas. Stitches are placed through the skin, starting from inside the nose and then exiting the skin at the level of the supraalar crease; the needle then returns through the same hole and finally enters the inside of the nose, where the sutures are tied (Figs. 8.20, 8.21, 8.22 and 8.23; see Figs. 6.32, 6.33, 6.34 and 6.35).

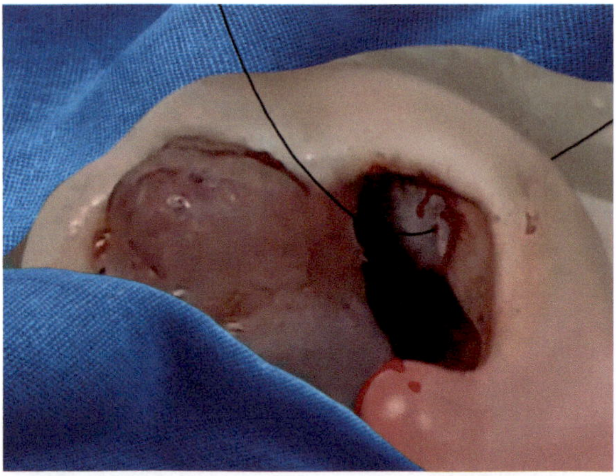

Fig. 8.20 Transcutaneous stitch. Second stitch of the recommended sequence coming inside the nose at the lateral segment of the rotational composite flap and coming out at the supraalar crease level

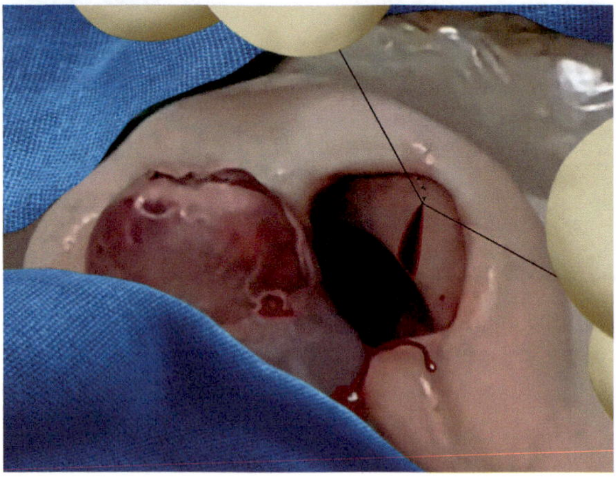

Fig. 8.21 Transcutaneous stitch. Stitch is tied

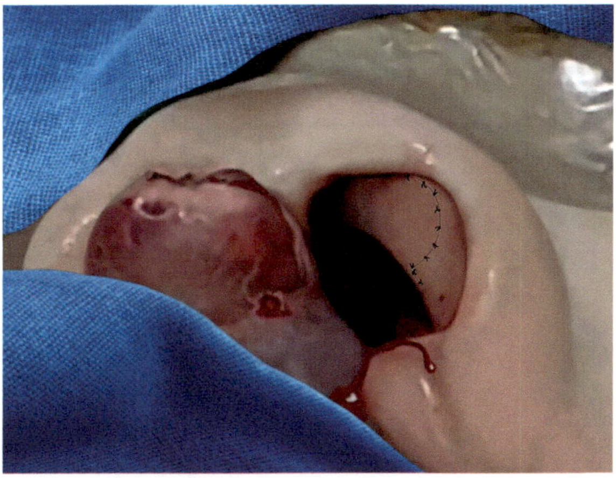

Fig. 8.22 Final closure of the rotational composite flap (left side)

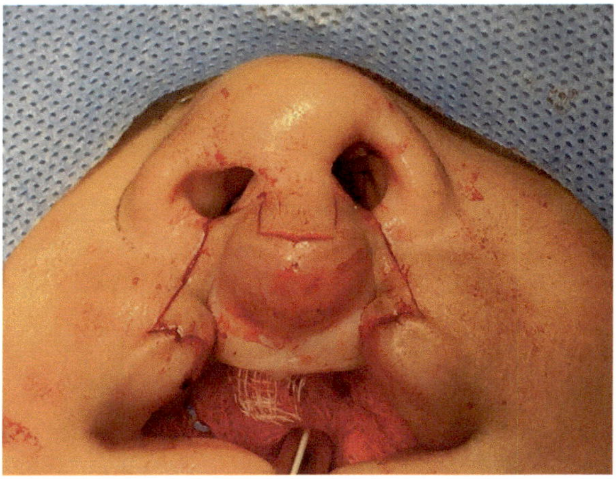

Fig. 8.23 Comparative view between both sides after using the rotational composite flap cleft rhinoplasty on the left side in a patient with incomplete bilateral cleft lip

This is the recommended sequence (Fig. 8.24).

First stitch: After identification of the alar dome in both sides, these are medially displaced and fixed using oblique transcutaneous stitch on each side. Then, the alar domes are placed in correct position in both sides. Special attention must be paid at the level of the soft triangle avoiding skin retraction due to the lack of cartilage in this area.

Second stitch: Placed at the level of the lateral border of the flap using a vertical stitch at the level of the supra alar crease in both sides. These two sutures mobilize the flap medially after rotation and leave a triangular donor site laterally.

Third stitch: Between the two alar domes using a transcutaneous stitch at the level of the anterior border of the alar domes.

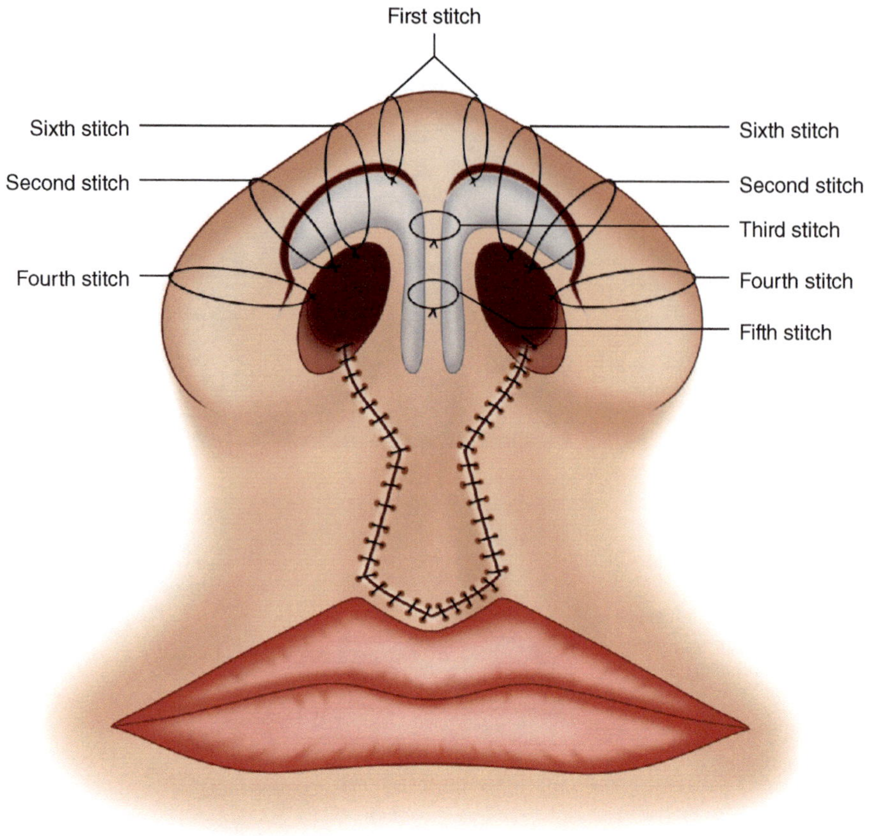

Fig. 8.24 Sequence of transcutaneous stitches used during rotational composite flap cleft rhinoplasty for bilateral cleft lip

Fourth stitch: Used to close the donor areas of the flaps. They are lateral triangular raw surfaces which are closed by advancement of the vestibular skin.

Fifth stitch: The suture enters through the caudal septum and exits at the same level on the opposite side, and then the needle enters through the columella (alar medial crus and skin) in both sides; finally the sutures are tied.

Sixth stitch: Necessary to correct the position of the alar cartilage in relation to the upper lateral cartilage of the nose. There is a luxation of the alar cartilage and requires a reposition over the upper lateral cartilage using a vertical transcutaneous stitch placed lateral to the internal nasal valve at the level of the supra alar

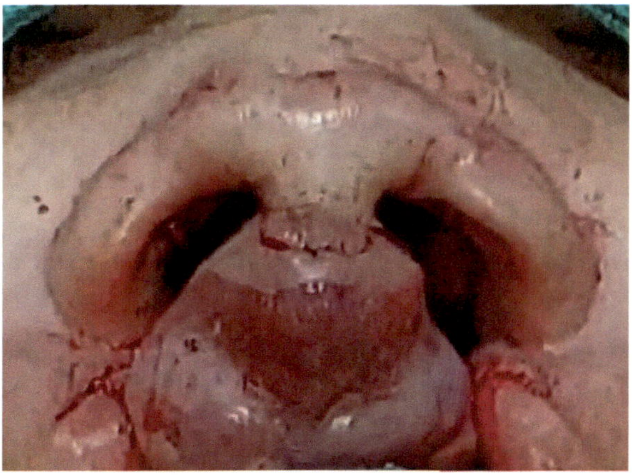

Fig. 8.25 Final appearance of the nose after using the rotational composite flap cleft rhinoplasty for bilateral cleft lip

crease in both sides. An important recommendation is not to exceed using these transcutaneous stitches because it may create a compromise of the vascular supply of the ala and develops necrosis and also may develop granulomas. Finally, few simple stitches may be used to align correctly the borders of the composite flap in both sides (Fig. 8.25).

Nasal Floor

The nasal floor reconstruction is performed during the cleft lip repair, and this is involving the use of two flaps: a medial cutaneous flap lateral to the base of the columella and a lateral flap, which is composed of the base of the ala in both sides. A suture of prolene 4/0 is used through the alar base dermis of each side, passing beneath the philtral flap and tied in midline narrowing the interalar distance and minimizing the postoperative nasal widening (Fig. 8.26). The lateral flaps (alar bases) are advanced and sutured side to end to the medial flap. During cheiloplasty, the levator labii superioris alaeque nasi and orbicularis oris muscles are identified and repaired at the midline using PDS suture supporting the final position of the nasal base in both sides (Fig. 8.27).

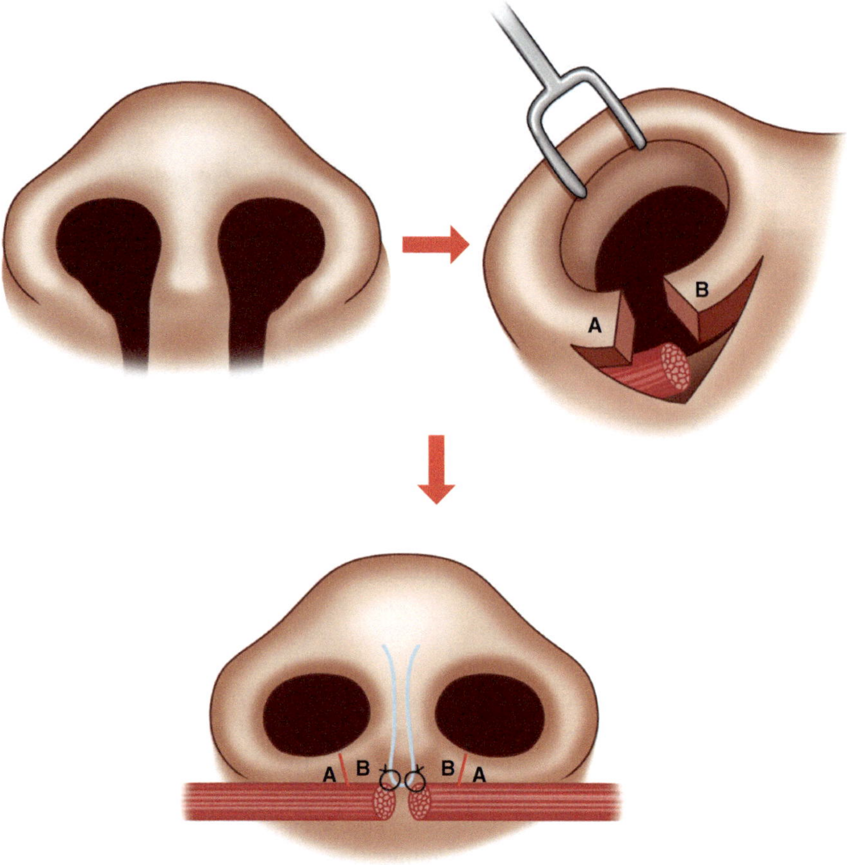

Fig. 8.26 A suture of prolene is used through the alar base dermis of each side and tied in midline narrowing the interalar distance during rotational composite flap technique for bilateral cleft lip nose repair

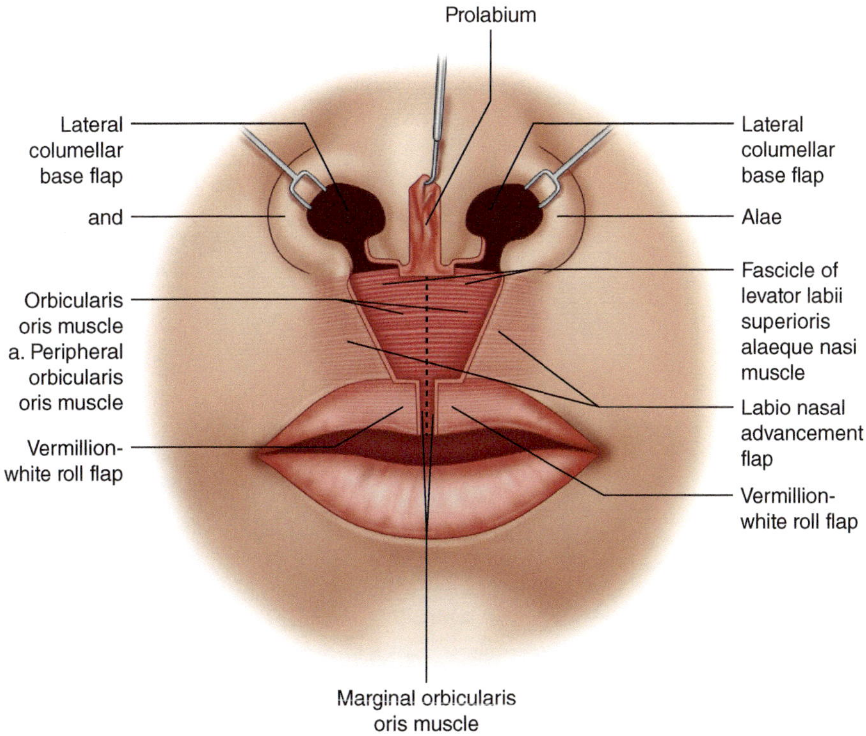

Fig. 8.27 Muscular reconstruction is providing support to the base of the nose during rotational composite flap for bilateral cleft lip nose repair

Cases (Figs. 8.28, 8.29, 8.30, 8.31, 8.32 and 8.33)

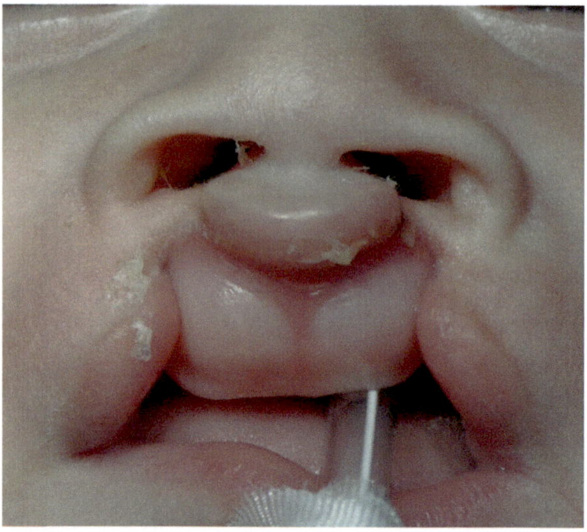

Fig. 8.28 Case 1. Preoperative view of a 3-month-old infant with incomplete bilateral cleft lip

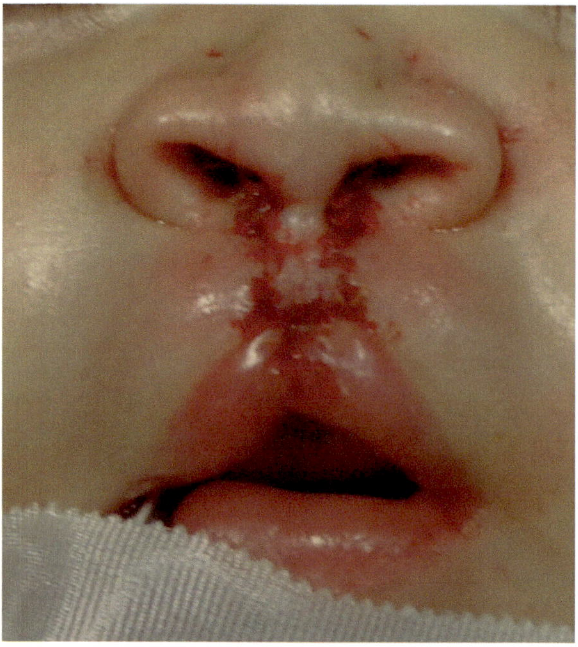

Fig. 8.29 Case 1. Immediate postoperative view of the infant shown in Fig. 8.28 after undergoing nasal repair using the rotational composite flap technique

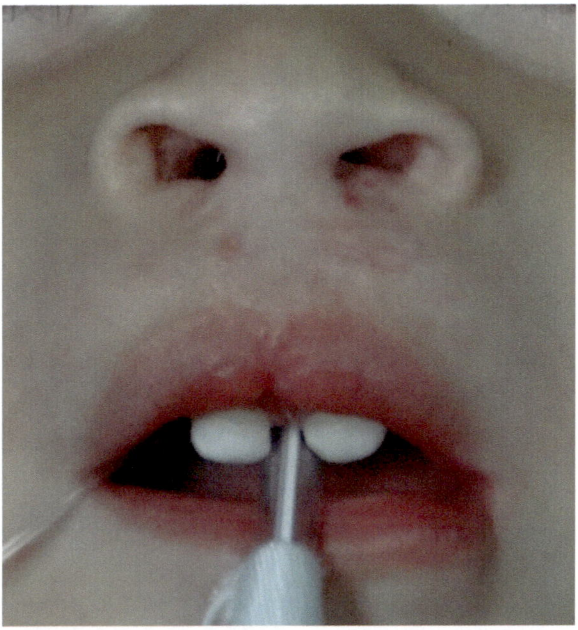

Fig. 8.30 Case 1. Long-term postoperative view of the infant shown in Fig. 8.28 after undergoing nasal repair using the rotational composite flap technique

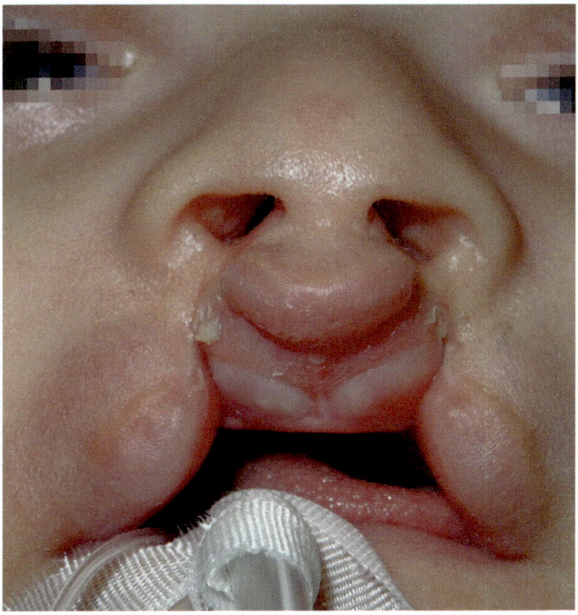

Fig. 8.31 Case 2. Preoperative view of a 3-month-old infant with incomplete bilateral cleft lip

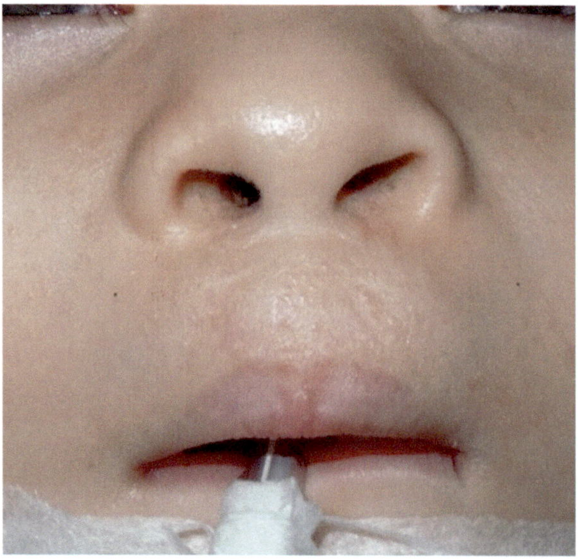

Fig. 8.32 Case 2. A 1-year postoperative view of the infant shown in Fig. 8.31 after undergoing nasal repair using the rotational composite flap technique without presurgical orthopedics (frontal view)

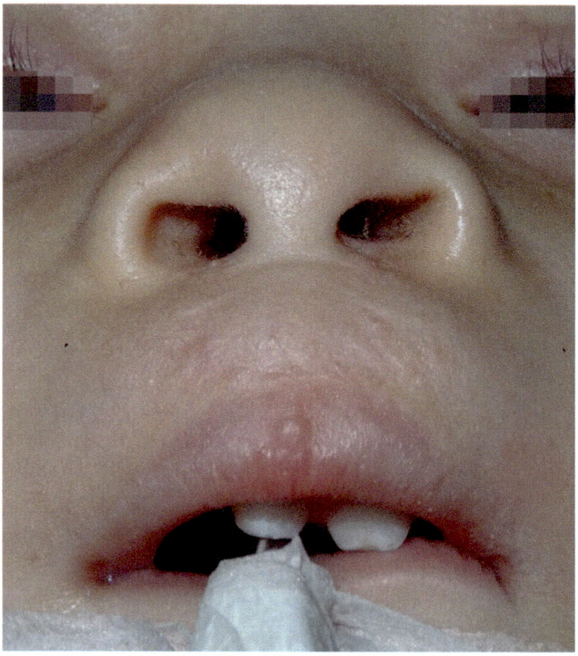

Fig. 8.33 Case 2. A 1-year postoperative view of the infant shown in Fig. 8.31 after undergoing nasal repair using the rotational composite flap technique (worm eye view)

The VYZ Technique in Complete Bilateral Cleft Lip Nose

The combination of the V-Y advanced flap and lateral Z plasty is an effective form of bilateral cleft lip nose repair based on our previous studies [3] (Figs. 8.34 and 8.35). The combination of these two techniques produces an expansion of the

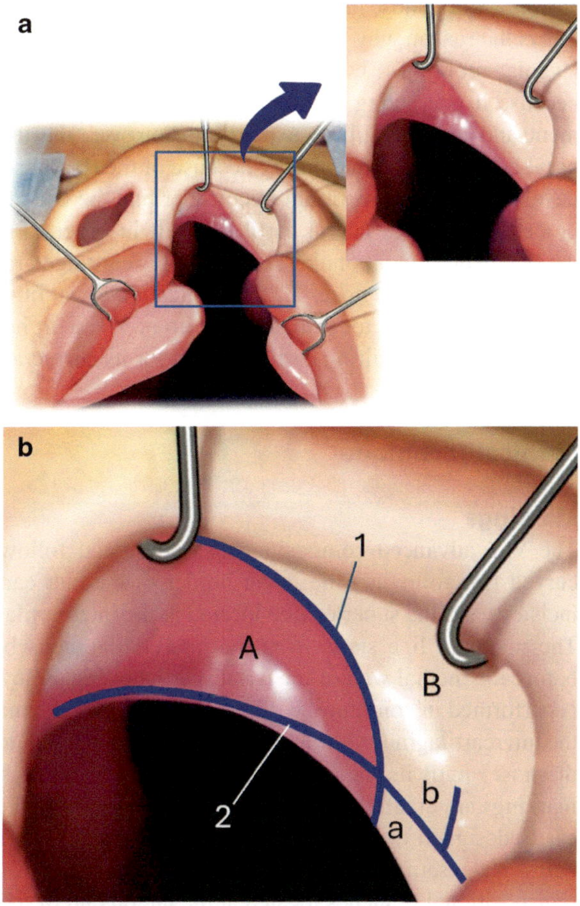

Fig. 8.34 The VYZ cleft rhinoplasty. Surgical marking diagram. 1. V composite flap. 2. Marginal incision. (**a**) and (**b**) Z plasty branch B. Nasal vestibule

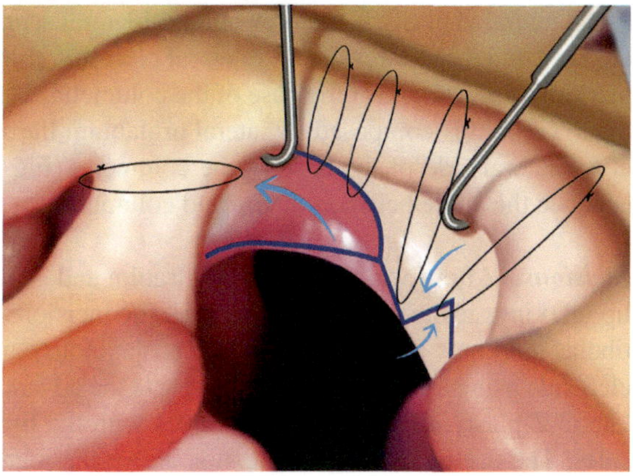

Fig. 8.35 The VYZ cleft rhinoplasty. Medial VY advancement and lateral Z plasty transposition using transcutaneous stitches

vestibule of the nose in a similar form as the presurgical orthopedic (NAM) is doing; this is the reason why the method was published by the author as the surgical naso-alveolar molding [3]. This is indicated for complete bilateral cleft lip nose cases because it is creating a columellar lengthening by alar cartilage medial displacement and nasal vestibule expansion; however, the use of bilateral postoperative nasal conformers is mandatory because of the risk of scar contracture and synechia development. It is important to consider that the use of this method as a secondary procedure requires lateral cartilage graft in order to replace the donor area after medial displacement of alar cartilage. This cartilage graft prevents the development of notch or pinched nose. This complication is not observed frequently after using the VYZ technique for primary cleft lip nose repair; however, it may be developed after long term requiring cartilage graft for its correction.

Surgical Technique

Markings

The V-Y advanced composite flap is designed following two lines: the inferior curved line following the lower border of the alar cartilage (line of the marginal incision) and the superior line located at the intercartilaginous border in both sides. The marginal line starts from the intercartilaginous border laterally and finishes before the medial wall of the nasal vestibule (Fig. 8.36). The intercartilaginous line is performed in continuity with the lateral side of the marginal marking and follows the intercartilaginous border (limit between the upper and lower lateral cartilages of the nose) until its medial end (before the internal nasal valve) (Fig. 8.37). Both markings are creating a V form advanced composite flap, and this triangular flap is easily designed observing the change of color; above the marginal line is red and below is the same color as the nasal skin. The lateral Z plasty is designed using two transpositional branches located at the lateral end of the V composite flap. This lateral design continues with the lip marking through the alar base. The main benefit of the lateral Z plasty is the prevention of lateral scar contractures. These markings are performed in both sides in bilateral cleft lips (Fig. 8.38). Finally, an additional marking is performed at the base of the columella, a Z plasty is designed bilaterally, the lower arm is composed by lateral prolabium flaps, and the upper arm is located at the lateral side of the base of the columella (Fig. 8.39). This Z plasty helps to enhance the angle between the lip and columella.

Incisions. After local anesthetic infiltration and superficial lip incisions following lip markings using an 11-blade scalpel, the incisions are performed following vestibular markings (marginal and intercartilaginous) around the alar cartilage of the cleft side using a 15-blade scalpel to create the advanced V composite flap. Then the lateral Z plasty is incised and continues with the lip through the alar base in both sides. The use of small skin excision above the marginal incision may be used in severe forms of nose deformity in bilateral cleft lips. Lateral Z plasties used to improve labial columellar angle are performed during prolabium incisions.

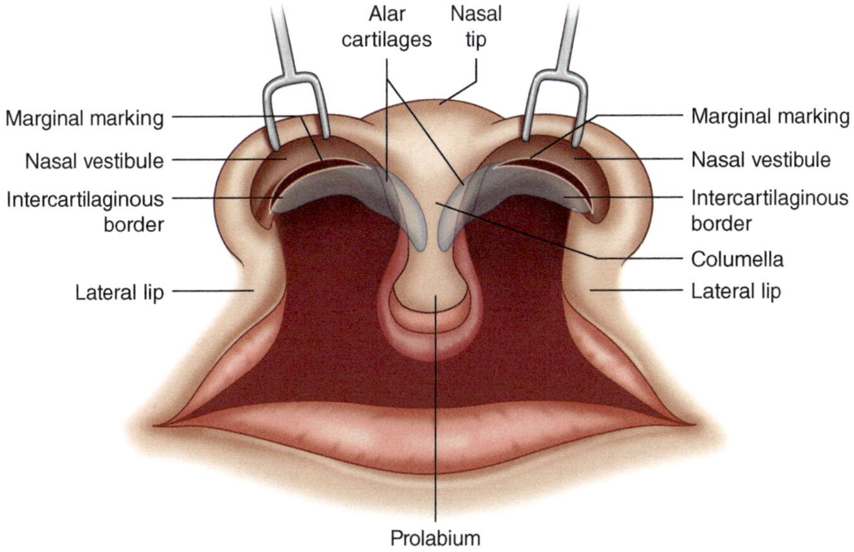

Fig. 8.36 Diagram of marginal marking during VYZ technique for bilateral cleft lip nose repair

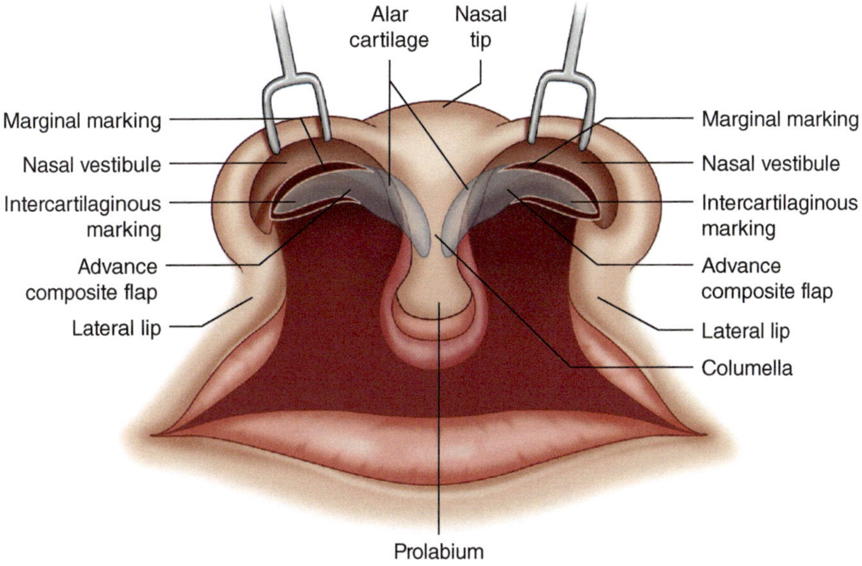

Fig. 8.37 Diagram of intercartilaginous marking during VYZ technique for bilateral cleft lip nose repair

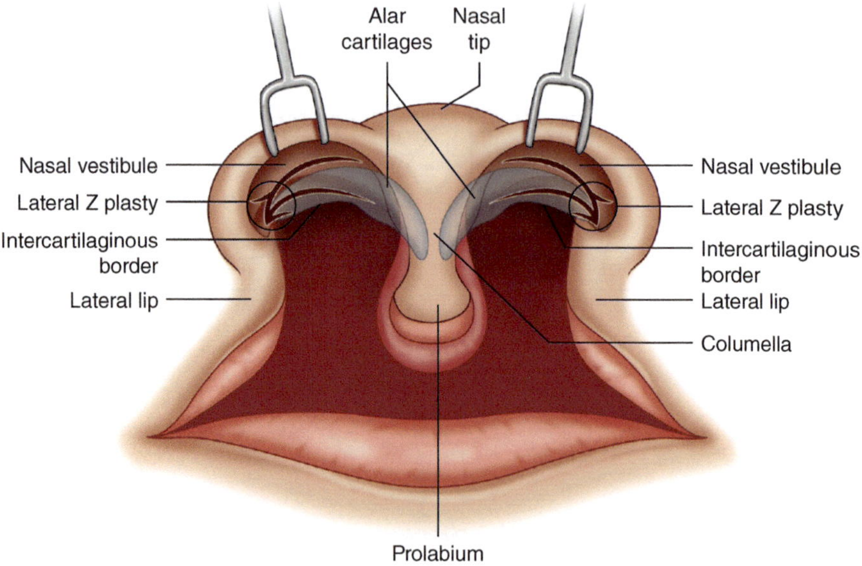

Fig. 8.38 Diagram of lateral Z plasty marking during VYZ technique for bilateral cleft lip nose repair

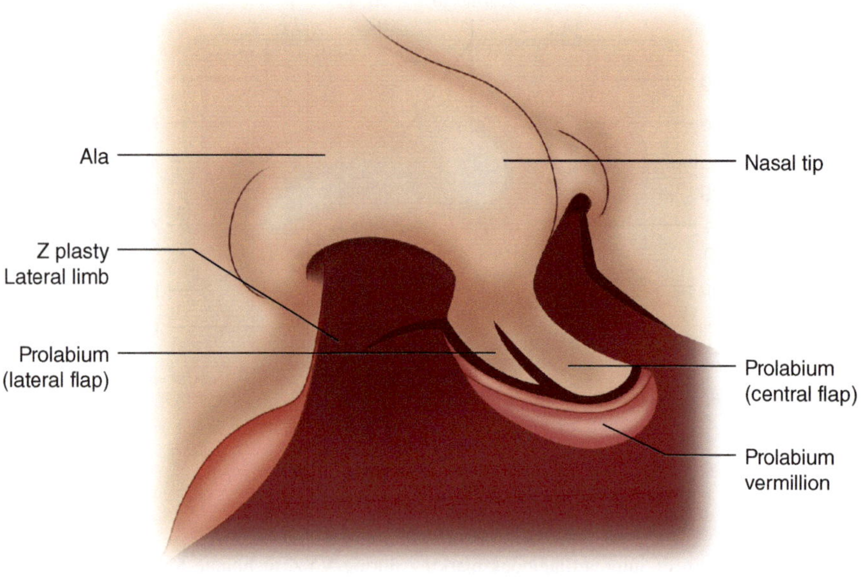

Fig. 8.39 Diagram of columellar base lateral Z plasty marking during VYZ technique for bilateral cleft lip nose repair

V Advancement Flap and Nasal Tip Dissection

Using a semiopen approach through the bilateral vestibular incisions the anterior surface of the alar cartilages is exposed on the supracartilaginous plane in both sides, elevating the advanced V composite flap which includes alar cartilage and vestibular skin. This dissection continues over the upper lateral cartilages (Figs. 8.40,

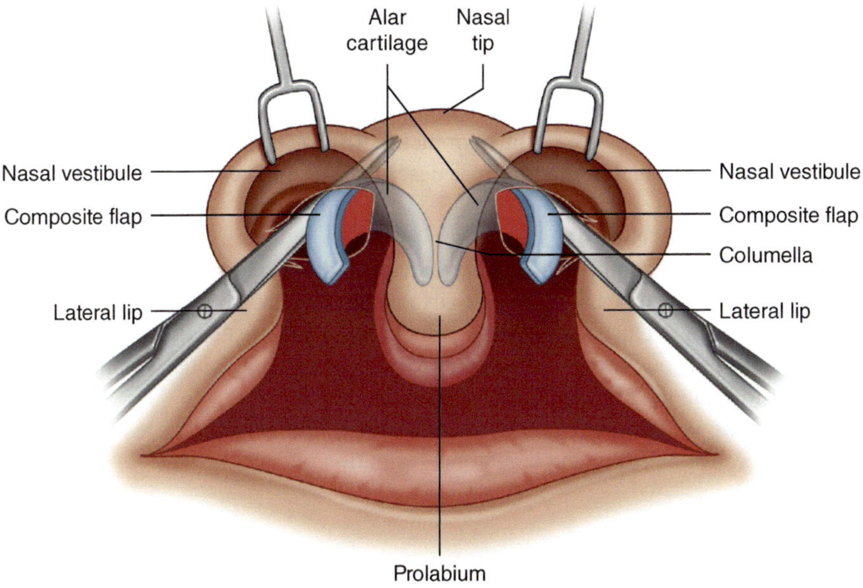

Fig. 8.40 Diagram of nasal tip dissection during VYZ technique for bilateral cleft lip nose repair

8.41 and 8.42). Both alar domes are separated from the overlaying skin in order to facilitate the reposition of the structures from the cleft side. Interdomal fatty tissue is preserved.

Lateral Z Plasty Dissection

Transpositional flaps are elevated at the subcutaneous level. Then the alar base is released using a supraperiosteal dissection in both sides.

Nasal Septum

The septal deviation associated with the bilateral cleft lips is less frequently observed in comparison with unilateral forms; therefore, its early correction is not necessary; however, it may be considered in asymmetrical forms. In these cases, the caudal septum is dissected in the same form as described for unilateral cleft lips.

Nasal Tip Reconstruction

After elevation, the composite flap is advanced medially and sutured using transcutaneous 5/0 PDS stitches. The medial advancement of the composite flap leaves a donor site which is closed using the vestibular skin and creates the V-Y form. The use of transcutaneous stitches allowed us to achieve the following two objectives:

1. Repositioning the alar cartilage at the cleft side
2. Decreasing the space created by surgical dissection, which reduces the risks of postoperative bleeding and hematoma formation.

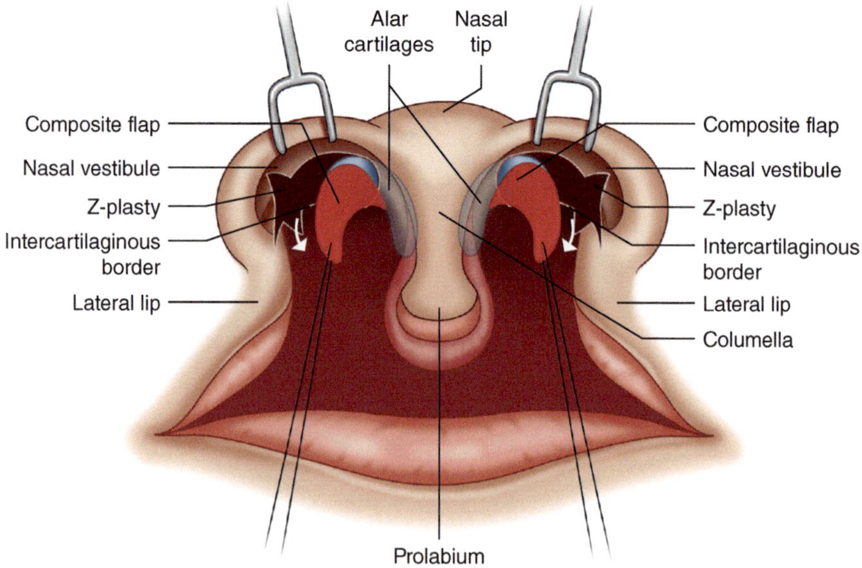

Fig. 8.41 Diagram of bilateral V composite flap elevation during the bilateral VYZ cleft rhinoplasty for the bilateral cleft lip

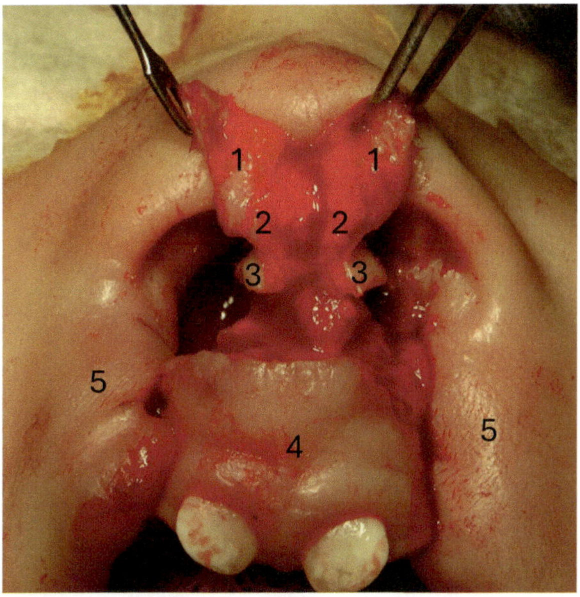

Fig. 8.42 Bilateral V composite flap elevation during VYZ cleft rhinoplasty for bilateral cleft lip. 1. V composite flap elevated. 2. Alar dome. 3. Alar medial crus. 4. Premaxilla. 5. Lateral lip segments

Stitches are placed through the skin, starting from inside the nose and then exiting the skin at the level of the supraalar crease; the needle then returns through the same hole and finally enters the inside of the nose, where the sutures are tied (Figs. 6.32, 6.33, 6.34 and 6.35).

This is the recommended sequence (Figs. 8.43):

First stitch: The alar cartilage dome of the composite flap is medially displaced and fixed using oblique transcutaneous stitch. All these sutures leave and return the skin at the level of the medial end of supraalar crease.

Second stitch: Placed at the level of the lateral corner of the triangular composite flap and using a vertical stitch at the level of the supraalar crease in both sides. These two initial stitches mobilize the flap medially and leave a triangular donor site laterally.

Third stitch: Between the two alar domes using a transcutaneous stitch at the level of the anterior border of the alar domes.

Fourth stitch: Used to close the donor area of the composite flap by advancement of the vestibular skin in a V-Y form finally.

Fifth stitch: The suture enters through the caudal septum and exits at the same level on the opposite side, and then the needle enters through the columella (alar medial crus and skin) in both sides; finally the sutures are tied.

Sixth stitch: Used to correct the position of the alar cartilage in relation to the upper lateral cartilage. This is repositioned using a vertical transcutaneous stitch placed lateral to the internal nasal valve in both sides.

Lateral stitches: They are placed to transpose the branches of the lateral Z plasty as in Fig. 8.43 in both sides. The suture enters through the lateral wall of the nasal vestibule and exits at the level of the alar facial groove returning and then through

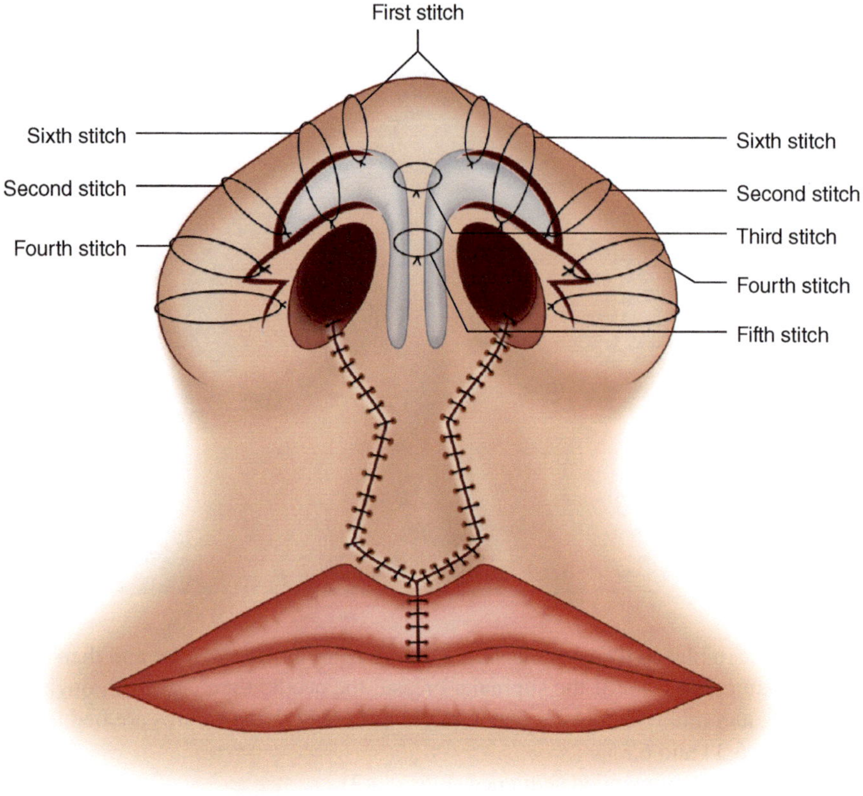

Fig. 8.43 Sequence of transcutaneous stitches used during cleft rhinoplasty for bilateral cleft lip

the same hole and exits at the lateral wall of the vestibule to be tied. Finally, few simple stitches may be used to align correctly the borders of the V-Y and lateral Z plasty (Figs. 8.44 and 8.45). A similar recommendation should be taken in consideration to prevent not to exceed the number of these transcutaneous stitches in order to prevent alar necrosis and also the development of granulomas.

Columellar Lateral Z Plasty

A z plasty is used in both sides of the columellar base to address the lack of definition of the labial columellar angle. This angle is not clearly defined and often obtuse in bilateral cleft lip in special in cases with more hypoplasia of the prolabium (Fig. 8.46). A cephalad rotation of the c flaps (lateral flaps of the prolabium) (Figure) is used as a Z plasty form to obtain a better definition of this angle. These flaps represent the lower arm of the Z plasty. These flaps are transposed into the nostril performing 90–120° of rotation and creating a more acute angle between the lip and the prolabium. The upper arm of the Z plasty is designed bilaterally from the lateral side of the base of the columella and transposed down resembling the medial base of the

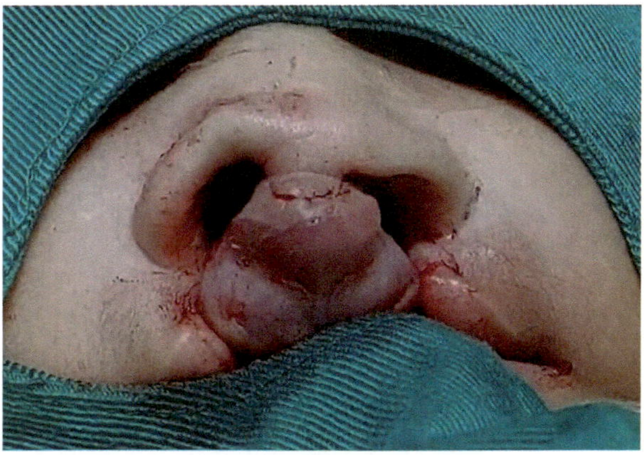

Fig. 8.44 Comparative view between both sides after using the VYZ cleft rhinoplasty on the right side in a patient with incomplete bilateral cleft lip

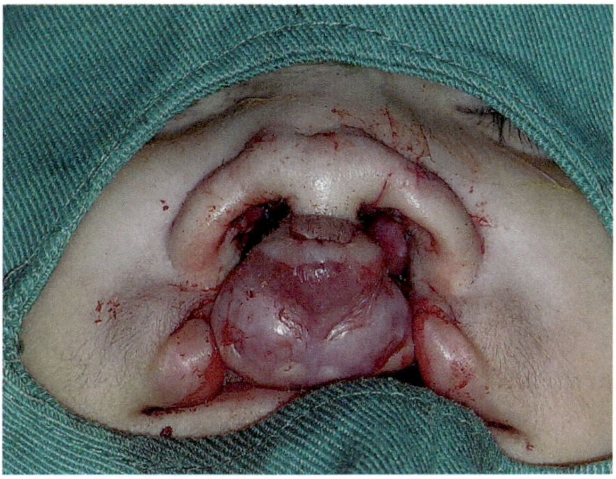

Fig. 8.45 Final appearance of the nose after using the bilateral VYZ cleft rhinoplasty for bilateral cleft lip

columella. This design may be limited to be used in cases with very small prolabium; however, these cases are more associated with complete bilateral cleft lips than incomplete cases.

Nasal Floor

The nasal floor reconstruction is performed during the cleft lip repair, and this is involving the use of two flaps: a medial cutaneous flap lateral to the base of the columella and a lateral flap, which is composed of the base of the ala in both sides. A suture of prolene is used through the alar base dermis of each side, passing beneath the philtral flap and tied in midline narrowing the interalar distance and minimizing the postoperative nasal widening. The lateral flaps (alar bases) are advanced and sutured side to end to the medial flap. The role of muscular repair in bilateral forms supporting the anterior nasal floor is less relevant because of the muscular hypoplasia observed in lateral cleft sides. Skeletal base is finally repaired using the alveolar bone graft later during mixed dentition period (Fig. 8.47).

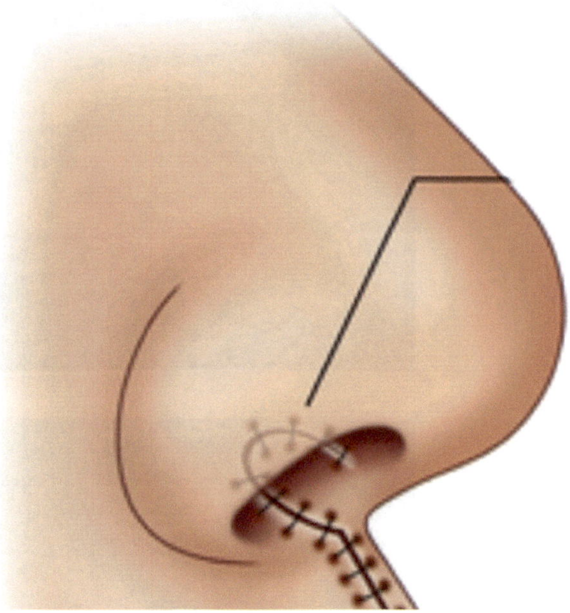

Fig. 8.46 Labio nasal columellar angle improvement after using columellar base lateral Z plasty transposition during VYZ technique for bilateral cleft lip nose repair [12]

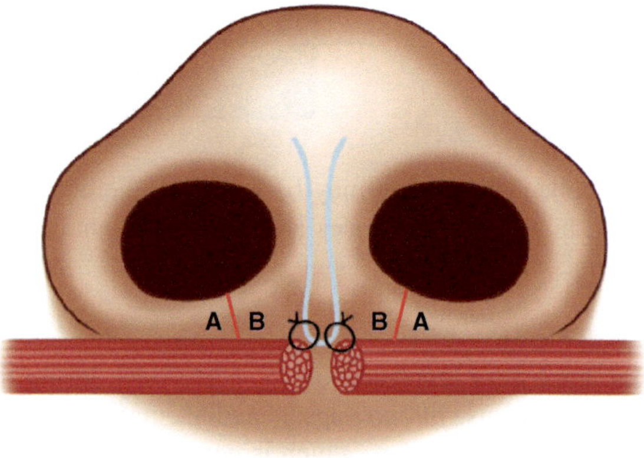

Fig. 8.47 Surgical technique for vestibular segment of nasal floor repair. Flap A (lateral): Alar segment of the lateral advancement cutaneous flap. Flap B (medial): Columellar base flap. The nasal fascicle of levator labii superioris alaeque nasi muscle is used to provide structural support for the vestibular nasal floor

Cases (Figs. 8.48, 8.49, 8.50, 8.51, 8.52, 8.53, 8.54, 8.55, 8.56, 8.57, 8.58, 8.59 and 8.60)

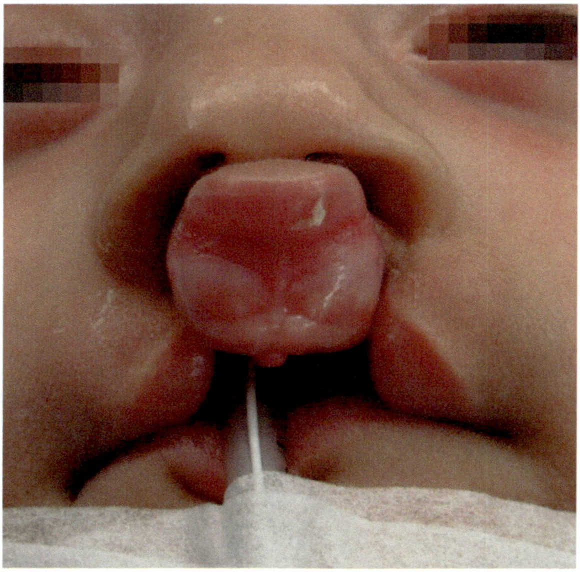

Fig. 8.48 Case 1. Preoperative view of a 3-month-old infant with complete bilateral cleft lip

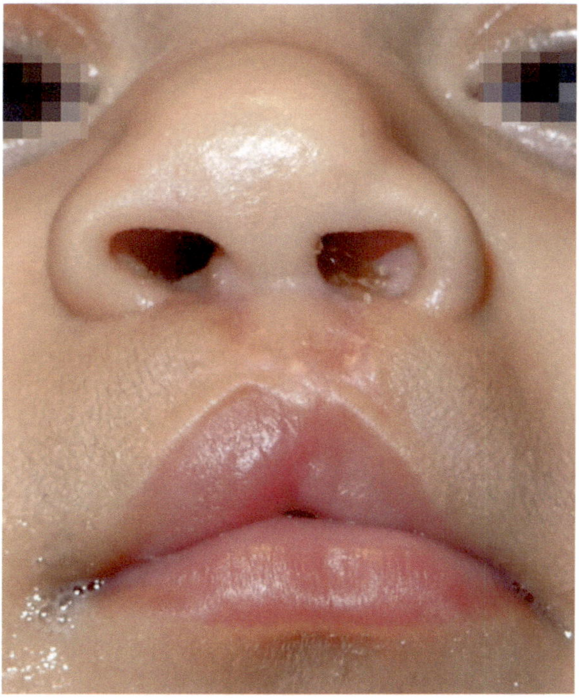

Fig. 8.49 Case 1. A 1-year postoperative view of the infant shown in Fig. 8.48 after undergoing nasal repair using the VYZ technique without presurgical orthopedics

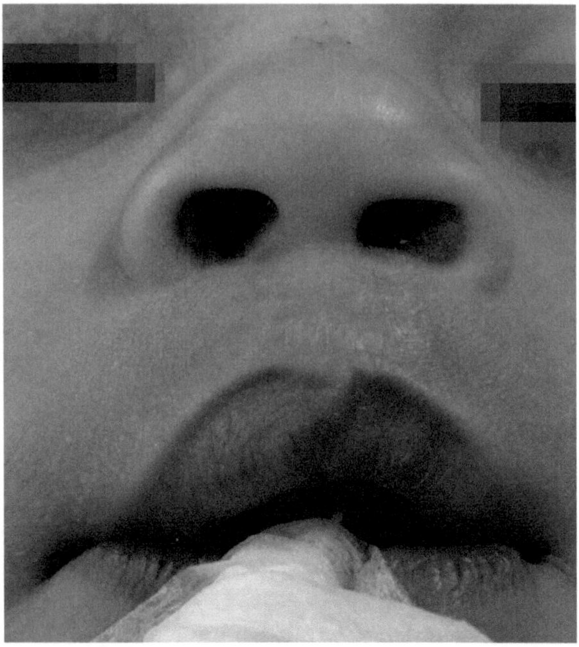

Fig. 8.50 Case 1. A 5-year postoperative view of the infant shown in Fig. 8.48 after undergoing nasal repair using the VYZ technique

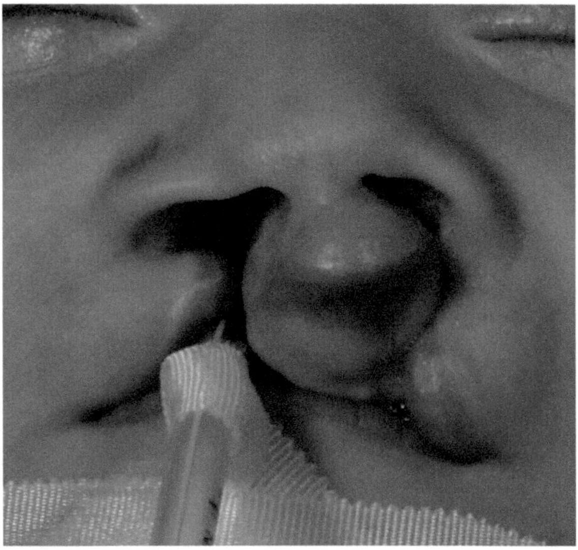

Fig. 8.51 Case 2. Preoperative view of a 3-month-old infant with complete bilateral cleft lip

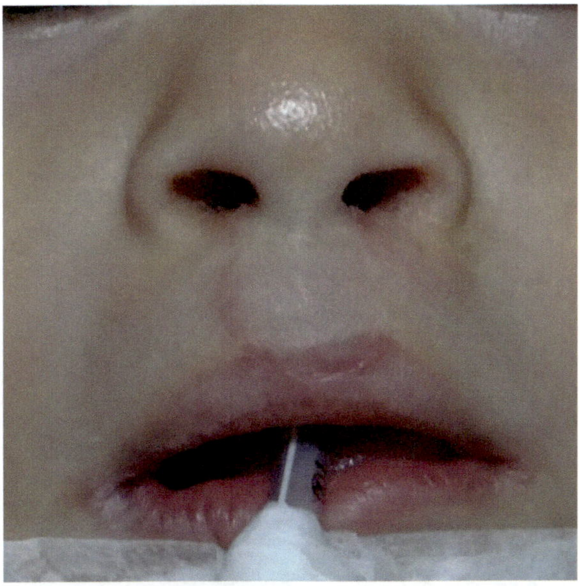

Fig. 8.52 Case 2. A 1-year postoperative view of the infant shown in Fig. 8.51 after undergoing nasal repair using the VYZ technique without presurgical orthopedics (frontal view)

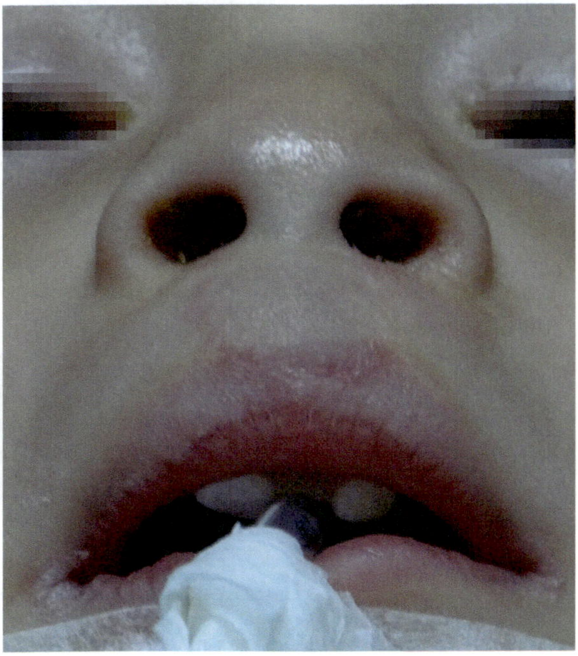

Fig. 8.53 Case 2. A 1-year postoperative view of the infant shown in Fig. 8.51 after undergoing nasal repair using the VYZ technique (worm eye view)

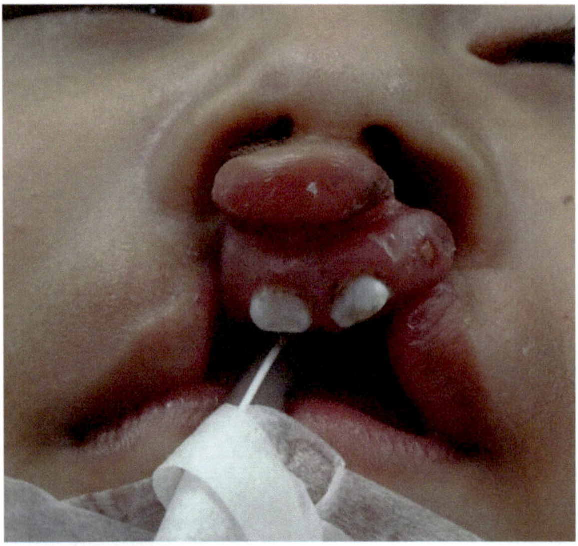

Fig. 8.54 Case 3. Preoperative view of a 3-month-old infant with complete bilateral cleft lip

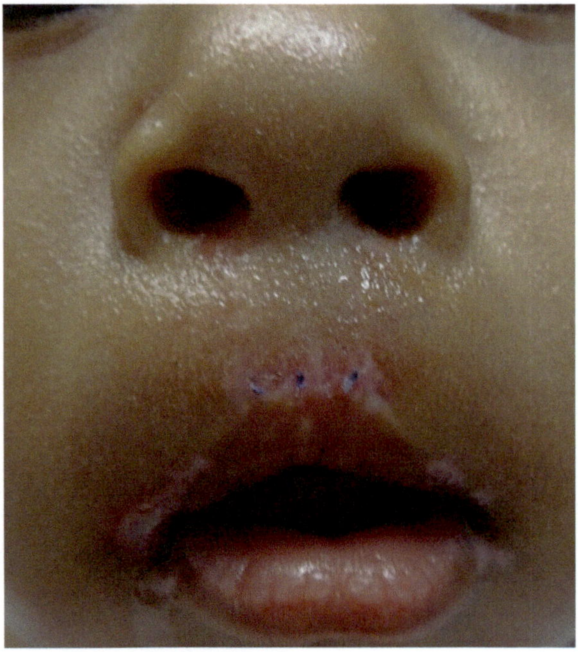

Fig. 8.55 Case 3. 1-year postoperative view of the infant shown in Fig. 8.54 after undergoing nasal repair using the VYZ technique without presurgical orthopedics (frontal view)

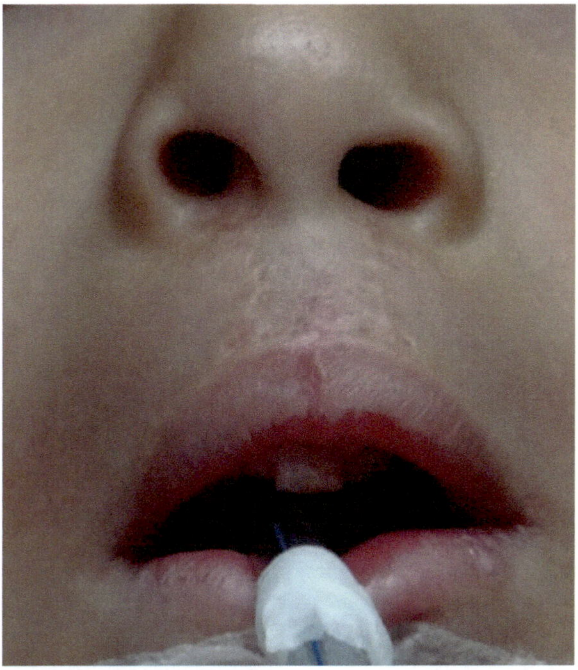

Fig. 8.56 Case 3. A 7-year postoperative view of the infant shown in Fig. 8.54 after undergoing nasal repair using the VYZ technique (worm eye view)

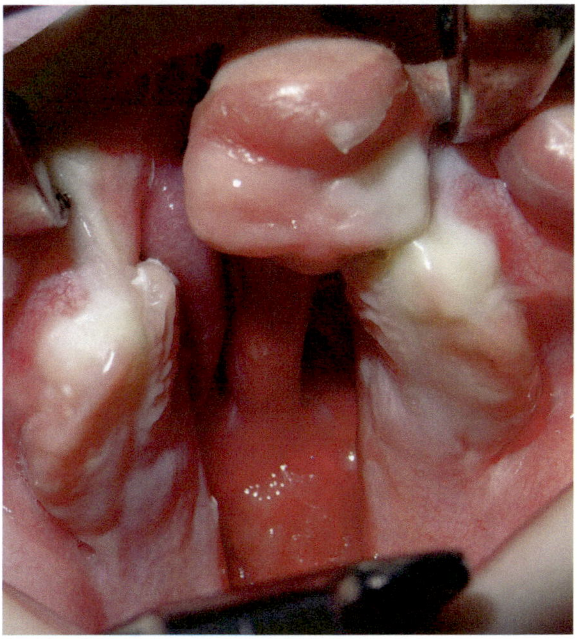

Fig. 8.57 Case 3. Preoperative view of a 3-month-old infant with severe complete bilateral cleft lip (premaxilla position intraoral view)

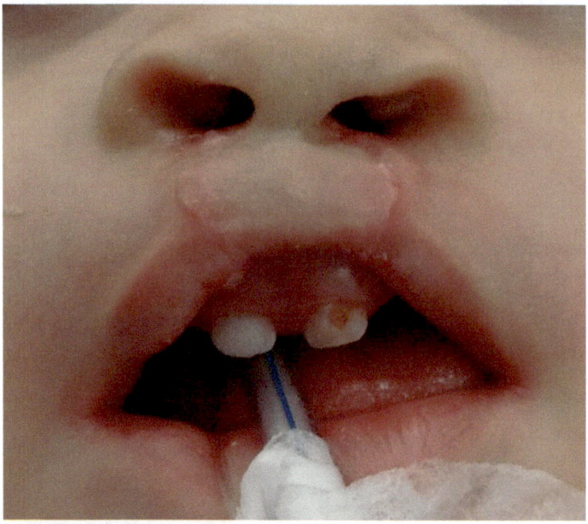

Fig. 8.58 Case 3. Postoperative view of the infant shown in Fig. 8.57 after undergoing bilateral surgical lip adhesion

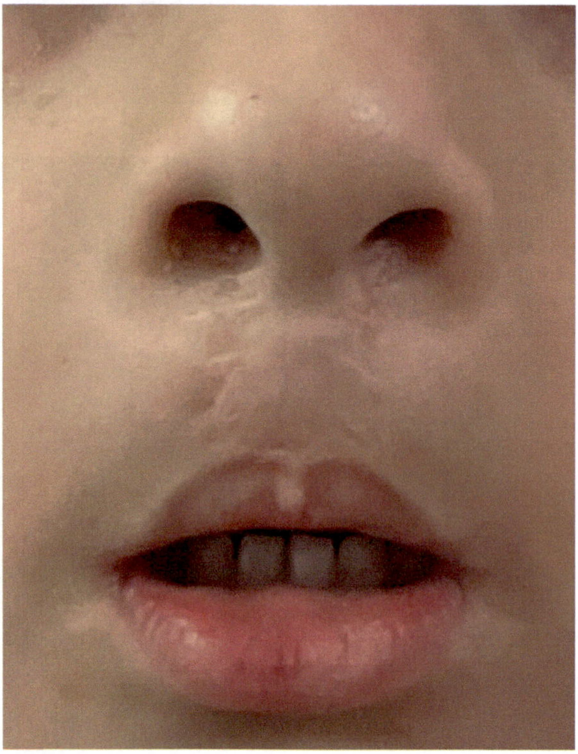

Fig. 8.59 Case 3. A 6-year-old postoperative view of the infant shown in Fig. 8.57 after undergoing nasal repair using the VYZ technique (frontal view)

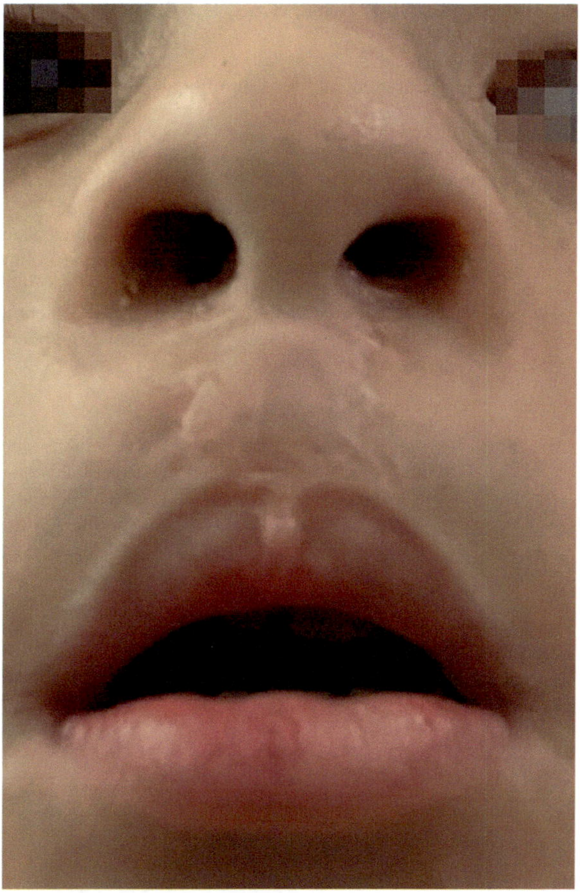

Fig. 8.60 Case 3. A 6-year postoperative view of the infant shown in Fig. 8.57 after undergoing nasal repair using the VYZ technique with surgical lip adhesion (worm eye view)

Surgical Treatment for Combined Bilateral Cleft Lip Nose

Bilateral cleft lip and associated nose deformity present in a wide spectrum including combination of complete or incomplete cleft lips and microforms. The lip and nose deformity is frequently asymmetric requiring a different management for each side. Commonly the degree of severity of the cleft lip correlates with the degree of severity of the nasal deformity being the most severe the one associated with complete cleft lip and protruding premaxilla. This type of cleft lip is the most difficult-to-achieve nose symmetry after the surgical repair because the "control side" (observed in unilateral cleft lips) is not normal and each side requires different surgical treatments. Nasal symmetry is the primary guiding principle during bilateral cleft lip and nose repair. Alternatives for primary cleft rhinoplasty in bilateral cleft lips are presented in Table 8.1 [11].

Cases (Figs. 8.61, 8.62, 8.63, 8.64, 8.65, 8.66, 8.67 and 8.68)

Table 8.1 Surgical protocol for repair of bilateral cleft lip nose

Type of cleft lip	Complete	Incomplete	Microform
Complete	Presurgical treatment + bilateral VYZ technique in both sides	Complete side: VYZ technique Incomplete side: rotational composite flap technique	Complete side: VYZ technique Microform side: nasal sill lenticular excision
Incomplete	Complete side: VYZ technique Incomplete side: rotational composite flap technique	Rotational composite flap technique in both sides	Incomplete side: rotational composite flap technique Microform side: nasal sill lenticular excision
Microform	Complete side: VYZ technique Microform side: nasal sill lenticular excision	Incomplete side: Rotational composite flap technique Microform side: nasal sill lenticular excision	Nasal sill lenticular excision in both sides

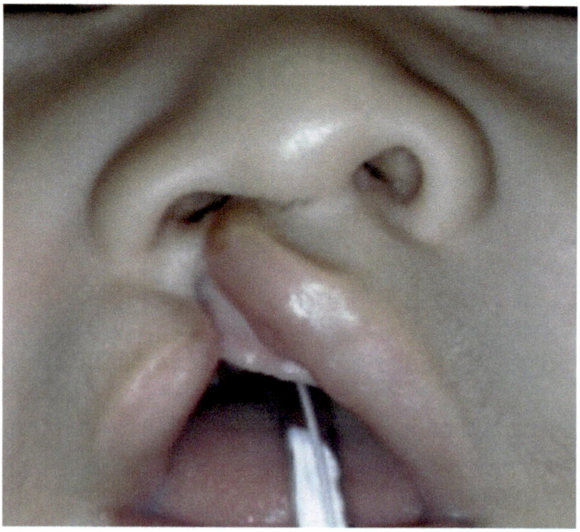

Fig. 8.61 Case 1. Preoperative view of a 3-month-old infant with combined bilateral cleft lip

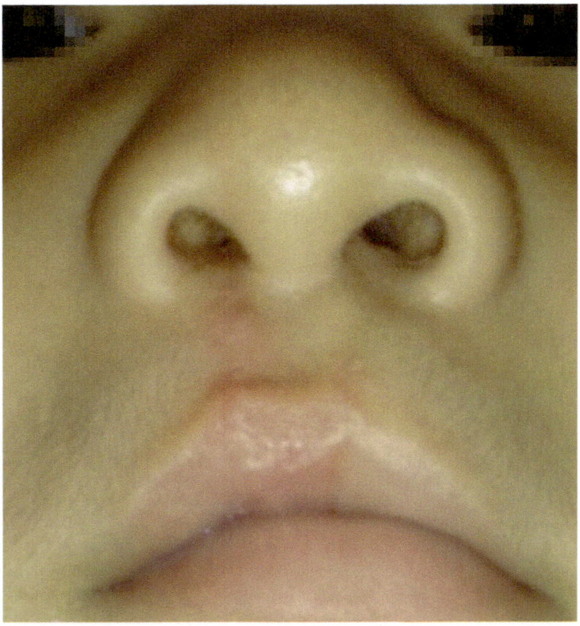

Fig. 8.62 Case 1. A 1-year postoperative view of the infant shown in Fig. 8.61 after undergoing nasal repair using combined techniques

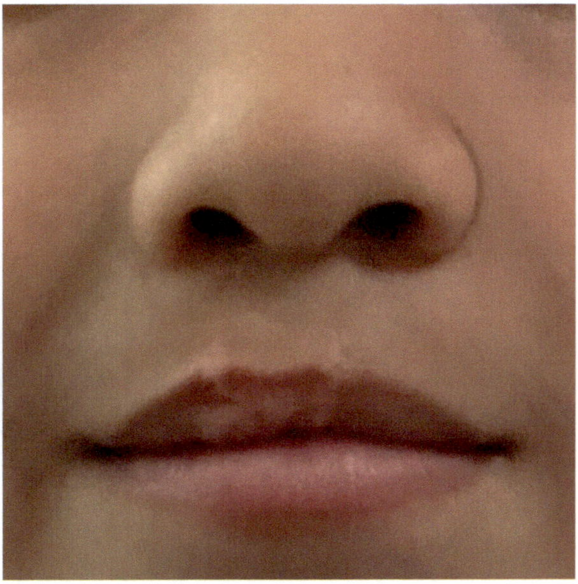

Fig. 8.63 Case 1. A 10-year-old postoperative view of the infant shown in Fig. 8.61 after undergoing nasal repair using combined techniques (frontal view)

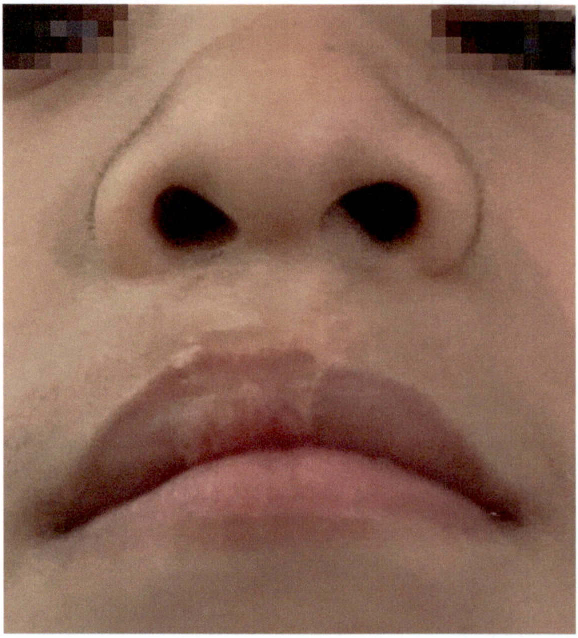

Fig. 8.64 Case 1. A 10 year-old postoperative view of the infant shown in Fig. 8.61 after undergoing nasal repair using combined techniques (worm eye view)

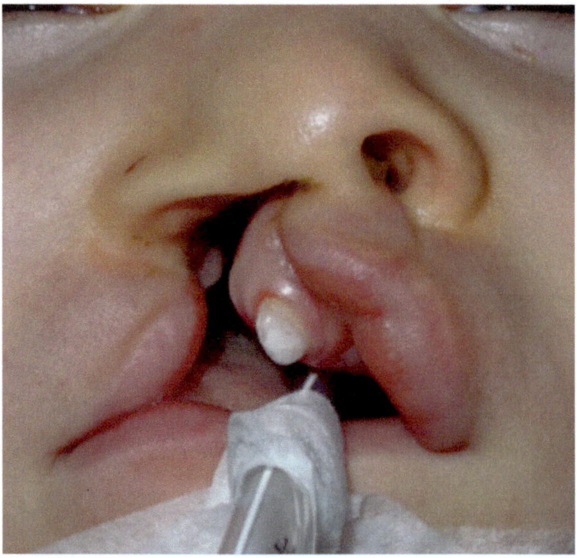

Fig. 8.65 Case 1. Preoperative view of a 3-month-old infant with combined bilateral cleft lip

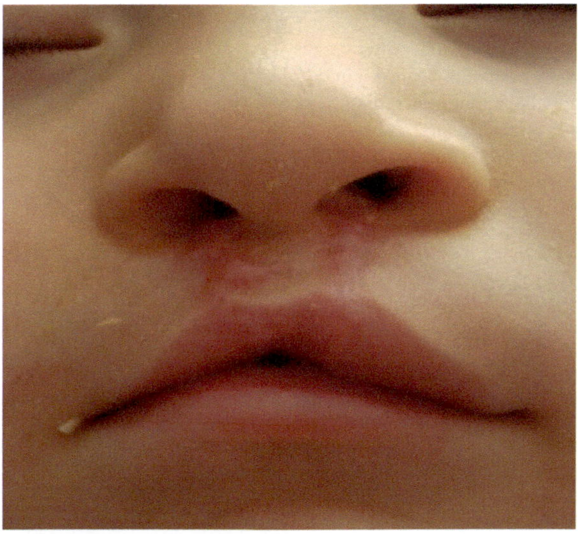

Fig. 8.66 Case 1. A 1-year postoperative view of the infant shown in Fig. 8.65 after undergoing nasal repair using combined techniques

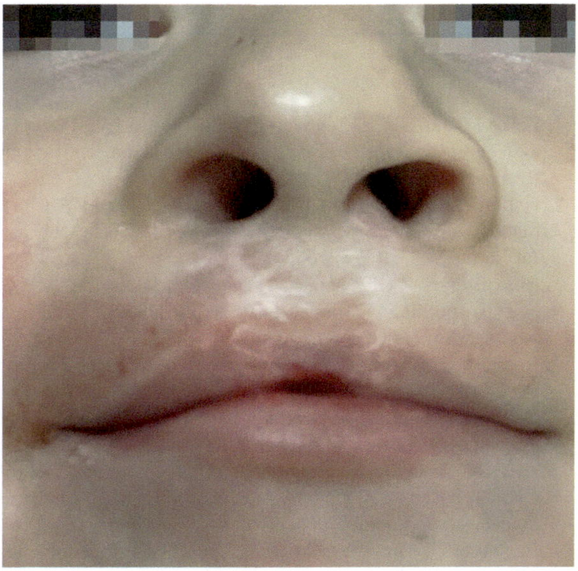

Fig. 8.67 Case 1. A 7 year-old postoperative view of the infant shown in Fig. 8.65 after undergoing nasal repair using combined techniques (frontal view)

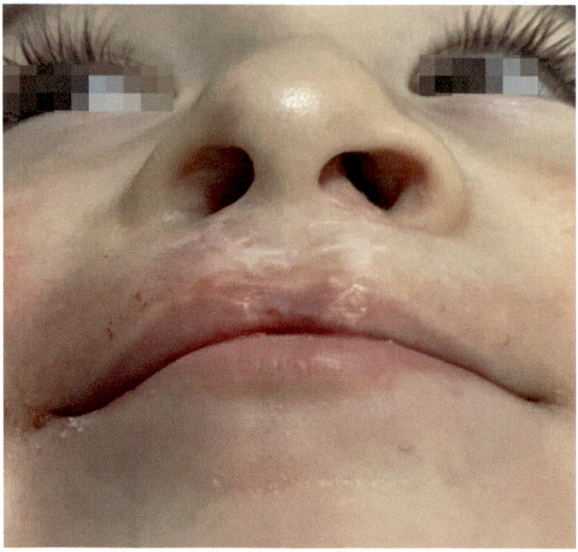

Fig. 8.68 Case 1. A 7-year-old postoperative view of the infant shown in Fig. 8.65 after undergoing nasal repair using combined techniques (worm eye view)

References

1. Zelko I, Zielinski E, Santiago CN, Alkureishi LW, Purnell CA. Primary cleft rhinoplasty: a systematic review of results, growth restriction, and avoiding secondary rhinoplasty. Plast Reconstr Surg. 2023;151(3):452e–62e.
2. Hattori Y, Pai BC, Saito T, Chou PY, Lu TC, Chang CS, Chen YR, Lo LJ. Long-term treatment outcome of patients with complete bilateral cleft lip and palate: a retrospective cohort study. Int J Surg. 2023;109(6):1656–67.
3. Rossell-Perry P, Olivencia-Flores C, Delgado-Jimenez MP, Ormeño-Aquino R. Surgical naso-alveolar molding: a rational treatment for bilateral cleft lip nose and systematic review. Plast Reconstr Surg Glob Open. 2020;8(9):e3082.
4. Rossell-Perry P. Rotational composite flap technique for primary incomplete cleft nose deformity. Plast Reconstr Surg Glob Open. 2020;8(6):e2870.
5. Doyle DJ, Hendrix JM, Garmon EH. American Society of Anesthesiologists Classification. [Updated 2023 Aug 17]. In: StatPearls [Internet]. Treasure Island: StatPearls Publishing; 2023. Available from: https://www.ncbi.nlm.nih.gov/books/NBK441940
6. Chow I, Purnell CA, Hanwright PJ, Gosain AK. Evaluating the rule of 10s in cleft lip repair: do data support dogma? Plast Reconstr Surg. 2016;138(3):670–9.
7. Raghavan U, Vijayadev V, Rao D, Ullas G. Postoperative management of cleft lip and palate surgery. Facial Plast Surg. 2018;34(06):605–11.
8. Bösenberg AT, Kimble FW. Infraorbital nerve block in neonates for cleft lip repair: anatomical study and clinical application. Br J Anaesth. 1995;74(5):506–8.
9. Feriani G, Hatanaka E, Torloni MR, da Silva EM. Infraorbital nerve block for postoperative pain following cleft lip repair in children. Cochrane Database Syst Rev. 2016;4(4):CD011131.
10. Rossell-Perry P. Modification of Reichert's technique based on natural landmarks and individual designs for unilateral repair of cleft lip. Scand J Plast Reconstr Surg Hand Surg. 2008;42(3):113–21.
11. Rossell-Perry P. Atlas of operative techniques in cleft lip and palate surgery. Cham: Springer; 2020.
12. Dhooghe NS, Chong DK. Reducing the Cleft Nose Deformity in Bilateral Cleft Lip Repair. Plast Reconstr Surg Glob Open. 2020;8(12):e3325.

Postoperative Management

9

Martha Mejia and Percy Rossell-Perry

Contents

Introduction

Interdisciplinary cleft care is essential for guaranteeing adequate outcomes, and the postoperative management represents an important period after primary cleft rhinoplasty. Complications observed after nose repair are associated with deficiencies in postoperative care; this attention is provided according to the short- and long-term moments, and more important topics are immediate postop monitoring, pain

M. Mejia
Department of Plastic Surgery, Nicklaus Children's Hospital, Miami, FL, USA

P. Rossell-Perry (✉)
Health of Science Faculty, School of Human Medicine, Peruvian University Union (UpeU), Lima, Peru
e-mail: percy.rossell@upeu.edu.pe

P. Rossell-Perry (ed.), *Atlas of Primary Cleft Rhinoplasty*,
https://doi.org/10.1007/978-3-031-68012-0_9

management, wound care, feeding, scar care, and the use of nasal stents. The use of postoperative nasal conformers remains controversial because of the need for high-level evidence to demonstrate their effectiveness; however, they are commonly used by surgeons worldwide after primary cleft rhinoplasty [1]. Our experience in the postoperative management of primary cleft rhinoplasty is described in detail in this chapter.

Immediate Postoperative Care

This period represents the first 24 h after surgery.

PACU Monitoring

Postanesthesia care unit monitoring is important for patient assessment after primary cleft lip and nose repair. This is based on continuous cardiorespiratory control and body temperature should also be controlled while keeping the baby warm.

It is important to note that an increase in the temperature may be observed frequently after cleft lip and palate surgery during the first day which is related mostly to physiological factors. Patients are used to be in this unit approximately 3 h after surgery; later when the vital signs are stable, they will be moved to a regular patient room, if hospitalization is indicated (when intolerance toward oral foods and/or uncontrollable pain exist). The author recommends at least an overnight stay to guarantee patient feeding and control of vital signs and bleeding. Ambulatory cleft lip surgery should be avoided considering these patient age and the impact of potential complications, even when some studies reported that the same day discharge is safe. If the patient is not in stable condition (steady vital signs) and develops respiratory symptoms or has persistent bleeding, the patient should remain hospitalized and be evaluated by the team until this condition is resolved.

Wound Care

This is represented by the wound care provided immediately after surgery. Once the surgery is finalized, the wound is cleaned using saline solution. The author does not use any kind of wound coverage; it is left uncovered to facilitate free drainage of fluids. We observed drain collection and increased wound inflammation using coverages such as Steri-strips or gauze; this situation may lead to wound infection. Instead of wound coverage, we use an antibiotic ointment (bacitracin) applied once or twice daily to the lip and nose surgical wound; ointments are usually free of preservatives, so they are suitable for sensitive skin. The antibiotic ointment is applied over the lip closure and over the nasal tip and ala including the supraalar crease and alar facial groove where the transcutaneous stitches are placed. Compared with the use of antiseptics or placebo, the use of topical antibiotic effectively recues the risk of infection in surgical wounds, but the absolute benefit is small [2]. There is a moderate quality evidence about the prevention of wound infection using topical antibiotics [3]; however, the application of skin ointment may protect the wound site from contamination and may reduce the inflammatory process of wound healing according to the author's observations. Scabbing on the wound is frequently observed (especially after rhinoplasty), and its removal is not recommended. This action is painful and may produce more bleeding and new scab formation. They may fall off on their own during wound cleaning or may be cleaned using a cotton swab soaked with hydrogen peroxide only if breathing problem exists. Bleeding is a common complication after rhinoplasty; therefore, nasal packing is mandatory after primary cleft rhinoplasty. However, this technique depends on the type of surgical technique, so techniques involving vestibular incisions (such as the rotational composite flap and VYZ) require nasal packing. This is why we did not use nasal stents after completing the surgery.

For this purpose, anterior nasal packing (vestibular) is performed and the technique used is described as follows:

1. The nasal pack is prepared by smearing it with antibiotic ointment. It is very important to use a long pack to avoid displacement outside or inside the nose.
2. The nasal vestibule is cleaned by removing fluids and clots.
3. Then, using the nondominant hand and a double skin hook, the ala of the operated side was pushed up to expose the nasal vestibule.
4. The pack is inserted placing it first medially against the caudal septum (medial wall of the vestibule) and then against the lateral wall in the horizontal plane, parallel to the nasal floor, and finally in the direction of the roof of the vestibule until the end of the pack, filling the nasal vestibule (Figs. 9.1 and 9.2).

The nasal packing is removed slowly the day before the surgery; some bleeding may appear, especially if the baby cries but rarely requires a new packing and stops spontaneously.

Feeding

It is initiated with IV administration of saline solution, and oral feeding is started 3 h after surgery using a small spoon to avoid the use of syringes because of the risk of aspiration. Even when the breastfeeding is possible during the immediate postoperative care, the use of a bottle and breast suction is not recommended during the first 24–48 h because of the risk of wound bleeding and hematoma [4]. There is no association with lip dehiscence, and breastfeeding or bottle-feeding may result in more weight gain facilitating wound healing [5]. The use of syringes for feeding is not recommended because of the risk of aspiration when syringes are not properly used. Breastfeeding may be initiated 2 or 3 days after surgery, and the use of special nipples is an alternative and not mandatory in our experience.

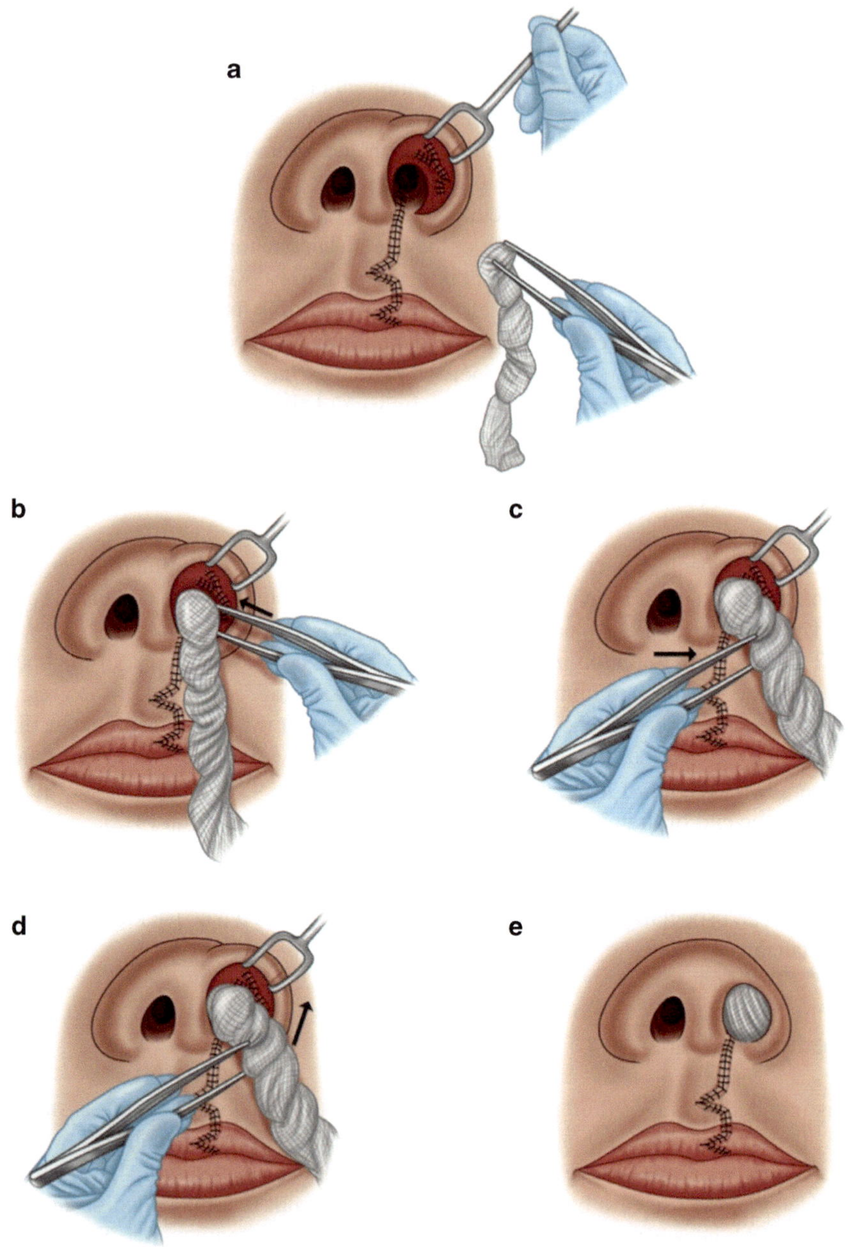

Fig. 9.1 Nasal packing technique. (**a**) The nasal pack is prepared by smearing it with antibiotic ointment and using a double skin hook; the nasal vestibule is exposed. (**b**) The pack is inserted placing it first medially against the caudal septum. (**c** and **d**) The pack is directed parallel to the nasal floor and finally in the direction of the roof of the vestibule until the end of the pack. (**e**) The pack fills the nasal vestibule

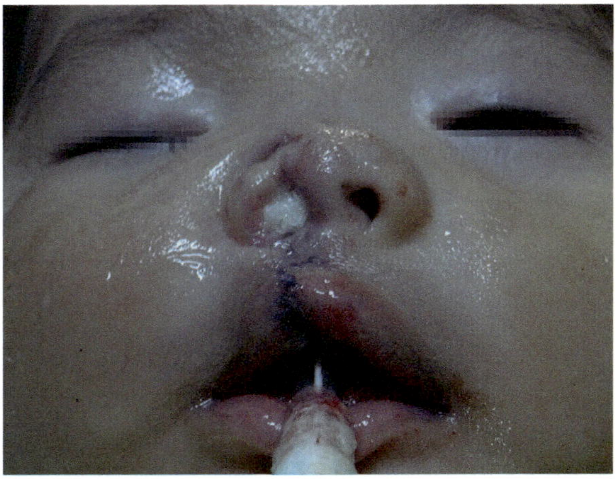

Fig. 9.2 Nasal pack after unilateral primary cleft cheilorhinoplasty

Pain Management

Multimodal pain management is actually recommended. A nerve block in combination with acetaminophen is sufficient for pain control. Opioids are not used in our practice due to the risk of undesirable side effects [6–8].

Agitation Control

Emergence agitation is a common complication and sedation may be necessary in selected patients after cleft lip nose repair [9]. The use of benzodiazepines is indicated when the baby is persistently crying under pain medication, and midazolam may be used for this purpose [10]. Dexmedetomidine is also effective in reducing the incidence of emergency agitation [11].

The medical discharge criteria for patients are stable vital signs, oral feeding restored, and surgical wounds without active bleeding. These are the medical indications: oral feeding including diet according to the patient's age and prophylactic antibiotics and analgesics conditional on pain.

Short-Term Postoperative Care

This period represents the first postoperative week.

Antibiotics and analgesics A prophylactic antibiotic is used orally for 3–5 days. Analgesics are indicated only conditional to pain, and a pediatrician should evaluate any persistent crying or discomfort as a probability of associated disease.

Feeding To guarantee normal restoration, a pediatrician should supervise oral feeding during this period.

Wound care Antibiotic ointment is used until the stitches disappear (1 or 2 weeks depending on suture type). The author prefers to use 6/0 catgut fast-absorbing sutures for skin closure of the lip, but nose correction requires different absorbing sutures, and 5/0 or 6/0 PDS (polydioxanone) is indicated for that purpose. Using nonresorbable sutures for skin closure requires their removal under sedation in the operating room. The transcutaneous stitches may develop reaction in tissues and increase the risk of bacterial colonization at the sites they occupied. These stitches may lead to infections (small suture abscesses can be observed) and granulomas. Both of them are temporary and resolve spontaneously when the suture is reabsorbed.

Scar care After the sutures are resorbable, we recommend keeping the scar clean, starting the massage protocol 3 weeks after surgery, and using silicone scar gel and silicone tapes at night during the first 6 months of healing (Fig. 9.3).

Hypertrophic scar formation is a frequent postoperative complication that impairs soft tissue form, function, or movement. Hypertrophic scars require special attention and treatment because they sometimes exhibit chronic inflammation and fibrosis that may impact facial growth [12].

Our massage protocol consists of two phases: First, putting one finger is placed inside the lip because massage requires support. Finding a place for the finger is a little tricky because you cannot find too much space; the other finger is up to the scar tissue, so the scar tissue is in the middle of the fingers, and you need to apply some pressure to break the collagen formation.

The second step involves proper rotation between the fingers to produce a circular massage, and the last step involves slight elongation to stretch the upper part of the scar to down. Massage must be performed five times during the day if babies tolerate it (Figs. 9.4 and 9.5).

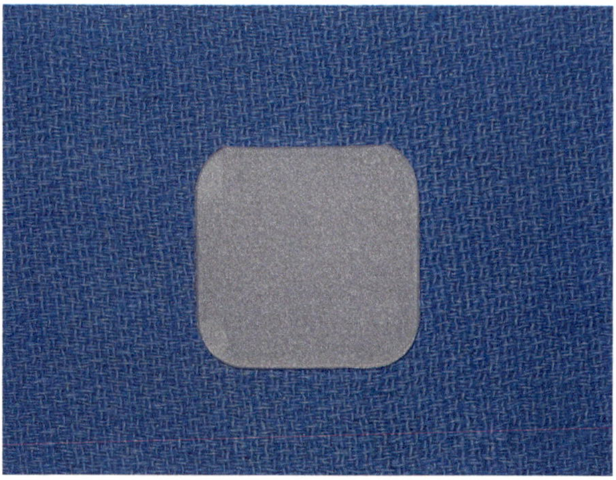

Fig. 9.3 Silicone tapes for hypertrophic scar prevention

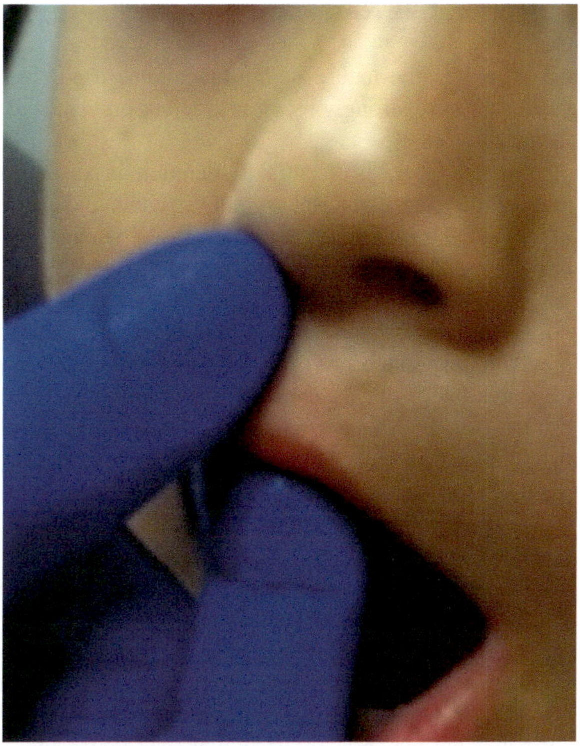

Fig. 9.4 Postoperative oral massages. Finger support and rotation between the fingers

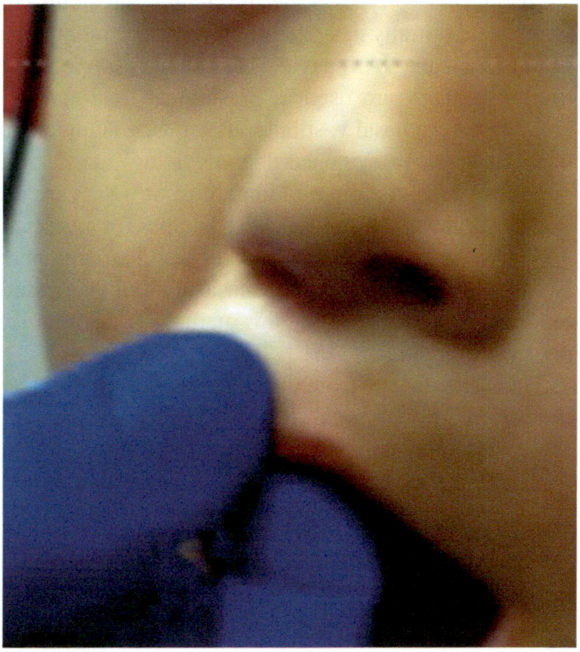

Fig. 9.5 Postoperative oral massages. Tension down with the upper finger

Postoperative Nasal Conformers

According to the nature of the techniques used (including vestibular incisions), nasal stents are strongly recommended to prevent scar contracture and synechia of the nasal vestibule.

After surgery, it is essential to maintain nasal structures in the correct position to prevent the relapse of nasal asymmetry and avoid cicatricial stenosis that may occur in the caudal most portion of the nasal vestibule in CLP patients, resulting in a micro or collapsed nostril [13].

An individual design is recommended and should be used early (second or third postoperative week) and least 6 months at least. Moisturizing cream is applied to prevent injury to the soft tissues which are fixed using tapes.

These devices have been used in combination with presurgical nasal molding and primary surgery, due to frequent nose deformity relapse after surgery, and different methods have been used for this purpose to guarantee long-term results. Postoperative nasal conformers may prevent the nose relapse because of wound contraction during healing process; however, the use of postoperative nasal conformers (stents) remains controversial, and there is a lack of evidence demonstrating its role after primary cleft rhinoplasty. To date, no randomized clinical trial has supported its efficacy.

A recent systematic review revealed that clear conclusions cannot be drawn because of the limited and low-quality evidence of the reviewed studies [1]. Another observational study concluded that the use of these devices does not improve nasal aesthetics but may prevent vestibular scar contracture and vestibular synechia [14]. For these purposes, different devices have been described in the literature, and they are based on two types of design: hooks and stents (Figs. 9.6, 9.7, and 9.8). Nasal stents were initially designed for nasal molding in combination with alveolar molding by Grayson (NAM device). The stent is supported using a wire fixed to the palatine plate. They are used as presurgical treatment. The stent molds the nose by pressure on the nasal vestibule. Its efficacy is under strong debate actually because there is a lack of evidence demonstrating its effect. Different hook devices have been designed for nasal molding, most of which are used empirically.

The Dynacleft system is based on tapes for alveolar molding and a hook attached to the forehead, which suspends the nasal structures only vertically. They can also be used also for postsurgical nasal treatment. A study published by Monasterio reported that the efficacy of this method was similar to that of the NAM device as a presurgical treatment [15].

Dr. Martha Mejia from the Nicklaus Children's Hospital in Miami Florida, USA, developed a postsurgical treatment using silicone Porex^{R} Stents for 3 weeks after surgery. Immediately after removal, the *Rhinoplastic Appliance System* (RAS) was used for 6 months for 24 h [16] (Figs. 9.9, 9.10, and 9.11).

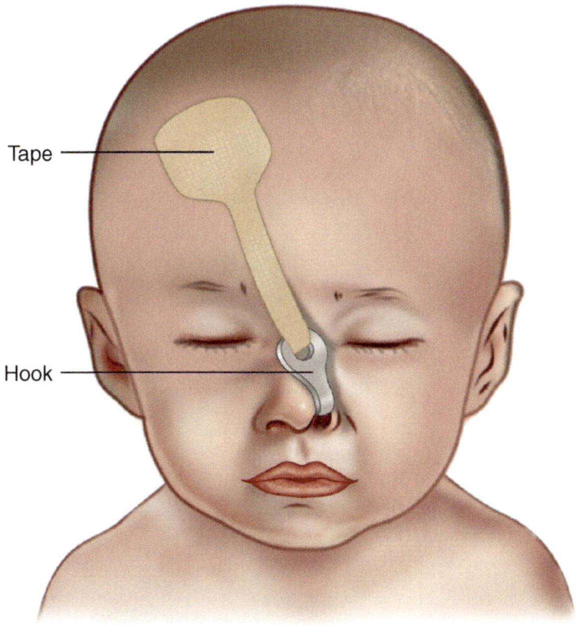

Fig. 9.6 Postoperative nasal hook type used in Dynacleft method

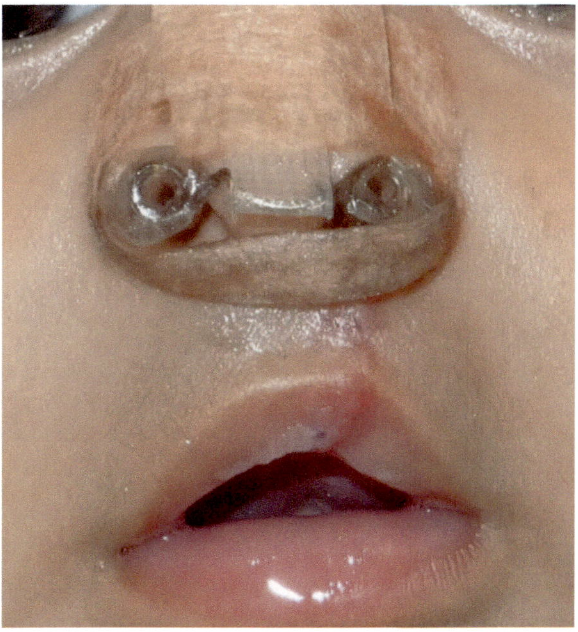

Fig. 9.7 Postoperative nasal stents in a patient after unilateral primary cleft rhinoplasty

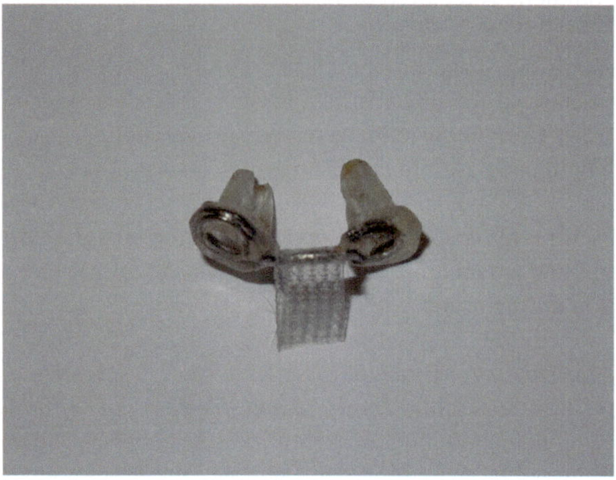

Fig. 9.8 Individualized acrylic custom-made postoperative nasal hook device

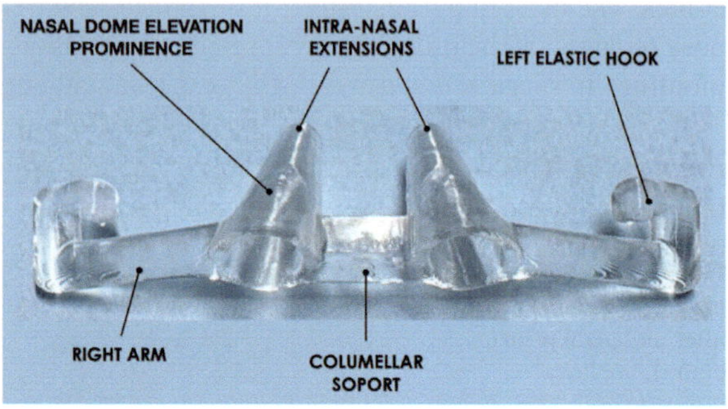

Fig. 9.9 Rhinoplastic Appliance System (RAS)

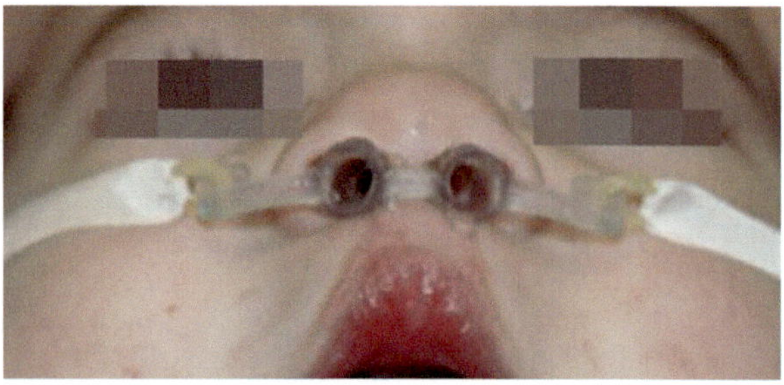

Fig. 9.10 Rhinoplastic Appliance System (RAS) in position

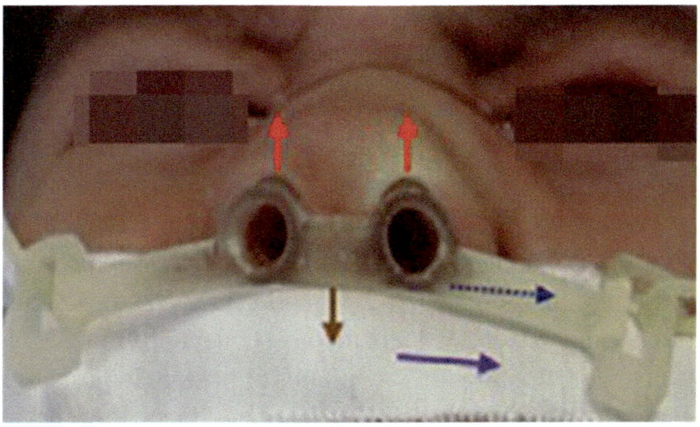

Fig. 9.11 Patient using the RAS illustrating the forces when the device is inserted

In postsurgical treatments, experience has shown that applying a dynamic nasal splint can contribute effectively to maintaining the surgical results by opposing forces of contracture. An alternative method is the use of individualized acrylic custom-made nasal stent used in our center in Lima, Peru. This is a less expensive method and represents an alternative for those sites where the manufactured devices (silicone, porex, etc.) are unavailable. This nasal conformer is recommended for at least 6 months and 8 h daily. Its utility has been studied in a recently published study [14].

Types of Postoperative Nasal Conformers

In the literature, many different clips, hooks, and silicone stents are used in postsurgical treatments. This chapter presents three alternatives to be used according to the sites. The first two alternatives are used immediately after surgery to preserve nasal correction; the last alternative is for older patients with some degree of nostril stenosis.

Acrylic Custom-Made Nasal Stent

This is an interesting device developed by the author (P.R.P) in association with Olga Figallo DDS in a center in Lima Peru for postoperative treatment of primary cleft rhinoplasty. This is a custom-made acrylic device which can be easily fabricated and used in middle- and low-income countries [14] (Figs. 9.7 and 9.8).

These devices should be applied 1 week after surgery to prevent any associated complication during the early process of wound healing. They are manufactured in a mold acquired by taking an impression of the nose, and then they are fashioned from acrylic material to create stents according to the patient's nasal anatomy. A central perforation is included in the stent that keeps the airway clear; this perforation is also designed bilaterally and supported using a wire framework through the aid of tapes. The appliance is adjusted according to the patient's progress by adding acrylic to the stent.

Three-Dimensional Printer Rhinoplasty Appliance System (RAS)

The RAS (Rhinoplasty Appliance System) is a three-dimensional system printer with previous nasal correction and consists of nasal stents inserted into the nostrils, with two lateral components that keep the appliance in position allowing for simultaneous manipulation of the nasal septum and nostril height horizontally and vertically. The device is placed with adhesive tape on the patient's cheeks. With the RAS appliance system, it is possible to maintain the correction of the nasal septum, projection of the nose, and nostril symmetry [17] (Figs. 9.9, 9.10, and 9.11). This is a digitally designed device manufactured using CAD/CAM technology sequentially applied. The appliances are sequentially exchanged monthly for 3–6 months of postop. In postsurgical treatments, experience has shown that applying a dynamic nasal appliance RAS device can contribute effectively to maintaining the surgical results by opposing forces of contracture. Postsurgical treatment is essential to maintaining the proper shape and size of the nostrils. Holding the position of the nasal septum and nares is also crucial since cartilage has memory and tends to return; however, this limitation may be improved by using an adequate surgical technique.

Unilateral and Bilateral Postsurgical Treatment

Materials

- The nasal appliance in a measure printed on a three-dimensional laser printer.
- Four orthodontic elastics of 3/16 or 4.7 mm (half 3 ounces).
- Steri-strip adhesive tape or similar.
- A lcohol and gauze.

Procedure

- Remove excess grease from the cheeks at the height of the nose with alcohol and dry.
- The nasal apparatus is inserted with the elastics attached to the side straps of the steri-strip (5 cm long) and rubber bands to the side of the lateral alar of the nose.
- The appliance will be used for 24 h for the first 6 months after surgery and then in the evening for 4–6-month retention.
- The device is removed twice daily to clean it with soap and water.

Recommendations

1. The location of the rhinoplastic appliance with the tension of the elastics and tapes. It is a frequent complication. For this reason, it is necessary to explain to the parents how to put the device and the tension of the elastics.

Soft Tissue Complications

2. It is very important to properly insert the device and lubricate it with petroleum jelly so as not to cause irritation and subsequent wounds in the tissue. Additionally, there is special care in cleaning the tissue free of accumulated secretions. These can be the first complications; to manage them, if there is a wound in the tissue, a small portion of triple antibiotic cream is used. The wound healed for 1 week. However, the device was continued for only 2 days if it was strictly necessary for damage to occur. Secretions adhering to the skin or that have accumulated should be cleaned with a swab (Q-tip) two times a day.

3. Irritation or redness of the insertion area or the area where the tapes are used to hold the device. A mixture of a cream containing zinc and hydrocortisone should be applied.

   This mixture was used for approximately 5 h and then cleaned and returned to the device.
4. Allergy to tapes. This complication is not frequent, but if it occurs, the same mixture described above is used, and elastics with Velcro can be used. A hat to avoid using tape or dealing with other hypoallergenic tapes that you tolerate better.

The primary reason for not using the device is that the patient has any respiratory problems (asthma, low oxygen saturation) or any condition or disease that produces excess secretions. The other reasons are the time it is used (if it is not enough), the discontinuation of treatment and, finally, the need for cleaning (infection).

Orthonostric Appliance

It is used when the patient is older and has nasal stenosis. This appliance was designed on the bases of experience gained with passive nasoalveolar molding devices for the presurgical treatment of children with cleft lips; we have developed a stent called an orthonostric appliance that addresses all these problems. The orthonostric device is custom made for each patient with a previous impression and contains a small screw similar to an orthodontist retainer. The patient can activate it at home. Minor degrees of nostril asymmetry or stenosis can be corrected using this stent alone. The stent has the following features:

1. It is custom fabricated for each patient.
2. It is expansile, and the direction of expansion can be oriented as desired.
3. The head of the screw for the drive mechanism can be accessed without removing the stent.
4. The stent is maintained comfortably by an adjustable wire flange, which wraps around the alar crease [18]. After alginate impressions of the nose are taken, the device is fabricated on a stone model, inserted, and the expansion is started on the second day. The increase of the device is performed daily in increments of 0.5–1 mm at a time. The addition can be continued at home, but adjustments must be made by the orthodontist or the surgeon at the office. The appliance is used initially 24 h per day for 4–6 months and then for an additional 4–6 months at night only. It is generally preferable to initially perform an overcorrection because the forces of contraction frequently cause the recurrence of stenosis. To treat nostril stenosis, "the orthonostric" approach is used to correct and maintain nostril stenosis and other nostril shape abnormalities. Lesser degrees of deformity can be corrected nonsurgically by using this device alone. More severe degrees of stenosis or nostril asymmetry require surgical correction: in these cases, a Porex^{R} stent is placed at the time of surgery and maintained in place for the first 2 weeks; an expansile stent of the exact dimensions of the silicone stent is fabricated in the meantime and inserted at the time of removal of the silicone stent. Further expansion, if necessary, may be started 2 weeks postoperatively.

We recommend a 2 mm over increase because the nostril contracts approximately 2 mm when treatment is finished. These cases require longer retention times (Figs. 9.12 and 9.13).

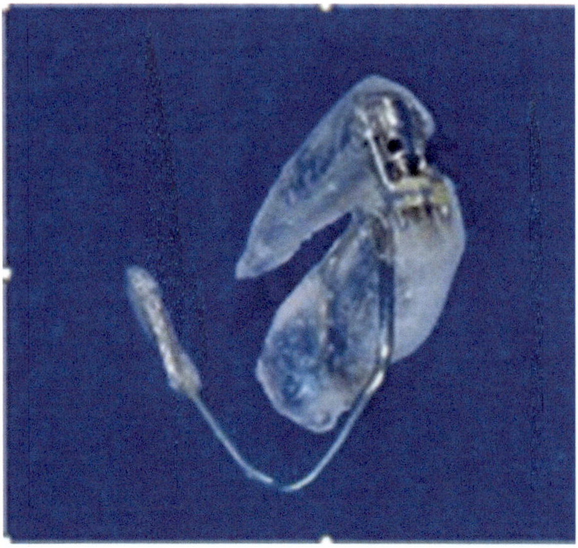

Fig. 9.12 Postoperative orthonostric appliance

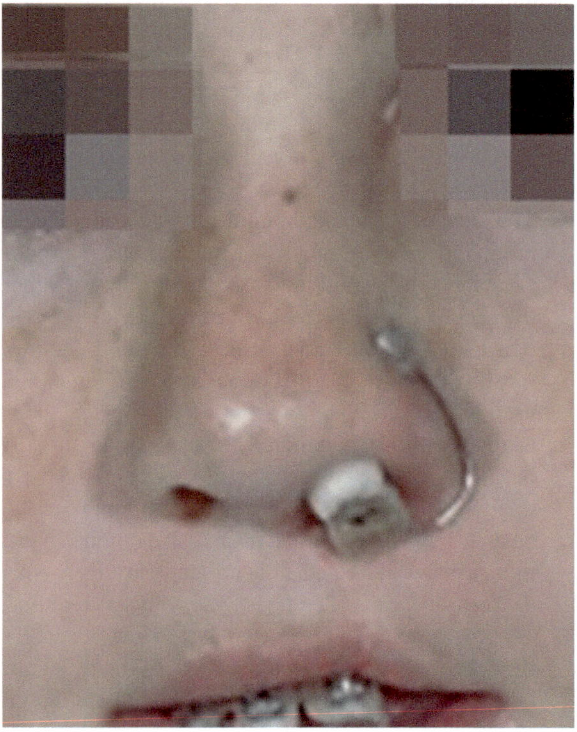

Fig. 9.13 Orthonostric appliance in position

Cases

Clinical Case 1

The patient was born with left unilateral cleft lip and palate consults for nostril stenosis on the left side at nine. The patient was treated with an orthonostric device 24 h for 6 months and for one-year retention with an acrylic stent used at nighttime (Fig. 9.14).

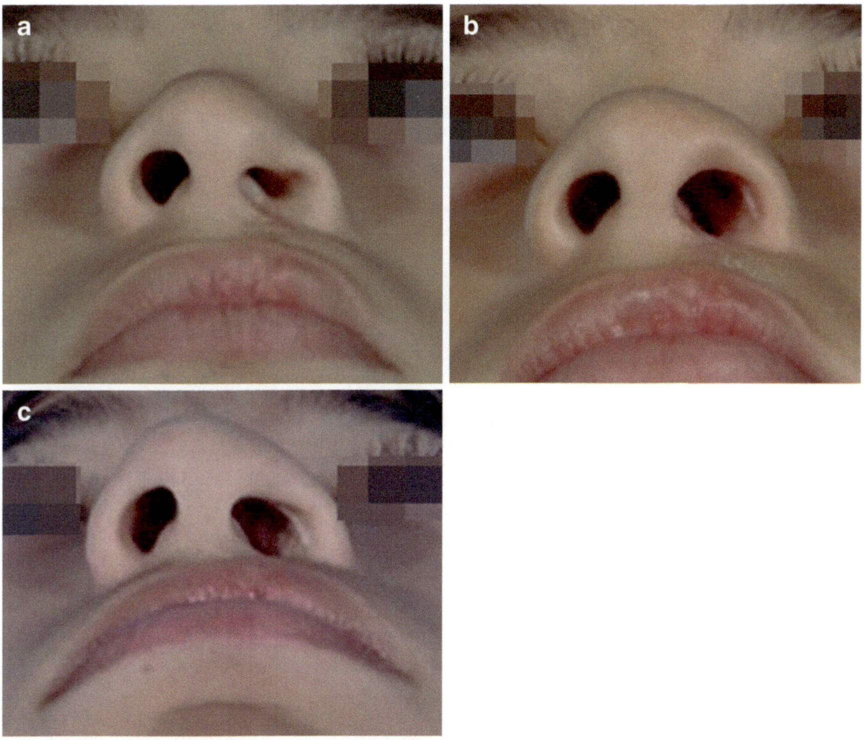

Fig. 9.14 Patient treated with an orthonostric. (**a**) Left nostril stenosis. (**b**) After orthonostric treatment. (**c**) Ten-year long-term follow up

Clinical Case 2

The patient was born with a complete unilateral cleft, lip, and palate on the left side at 8 years of age. The patient had severe stenosis in his left nostril. The stenosis was corrected twice with previous surgeries with no success. Patients came for a different approach with a combination of surgery, silicone stent, and orthonostric device. The patient used a silicone stent with suture for 3 weeks, and the day it was removed, the orthonostric device was inserted into the nostril, and the patient used it for 8 months, 24 h, and 1 year at nighttime for retention (Fig. 9.15).

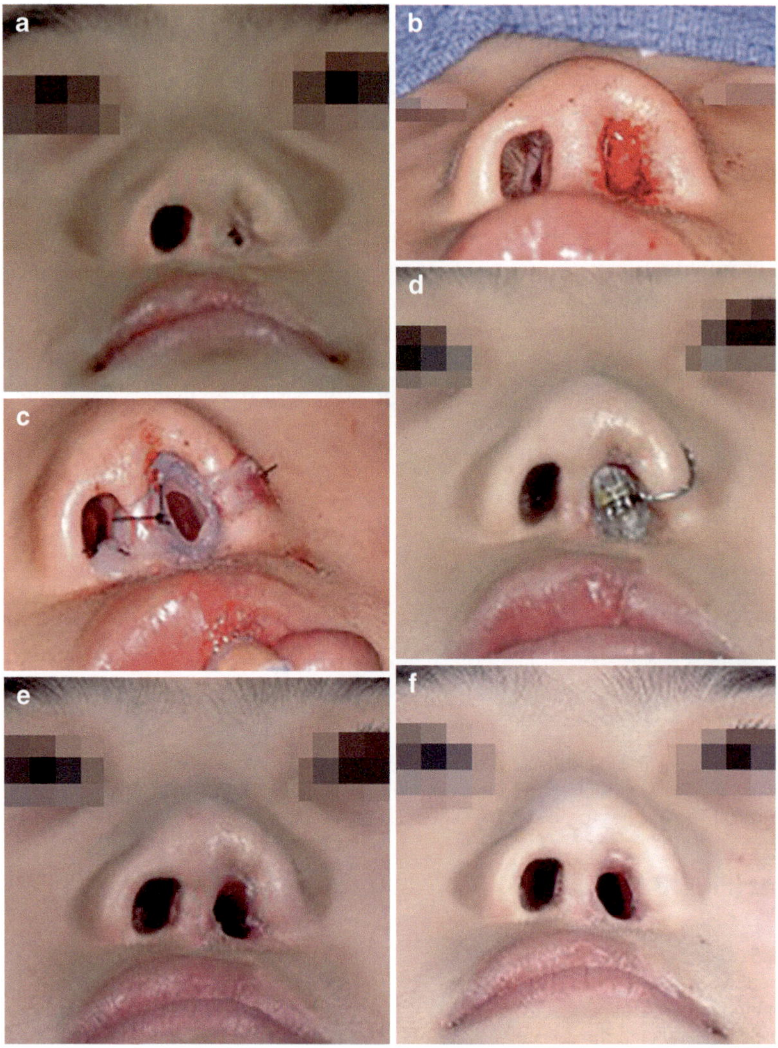

Fig. 9.15 (**a**) Severe left nostril stenosis. (**b**) Open surgically. (**c**) Silicone stent used during 3 weeks. (**d**) Orthonostric device applied. (**e**) Photo after treatment. (**f**) Long-term follow-up

Clinical Case 3

This was an infant with an incomplete bilateral cleft lip started with presurgical orthopedics at 4 weeks old for 18 weeks and underwent surgery at 6 months of age. After surgery, the patient received a Porex^{R} silicone stent with sutures for 3 weeks, and after it was immediately removed, the RAS appliance was inserted and used. This appliance is removable and needs to be cleaned daily and held in place with rubber bands and tape. The patient used the RAS for 6 months after surgery (Fig. 9.16).

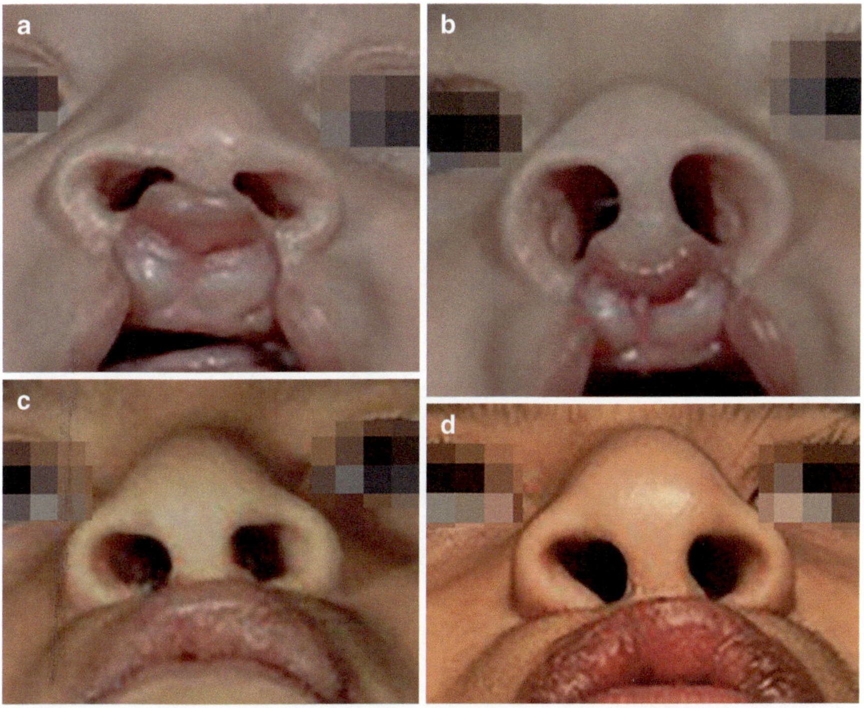

Fig. 9.16 (**a**) Incomplete bilateral cleft lip before presurgical orthopedic treatment. (**b**) After presurgical orthopedics. (**c**) After primary bilateral cleft lip nose repair. (**d**) A 15 year long-term follow-up

Clinical Case 4

An infant with complete bilateral cleft, lip, and palate. The baby started with presurgical orthopedics at 6 weeks old for 18 weeks and underwent surgery at 6 months of age. The patient initially used a maxillary plate for 6 weeks to rotate the premaxilla, reduce the gap between the segments, and start the nasal molding for 12 weeks. After surgery, the patient used the silicone PorexR stents for 3 weeks and an RAS device for 6 months (Fig. 9.17).

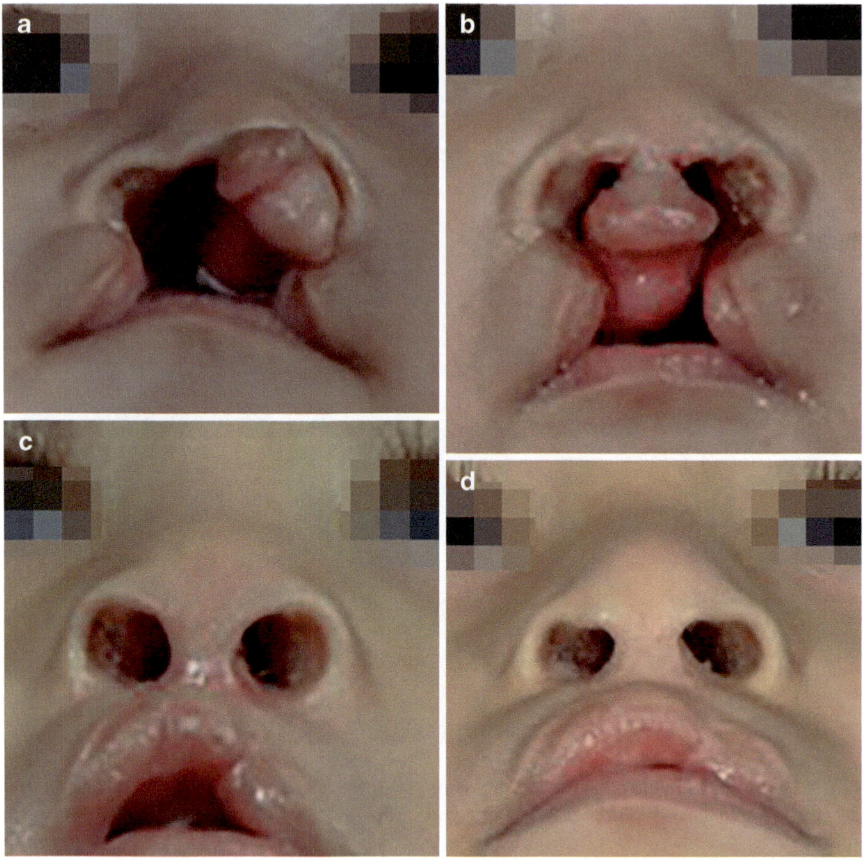

Fig. 9.17 (**a**) Complete bilateral cleft lip and palate before presurgical orthopedic treatment. (**b**) After presurgical orthopedic treatment. (**c**) After primary bilateral cleft lip nose repair. (**d**) A 5-year long-term follow-up

Clinical Case 5

This is an incomplete unilateral cleft lip and palate. The baby started with PSO at 2 weeks old and underwent surgery at 4 months of age. The patient used the RAS system 4 months after surgery (Fig. 9.18).

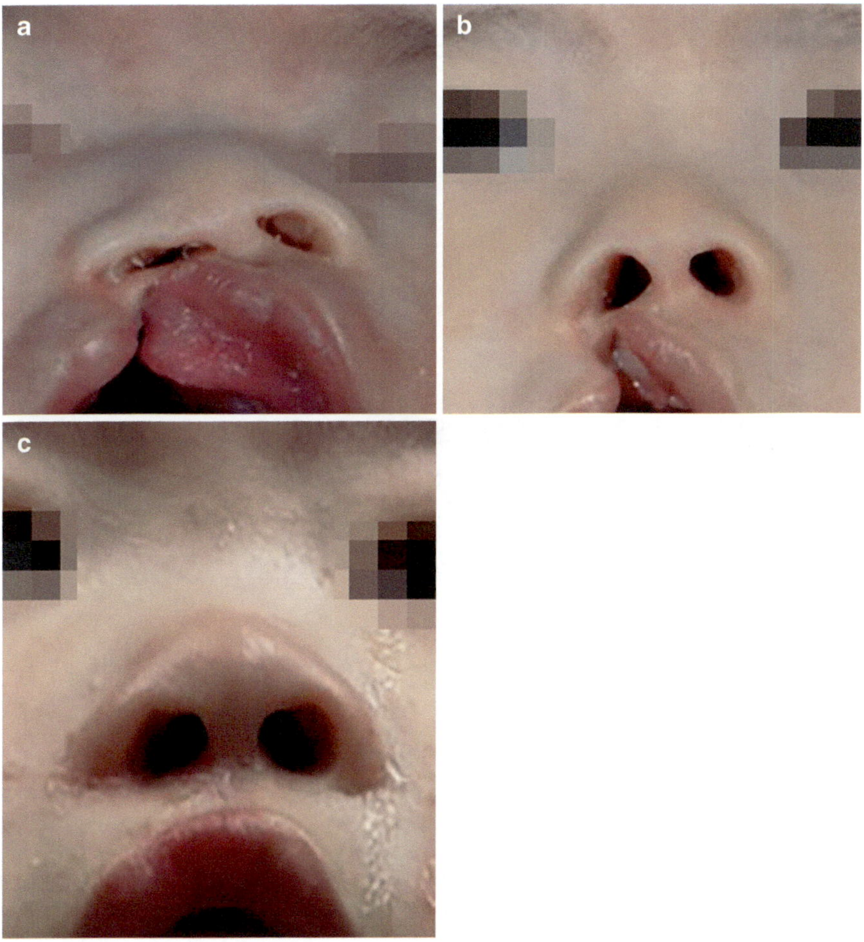

Fig. 9.18 (**a**) Incomplete unilateral cleft lip before presurgical orthopedic treatment. (**b**) After presurgical orthopedic treatment. (**c**) Eight months after primary unilateral cleft lip nose repair

Clinical Case 6

Patient was born with a complete right unilateral cleft lip and palate and used an individualized custom-made acrylic device starting 1 week after primary cleft lip and nose surgery and during 6 months (Fig. 9.19).

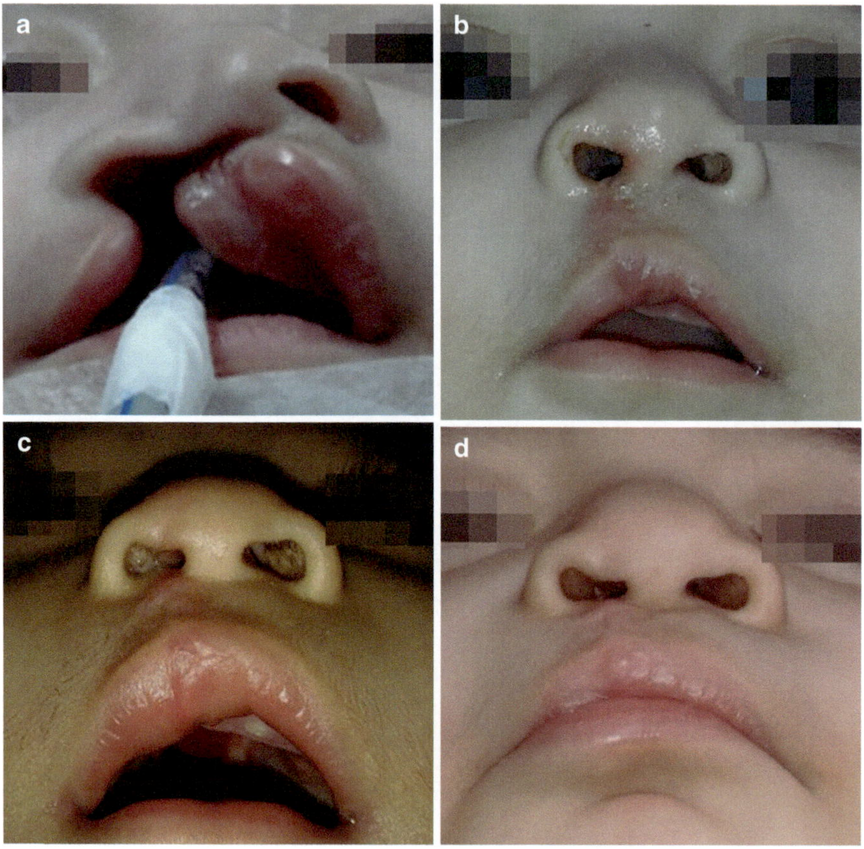

Fig. 9.19 (**a**) Complete unilateral cleft lip before surgical treatment. (**b**) One month using nasal stent orthopedic treatment. (**c**) One year after nasal stent orthopedic treatment. (**d**) Three-year long-term follow-up

References

1. Rossell-Perry P, Romero-Narvaez C, Marca-Ticona R, Figallo-Hudtwalcker O. Are the post-operative nasal conformers in cleft rhinoplasty efficacious?: a systematic review. Cir Plast Iberolatinoam. 2023;49(2):161–6.
2. Tong QJ, Hammer KD, Johnson EM, Zegarra M, Goto M, Lo TS. A systematic review and meta-analysis on the use of prophylactic topical antibiotics for the prevention of uncomplicated wound infections. Infect Drug Resist. 2018;11:417–25.
3. Heal CF, Banks JL, Lepper PD, Kontopantelis E, van Driel ML. Topical antibiotics for preventing surgical site infection in wounds healing by primary intention. Cochrane Database Syst Rev. 2016;11(11):CD011426.
4. Burianova I, Kulihova K, Vitkova V, Janota J. Breastfeeding after early repair of cleft lip in newborn with cleft lip or cleft lip and palate. J Hum Lact. 2017;33(3):504–8.
5. Matsunaka E, Ueki S, Makimoto K. Impact of breastfeeding or bottle-feeding on surgical wound dehiscence after cleft lip repair in infants: a systematic review protocol. JBI Database System Rev Implement Rep. 2015;13(10):3–11.
6. Rossell-Perry P, Romero-Narvaez C, Rojas-Sandoval R, Gomez-Henao P, Delgado-Jimenez MP, Marca-Ticona R. Is the use of opioids safe after primary cleft palate repair? A systematic review. Plast Reconstr Surg Glob Open. 2021;9(1):e3355.
7. Do A, Rorison E, Borucki A, Shibata GS, Pomerantz JH, Hoffman WY. Opioid-free pain management after cleft lip repair. Plast Reconstr Surg Glob Open. 2023;11(9):e5259.
8. Pfaff MJ, Nolan IT, Musavi L, Bertrand AA, Alford J, Krishna V, Arowojolu OA. Zhu X perioperative pain management in cleft lip and palate surgery: a systematic review and meta-analysis of randomized controlled studies. Plast Reconstr Surg. 2022;150(1):145e–56e.
9. Shi Y, Zhang X, Sun Y, Mei E, Wan X, Tian L. Emergence agitation after the cleft lip or palate surgery in pediatric patients: a prospective study. J Stomatol Oral Maxillofac Surg. 2021;122(6):539–43.
10. Cho EJ, Yoon SZ, Cho JE, Lee HW. Comparison of the effects of 0.03 and 0.05 mg/kg midazolam with placebo on prevention of emergence agitation in children having strabismus surgery. Anesthesiology. 2014;120(6):1354–61.
11. Liu D, Pan L, Gao Y, Liu J, Li F, Li X, Quan J, Huang C, Lian C. Efficaciousness of dexmedetomidine in children undergoing cleft lip and palate repair: a systematic review and meta-analysis. BMJ Open. 2021;11(8):e046798.
12. Papathanasiou E, Trotman C, Scott A, Van Dyke T. Current and emerging treatments for post-surgical cleft lip scarring. J Dent Res. 2017;96(12):1370–7.
13. Loftus J, Neale H. Cleft lip micronostril: the problem and proposed solution. Cleft Palate Craniofac Surg J. 1996;33(4):348–51.
14. Rossell-Perry P, Romero-Narvaez C, Gavino-Gutierrez A, Figallo-Hudtwalcker O. Postoperative nasal conformers in cleft rhinoplasty: are they efficacious? J Craniofac Surg. 2023;34(5):1416–9.
15. Monasterio L, Ford A, Gutiérrez C, Tastets ME, García J. Comparative study of nasoalveolar molding methods: nasal elevator plus DynaCleft® versus NAM-Grayson in patients with complete unilateral cleft lip and palate. Cleft Palate Craniofac J. 2013;50(5):548–54.
16. Zhang S, Yang C, Wu M, Yin J, Zeng N, Shi B, et al. Application of a novel nasal clip for nostril retention after primary unilateral cleft rhinoplasty. Cleft Palate Craniofac J. 2023;60(7):851–7.
17. Mejia ML, Pablo Gomez J, Moon SL, et al. 3D infant orthopedic nasal molding system for improved outcomes in cleft nasal deformity. FACE. 2023;4(2):141–7.
18. Wolfe SA, Podda S, Mejia M. Correction of nostril stenosis and alteration of nostril shape with an orthonostric device. Plast Reconstr Surg. 2008;121(6):1974–7.

Cleft Rhinoplasty-Related Complications and Management

10

Percy Rossell-Perry

Contents

P. Rossell-Perry (✉)
Health of Science Faculty, School of Human Medicine, Peruvian University Union (UpeU), Lima, Peru
e-mail: percy.rossell@upeu.edu.pe

P. Rossell-Perry (ed.), *Atlas of Primary Cleft Rhinoplasty*,
https://doi.org/10.1007/978-3-031-68012-0_10

Introduction

The expected results of a nasal surgical intervention cannot be 100% guaranteed because of the multifactorial nature of the tissue response and related perioperative events, which make it difficult to predict the disease evolution with certainty.

Three main factors are associated with the quality of surgical outcomes after cleft rhinoplasty; they are the surgeon, the surgical technique, and the patient. Most likely, the most important of these three is the surgeon's skills, experience, and performance [1]. Regarding the surgical technique, there is not enough evidence about which technique is better than other for primary nasal correction in cleft lip patients. There is a lack of scientific evidence for how to compare different methods of nasal correction in these patients. The patient is the third component, and there is a wide spectrum of characteristics, and the severity of the deformity should be well considered in order to select an adequate treatment. A common cause of poor outcomes is the use of an inadequate surgical technique to repair certain forms of cleft's severity. Certainly, there are other related complications that should be considered as a deficient care of postoperative wounds such as trauma due to falls or a child's ability to handle the wound. In addition, feeding-related events are important, and the aspiration of food is the leading cause of serious postoperative complications during this period, and it is associated with respiratory distress. According to the Smile Train database, postoperative aspiration is the most frequent cause of "sentinel events" (serious complications). With more than 30 years of experience in Lima, Perú, the rates of unilateral cleft lip revision were 10.1% and 21.6%, respectively, for bilateral cleft lip [2]. In a study published by the author including 1640 operated cases between 2001 and 2017, 7.22% of major nasal revisions were unilateral cleft lip surgeries and 19.40% of major nasal revisions were in bilateral cleft lip surgeries [3] (Figs. 10.1 and 10.2). The first step in the interdisciplinary management of the nasal secondary deformities is the physical examination and diagnosis as well as the adequate time for its correction. The most important aspects of the reconstructed nose to be considered are as follows:

(a) Projection of the nasal tip
(b) Symmetry of the nose
(c) Nasal columellar characteristics
(d) Symmetry and width of the nasal bases
(e) Vestibule of the nose characteristics
(f) Presence of scar contractures and synechiae
(g) Nasal septum characteristics
(h) Nasal valve function

It has been considered that better outcomes can be achieved at an early age, allowing the rehabilitation of patients who are integrated into society. The author suggested that the secondary correction of the nose should be performed before school age to avoid the psychological impact of the deformity during that age. This is in contrast to conventional protocols that recommend waiting for skeletal maturity in patient to

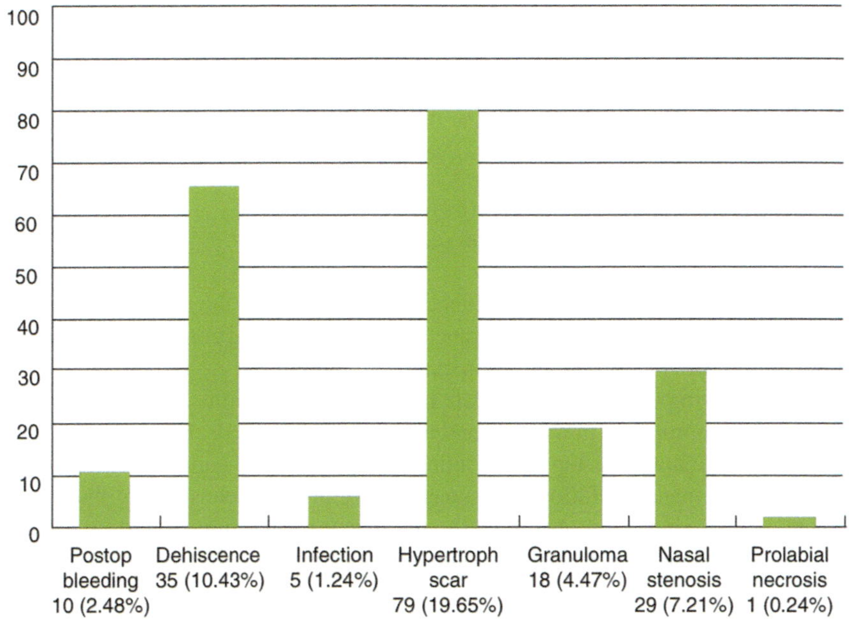

Fig. 10.1 Bad outcomes in bilateral cleft lip nose repair (n:183/623–29.37%)

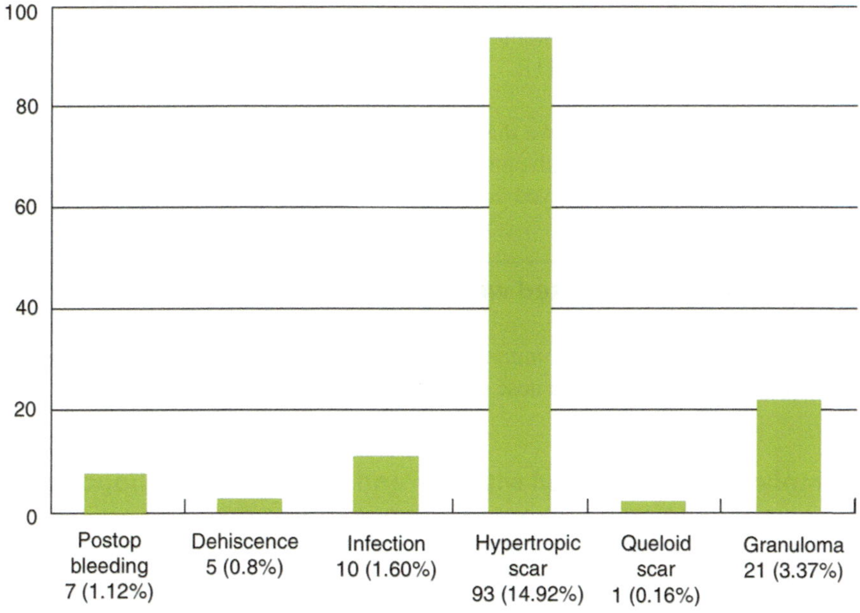

Fig. 10.2 Bad outcomes in unilateral cleft lip nose repair (n:207/402–51.49%)

correct these sequelae; therefore, there is no consensus regarding the ideal age. However, the time when the patient should be treated may depend on the following:

(a) Anesthetic evaluation
(b) Severity of the secondary aesthetic deformity
(c) Associated functional disorder
(d) Psychological impact
(e) Impact of the surgery on facial growth
(f) Complications associated with the secondary treatment

Although there is frequently a functional component, the nose deformity is closely related to the aesthetic appearance and psychological complications associated with the patient's social inclusion and development.

Finally, it is important to differentiate between complications and poor outcomes to determine appropriate prevention and management methods. For example, nasal scar contracture may develop due to a predisposition of the patient (complication) and should be managed following a conservative protocol considering that a new surgery is contraindicated. Additionally, nasal scar contracture caused by a badly positioned incision (a poor outcome) may require surgical correction.

Complication Complication is an event that occurs in the course of a surgical act and is different from the usual manifestations of this complication and is a consequence of the associated effects [1].

Poor Outcome This is an unwanted effect of the surgery that does not achieve the objectives set before surgery [1].

Based on these concepts, we may also consider that also the bad outcomes can be prevented but not all complications can be prevented. I described here the most common complications observed during 30 years of experience as a cleft surgeon.

Complications Associated with Primary Cleft Rhinoplasty

The following are the most common associated complications observed during our experience managing cleft lip nose deformity.

Complications Associated with Pre- and Postsurgical Orthopedics

Presurgical orthopedics are an alternative for cleft lip surgery management used to position the alveolar segments and premaxilla and also the nose is also molded by nasal stents or hooks depending on the device used. One of the most currently used methods is the nasoalveolar molding (NAM) described by Grayson [4]. This method is not free from complications among which the following have been reported.

Aspiration of the Impression Material

This is one of the most serious complications although it is infrequent. When this procedure is indicated, the parents must sign an informed consent form where related complications are described. If this complication occurs, the patient requires urgent attention due to respiratory distress and may require ventilatory support in the ICU. The use of three-dimensional technology for the design of the plates allows us to avoid this complication [5].

Skin Irritation and Pressure Sores

This is the most frequently associated complication (up to 36%) [6, 7]; using this technology and contact dermatitis may be observed with the concomitant use of tapes. Cases of skin ulcers due to pressure sores caused by the action of the nasal stent have also been reported (Fig. 10.3).

Nasal Bleeding

It is associated with pressure ulceration and skin damage of the nasal conformer.

Associated Infections

Candidiasis and a greater risk for dental caries development have been associated with the use of the presurgical nasoalveolar molding appliances. In a study published by Yilmaz et al., they observed that the appliance might not only cause an increase in the colonization of *C. albicans* but also provide the continuation of the colonization [8, 9]. Plates should be removed daily and cleaned.

Children's Stress

These are associated with the complications mentioned above which leads to stress in children whose impact on their health has not been well estimated [7].

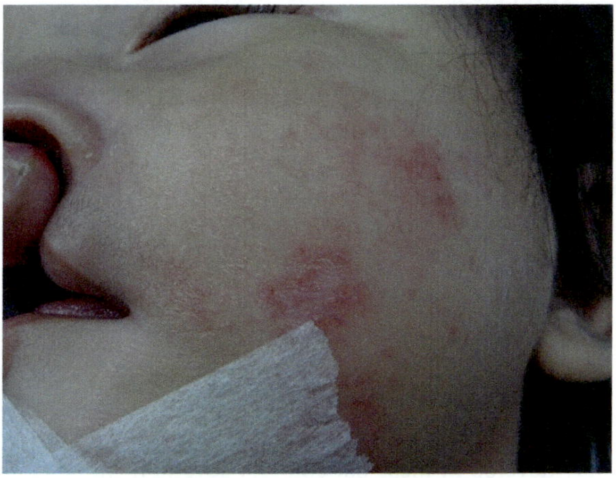

Fig. 10.3 Skin irritation during using NAM

Complications in Primary Cleft Rhinoplasty

The following are the most common complications associated with primary cleft rhinoplasty.

Postoperative Bleeding

The nose has a rich blood supply; therefore, this complication should be considered. In primary cleft lip nose surgery, we observed a rate of 1.12% (unilateral) and 2.48% (bilateral), and these complications may be associated with the surgeon's experience and surgical technique [2]. Fillies reported an average of 21 ml of blood loss and 0.2% of reported cases in relation to cleft lip and nose surgery [6]. Doyle and Hudson reported the need for blood transfusion in approximately 10% of the operated cleft lip and nose patients [10]. The common causes of postoperative bleeding after primary cleft rhinoplasty are poor hemostasis, excessive and persistent crying, lack of nasal packing, coagulopathy, infection, associated primary septoplasty, and uncontrolled pain [1]. The most common issue is probably patient agitation after surgery; for this reason, pain control is essential, and in some cases, associated sedation and the use of dexmedetomidine are indicated [11]. Postoperative nasal bleeding may be associated with other complications such as bruising, hematomas, aspiration, and vomiting. The recommended treatment of bleeding is usually conservative; doing gentle compression and hemostasis in the operating room is rarely necessary. Prevention is also important and nasal packing after surgery is strongly recommended [1]. Anterior nasal packing (vestibular) is performed after surgery and the technique used is described as follows:

1. The nasal pack is prepared by smearing it with antibiotic ointment. It is very important to use a long pack to avoid displacement outside or inside the nose.
2. The nasal vestibule is cleaned by removing fluids and clots.
3. Then, the nondominant hand and a double skin hook are used to push the tip of the nose to expose the nasal vestibule.
4. The pack is inserted first medially against the caudal septum (medial wall of the vestibule) and then against the lateral wall in the horizontal plane, parallel to the nasal floor until the end of the pack, filling the nasal vestibule.

The nasal packing is removed slowly the day before the surgery, and some bleeding may occur if the baby cries but rarely requires new packing and stops spontaneously.

If bleeding occurs and the patient does not have a nasal pack, it is recommended that the patient be placed under anesthesia in the operating room.

Hypertrophic Scarring

This is another common complication and severe aesthetic and functional problems may develop in these patients. Its development (as a complication) depends on the patient's idiosyncratic reaction and is also associated with scar disorders and the use of vestibular incisions during primary rhinoplasty (Figs. 10.4, 10.5, 10.6 and 10.7).

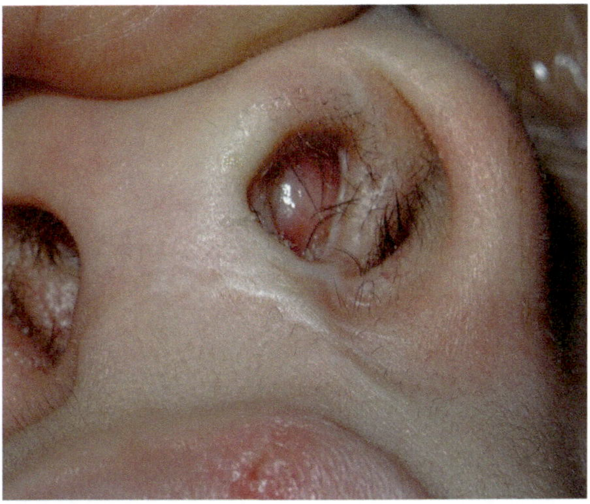

Fig. 10.4 Vestibular scar contracture left nostril after primary cleft rhinoplasty

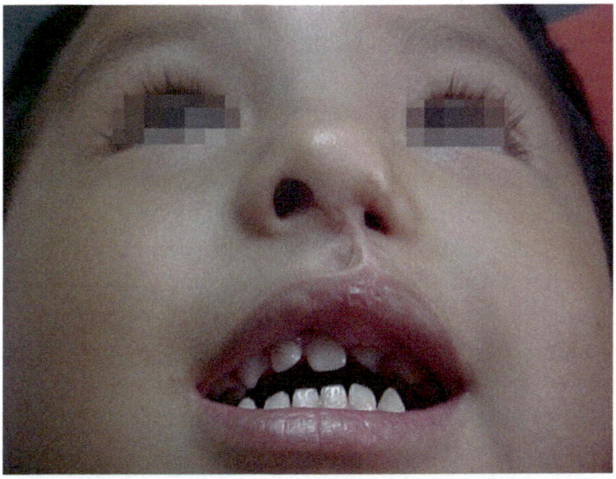

Fig. 10.5 Severe scar contracture of the nose and lip after primary cleft cheilorhinoplasty

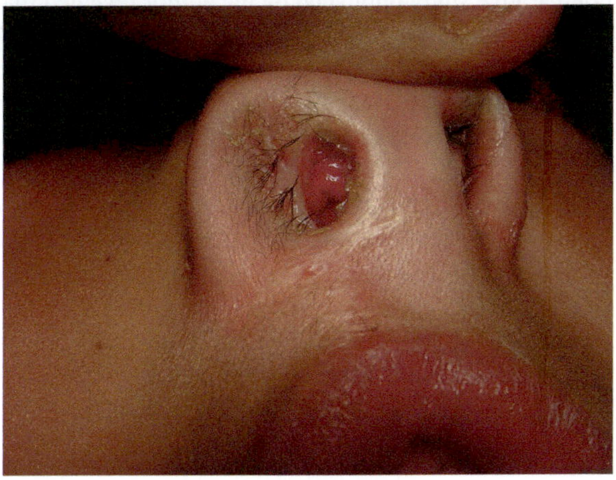

Fig. 10.6 Postoperative scar contracture after primary cleft rhinoplasty (preoperative view)

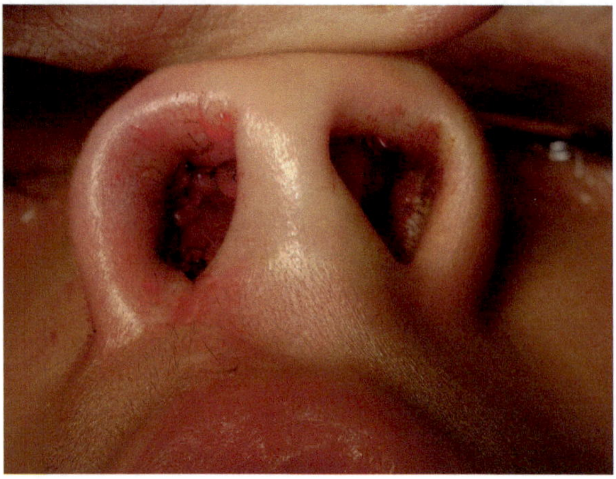

Fig. 10.7 Immediate postoperative view in case in Fig. 10.6 after correction of the scar contracture using the V-Y-Z surgical technique

This complication can occur more frequently because of the increased popularity of primary nasal surgery in cleft patients. The development of keloids after primary cleft rhinoplasty is quite rare in these patients. In severe forms, nostril stenosis and vestibular synechia can occur creating nasal obstruction and breathing problems. A study published by the author comparing different techniques for primary nasal repair in cleft lip patients concluded that the development of this complication is associated with the type of surgical technique used [3]. The following factors must be considered: the severity of the skeletal deformity, the functional nature of the scar (nasal vestibule synechia requires early care), and the severity of the aesthetic deformity (early correction may prevent the development of psychological sequelae). In addition, an increased risk of hypertrophic reaction of the scar was observed in patients after 8 years of age [12]. Based on my personal experience, any hypertrophic scar that generates functional retraction and aesthetic deformity must be treated at early before school time, so it does not affect the psychosocial development of the child during that time. Prevention of this complication is essential, and the use of postoperative nasal conformers must be used after primary cleft rhinoplasty. Another comparative study published by the author revealed that the group using postoperative conformers developed fewer scar contracture problems [3]. Early conservative treatment is indicated because this complication is mostly related to the patient's condition; however if the problem persists, surgery is indicated.

The basic principles of the treatment of this sequela are as follows:

- A period of time must be allowed (at least 1 year). Conservative treatment is always the first line of treatment. Silicone gel or patches work well. Infiltration using intralesional corticoids is performed in patients who are refractory to the silicone treatment.
- Surgical treatment is indicated only for patients who are refractory to conservative treatment and after 1 year postoperatively.

We used the V-Y-Z technique to release the retraction produced by the scar [13]. The incisions should be limited as much as possible to the scar tissue preserving healthy tissue and preventing a more severe recurrence of the scar disorder (Figs. 10.6 and 10.7).

Nonsurgical treatments such as dermabrasion, pulsed light, or lasers appear to be useful for correcting cleft lip scars; however, more studies are required to demonstrate their efficacy.

The author published a recent study to evaluate long-term follow-up after primary cleft rhinoplasty during the mixed dentition period and reported that 12.5% of patients had scar contracture and 6.25% had synechia [14].

Postoperative Wound Infection

This is not a common complication. Alef et al. observed 4.6% of infection after primary rhinoplasty [15]. These events occur 3–5 days after surgery and include inflammation, bleeding, and pain. Late infections can generally occur in association with a foreign body. Infection is caused by the breakdown of the balance between the tissue response and the pathogen. In review of more than 3000 patients in India, it revealed an infection rate of 1.1% after surgery [16]. A study published by Nagy in 2011 reported 2.6% infection [17].

The infected wound presents fever, a local inflammatory reaction, and edema that begins after 3–4 days postoperatively and evolves with purulent drainage and dehiscence of the operative wound. Most of cases evolve well with conventional treatment, and this complication should be managed promptly since severe cases can be associated with serious complications such as venous sinus thrombosis, meningitis, and sepsis [18]. Infected stitches are caused mostly by bacteria and common types of bacteria that can infect surgical wounds are *Streptococcus*, *Staphylococcus*, and *Pseudomonas* species [19]. Factors that may increase the risk of infection include inadequate wound cleaning after surgery, weakened immune system, and accidental trauma (Fig. 10.8).

Routinely I use amoxicillin or dicloxacillin for the initial treatment of the infection. If an antibiogram reveals an infection caused by a MRSA (methicillin-resistant *Staphylococcus aureus*) bacterium, a specific antibiotic treatment should be initiated [20]. The parenteral route is reserved for patients with oral intolerance. Prevention of the wound infection is based on an adequate surgical technique that provides good blood supply for the operated tissues. Postoperative antibiotic prophylaxis antibiotics are commonly used during that period; however, there is no scientific evidence to support this practice. The antimicrobial protocol review from the Greater Glasgow and Clyde Committee recommends the use of 5 days of postoperative antibiotics with amoxicillin clavulanic acid or clindamycin (in allergic patients) [21].

Suture abscess is a more common type of infection after primary cleft rhinoplasty. These abscesses develop as a result of suture infection. The suture material reacts with connective tissue, generating an inflammatory process and initial adhesion around the stitch. Then, increased redness around the wound or skin color changes and pus or bleeding from the wound occurs. Treatment is usually

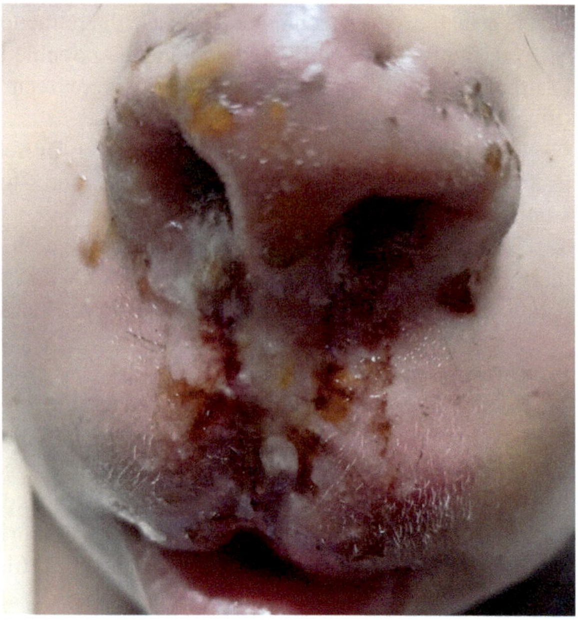

Fig. 10.8 A 3-year-old female patient who developed wound infection after primary bilateral cleft lip and nose repair

conservative and lesions resolve spontaneously after suture resorption. Abscess drainage and antibiotics are indicated for major and persistent lesions (Fig. 10.9).

Preoperatory use of antibiotics is also under discussion. A common protocol is the use of a single dose of first-generation cephalosporin 1 h before the operation, and cefazolin is recommended (25 mg/Kg). In allergic patients, vancomycin is an alternative (15 mg/Kg) [21]. A recent literature review and meta-analysis concluded that more studies are required to understand the utility of antibiotic prophylaxis in plastic surgery [21–23].

Granulomas

This complication is generated by a reaction to the use of surgical sutures. It is characterized by a bright red bleeding tumor at the suture site and is composed of granulation tissue (collagen fibers, fibroblasts, and blood vessels) [24]. Treatment is usually conservative since the granuloma disappears when the suture is reabsorbed although the need for removal is rare. Only when the suture is nonabsorbable, its removal is mandatory (Figs. 10.10, 10.11 and 10.12). As an alternative, the use of silver nitrate bars may be useful for cauterizing the granuloma by reducing the bleeding until the lesion resolves. The author published a recent study evaluating long-term follow-up after primary cleft rhinoplasty during the mixed dentition period and reported that 15.6% were granuloma [14].

Foreign Body

Foreign body complications after primary cleft rhinoplasty are usually related to the use of sutures (mentioned previously) and packs during surgery. They may remain inside the nose unnoticed during some time. Surgical bleeding can mask the gauze

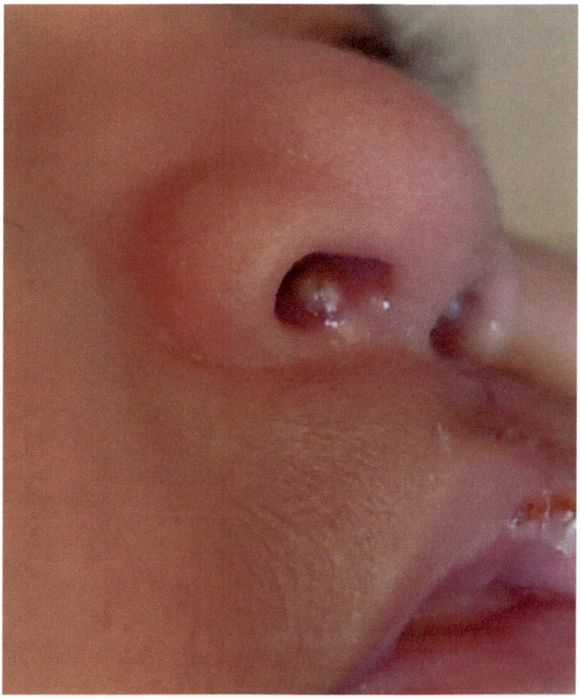

Fig. 10.9 Suture abscess developed after primary cleft rhinoplasty in a 3-month-old patient with unilateral cleft lip. Lesion resolved spontaneously after suture absorption

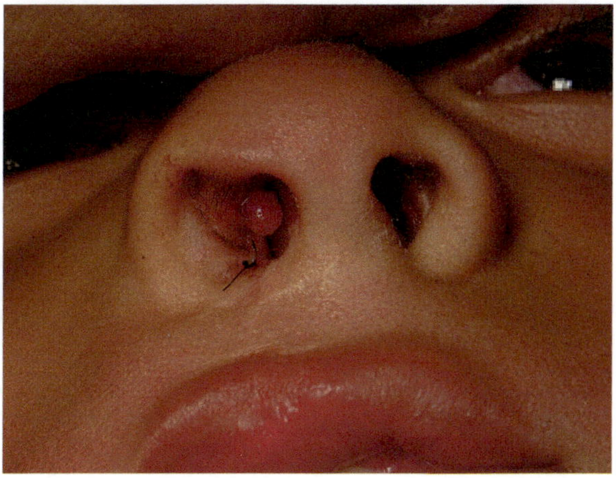

Fig. 10.10 Development of granuloma at the nasal vestibule after unilateral primary cleft rhinoplasty associated with the use of nonabsorbable sutures

and cannot be detected by the surgeon. This complication is characterized by a bad smell through the nose and may be associated with infection and bleeding. The diagnosis is sometimes difficult and may require the use of a rhinoscope. Treatment is based on foreign body removal which can be performed easily when the detection is performed early. For long-term foreign bodies, removal is more difficult because of the strong tissue adhesion. Its removal is associated with bleeding, and this procedure should be performed in operating room under general anesthesia. Antibiotic

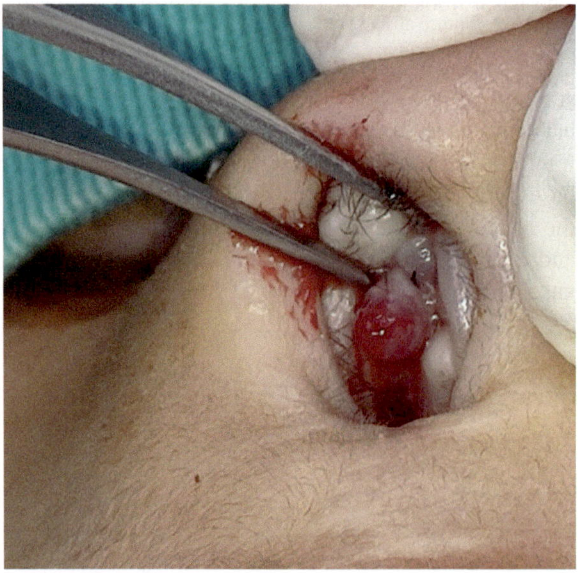

Fig. 10.11 Skin granuloma in the nasal vestibule developed after primary cleft rhinoplasty

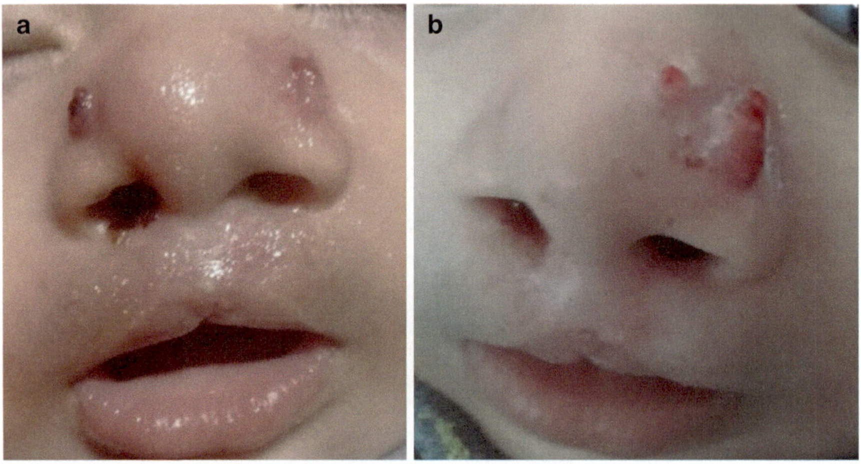

Fig. 10.12 Development of severe skin granulomas after primary cleft rhinoplasty. The lesions resolved spontaneously after suture resorption. (**a**) Frontal view. (**b**) Lateral view

treatment is recommended for 5–7 days. Other complications include synechiae, septal perforation, sinusitis, and local infections.

Skin Necrosis

It is a rare complication after primary cleft rhinoplasty and related to tissue compression or use of excessive alar transcutaneous stitches. The use of adhesive tape over the nasal tip or postoperative nasal shapers may create some pressure on the nasal tissues involved in surgery, affecting their blood supply. In addition, when excessive transcutaneous stitches are used, alar necrosis may develop. Another factor associated with this complication is the postoperative infection although nasal skin necrosis which is rare is characterized by columellar, tip, or alar skin paleness and later darkening resulting in severe aesthetic and functional sequelae. The recommended treatment is conservative and involves the use of topical antibiotics until the lesion is delimited and is reduced later by scar contracture. After this, the reconstructive strategy can be properly planned.

Suture Allergic Reaction

Another rare complication. Suture hypersensitivity is associated with the duration of suture absorption. Treatment is based on topical creams and oral antihistamines to reduce inflammation and symptoms. In severe cases, corticoid injections and suture removal may be necessary. PDS (polydioxanone), the suture used by the author for primary cleft rhinoplasty, is completely absorbed after 180 days and may be associated with granuloma and allergic reactions. In our experience, increased rate of hypersensitivity, granuloma, and infection have been observed in patients treated with vicryl.

The following complications may also be considered poor outcomes and are frequently observed after primary rhinoplasty using transcutaneous stitches and vestibular lengthening.

Dimples

This is produced by skin traction of the transcutaneous stitch when the needle does not return through the same cutaneous hole. Even a temporal defect, this may be associated with the development of granulomas. Both are resolved when the suture is reabsorbed and mostly represent a common parental complaint during the early postoperative period. This complication rarely creates a permanent problem.

Notching (Pinched nose)

Commonly, this is observed after cosmetic rhinoplasty when excessive amounts of alar cartilage are removed from the tip of the nose; however, this is not a conventional maneuver during primary cleft rhinoplasty because the cartilage is preserved. Notching after primary cleft rhinoplasty can occur secondary to wound contraction of the nasal tissue or postoperative associated complications such as infections (Fig. 10.13). This problem may also occur after primary cleft rhinoplasty in association with vestibular lengthening techniques (such as VYZ rhinoplasty and Potter's). The medial displacement of the alar cartilage used in these methods creates a lateral structural deficiency similar to that of cartilage resection during rhinoplasty. This problem requires cartilage grafts for its correction (Figs. 10.14, 10.15 and 10.16).

Lateral Web

Lateral vestibular webbing is a common problem after primary cleft rhinoplasty and may be considered as a poor outcome compared with surgical complication. The lateral web observed after nasal correction in patients with cleft lip is in fact a soft tissue

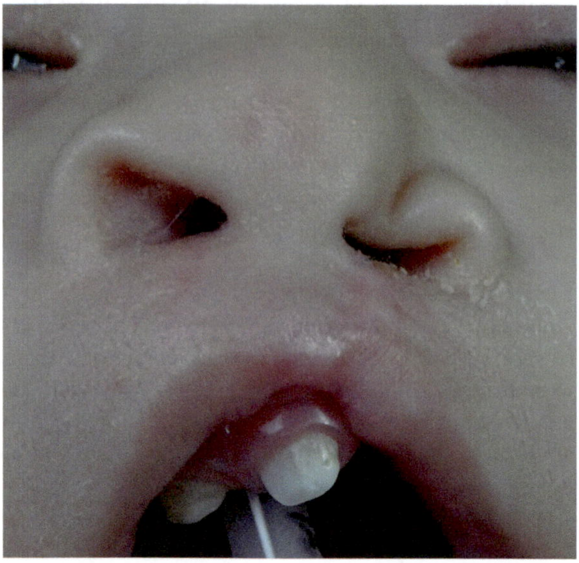

Fig. 10.13 Pinched nose after primary cleft rhinoplasty using the V-Y technique

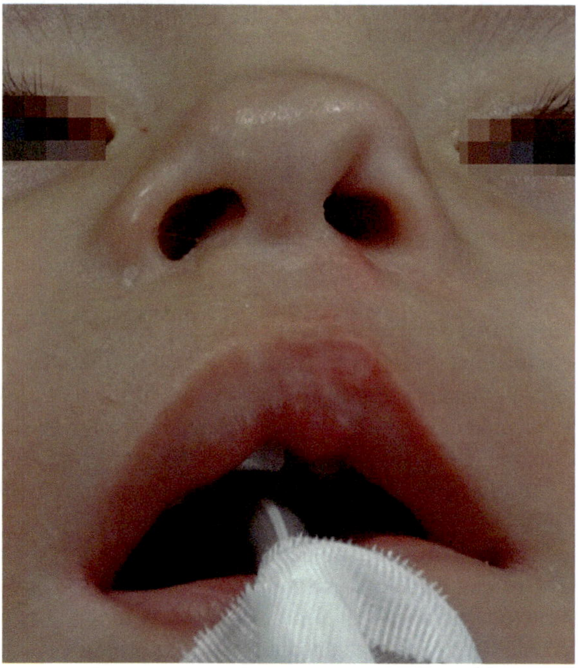

Fig. 10.14 Nasal tip notching after primary cleft rhinoplasty using the V-Y-Z technique

deficiency rather than tissue excess as some authors propose (Figs. 10.17 and 10.18). A migration and caudal overgrowth of the alar cartilage is also produced in this problem; the prolapsed alar cartilage overhangs the nasal vestibule. This is associated with scar contracture of the skin nasal vestibule and may explain the nose relapse after primary correction; however, it is important to differentiate the skin lateral web from

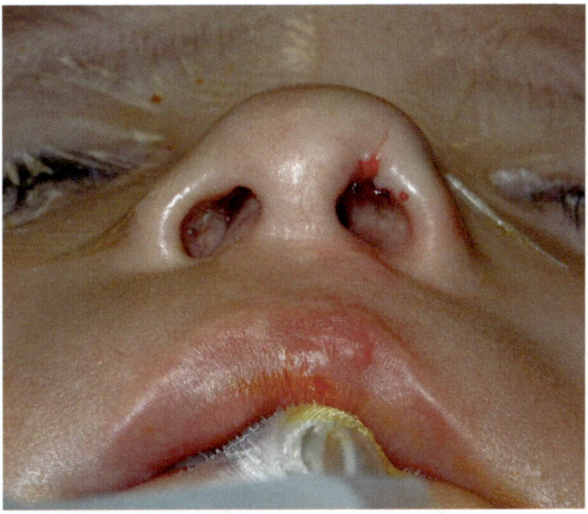

Fig. 10.15 Immediate postoperative view after nasal tip notching correction using auricular cartilage graft

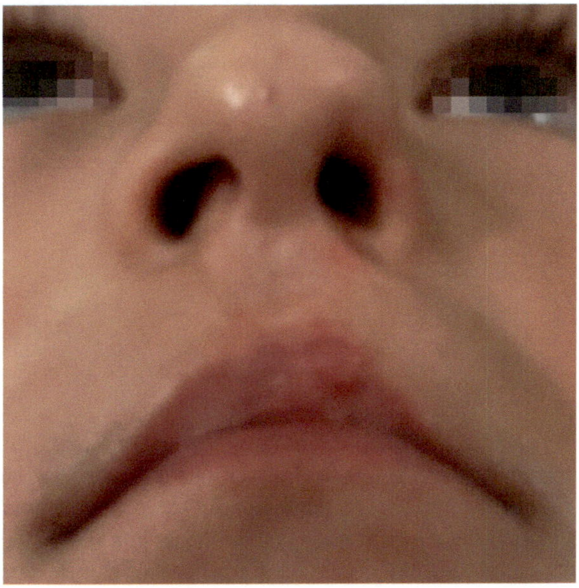

Fig. 10.16 A 5-year long-term follow-up of the patient's corrected nose presented in Fig. 10.14

the nasal deformity relapse which requires skin and cartilage reposition. Some authors reported different methods as the direct skin excision, Z plasty, and reverse U incisional plus V-Y advancement. Agarwal and Chandra [25] consider the existence of hypertrophied caudal border of the alar cartilage as an additional component of the deformity; therefore, they recommend cartilage excision to correct the web and prevent relapse during the growth. However, there is not a consensus regarding the hypertrophied nature of the cleft side alar cartilage, and this method may produce a lack of structural support developing another complication like pinched nose. Other authors like Mulliken recommend the skin excision of the lateral web; however, he does not

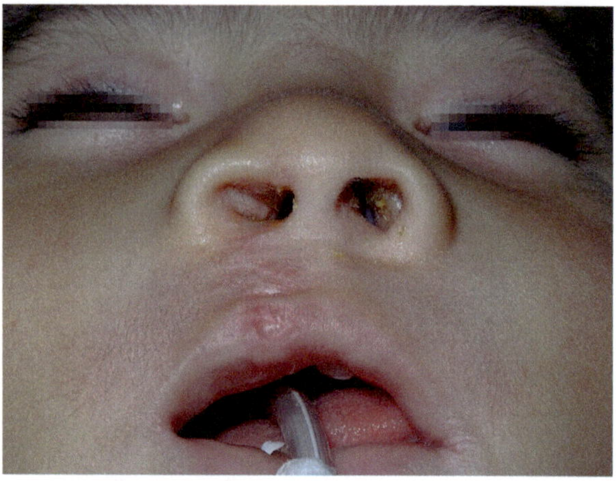

Fig. 10.17 Right nostril lateral web developed after primary unilateral cleft rhinoplasty using Mc Comb modified technique

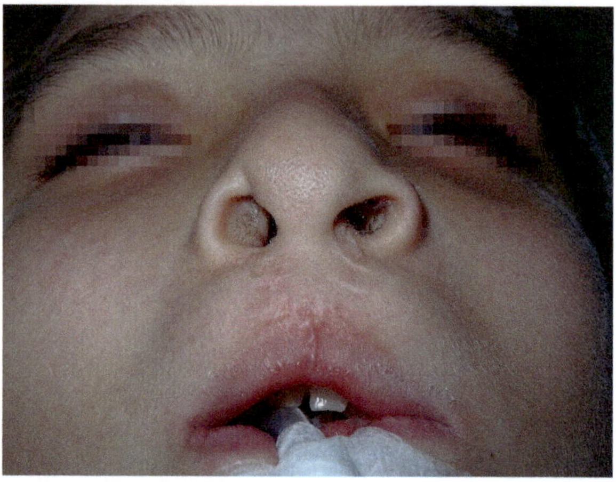

Fig. 10.18 Right nostril lateral web developed after primary bilateral cleft rhinoplasty using Mc Comb modified technique

support this method with long-term outcomes [26]. Cho [27] performed a reverse U incision plus V-Y advancement of the alar cartilage. The alar web is observed more frequently after using the Mc Comb-type techniques and may be prevented by lengthening of the nasal vestibule [3]. In the author's consideration, its treatment should be based on vestibular lengthening instead of skin resection which only worsens this condition. The VYZ primary cleft rhinoplasty lengthens the nasal vestibule (the surgical nasal molding effect) preventing the lateral web and explaining the low rate of this complication using this method. In addition, the use of nasal stents (i.e., orthonostric device) helps prevent the relapse of the lateral web.

Poor Outcomes Associated with Unilateral Primary Cleft Rhinoplasty

The characteristics of the secondary deformity of the nose depend on many factors including the nature of the primary surgery, the surgeon's performance, cleft lip severity, and the antecedents of postoperative complications. Adequate primary correction of the nose will reduce the need for secondary surgeries, and actually, there is a consensus regarding the efficacy and safety of primary correction of the nose during cleft lip repair. The psychosocial impact of facial deformities in children must be well considered during early life.

The secondary unilateral cleft lip nasal deformity presented the following characteristics (Figs. 10.19, 10.20 and 10.21):

- Malposition of the affected alar cartilage with the consequent asymmetry and lack of nasal tip projection. It is important to understand that there is no a cartilage deficiency; it is only displaced.
- Columellar shortening and malpositioning. "Short" columella on the cleft side as a result of the lateral displacement of the affected alar cartilage. In fact, this is not short; it is "hidden in the nose" as Mulliken noted for bilateral cleft lips. The same condition is observed in unilateral cleft lips; therefore for surgical planning, it is important to consider that lengthening of the columella is not necessary, only the alar cartilage repositioning.
- Ectopic insertion of the labial nasal muscles.
- Nasal septum deviation.
- Maxillary hypoplasia and malocclusion.

As I mentioned before, I believe that any severe aesthetic or functional affection should be treated at an early age, that is, before school age, to prevent the psychosocial impact of these conditions. This position contrasts with conventional conservative management which delays the treatment after skeletal correction (bone

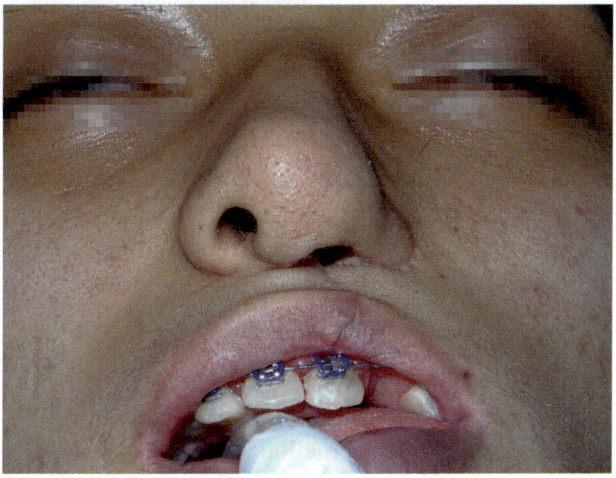

Fig. 10.19 Secondary nasal deformity of the unilateral cleft lip

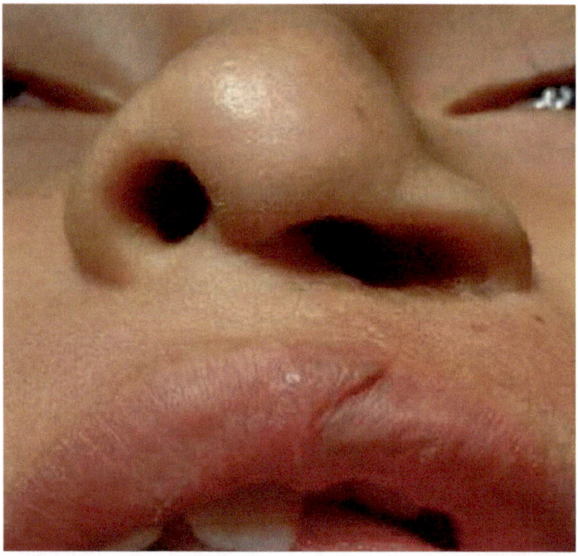

Fig. 10.20 Secondary nasal deformity of the unilateral cleft lip

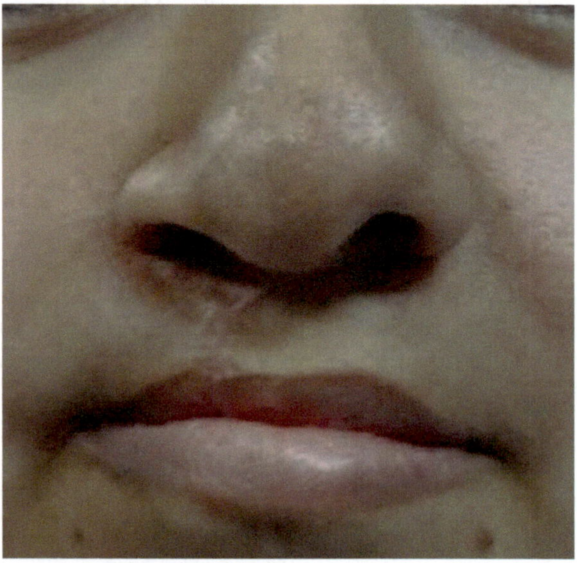

Fig. 10.21 Secondary nasal deformity of the unilateral cleft lip

maturity completion age). Any minor deformity may be delayed in order to avoid the negative effect of the anesthesia on the development of the child.

The main objective of secondary cleft rhinoplasty is to correct nasal asymmetry and function, which may be achieved following these principles:

- Alar cartilage reposition
- Correction of the alar base position
- Correction of the nasal septum deviation
- Alveolar cleft reconstruction

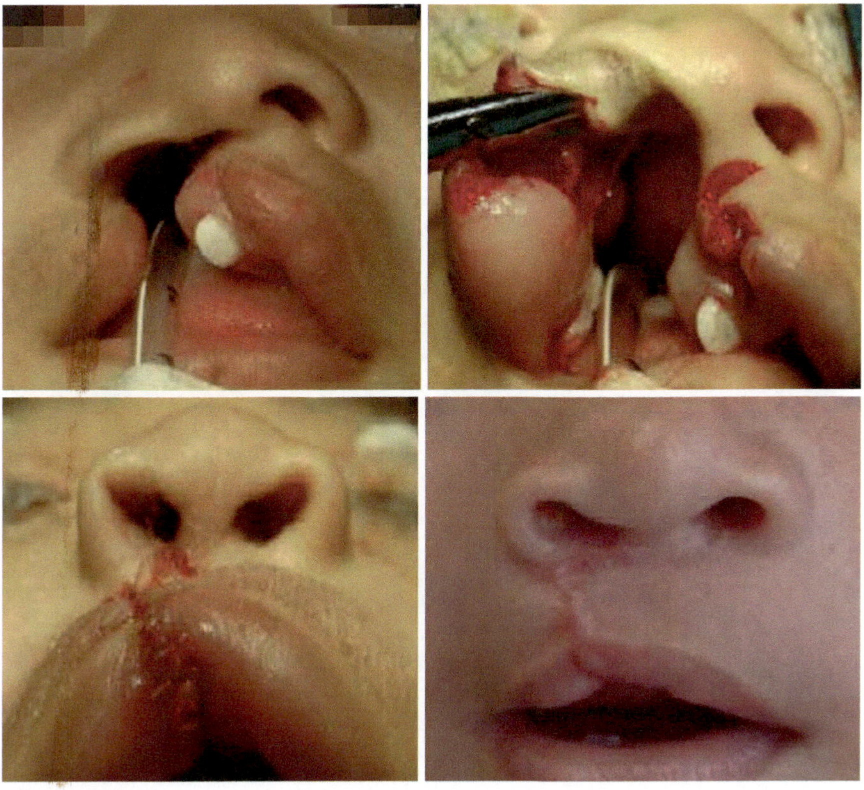

Fig. 10.22 Nose relapse after primary cleft rhinoplasty using Mc Comb modification technique. Upper left: Unilateral complete cleft lip and palate. Upper right: Nasal tip dissection using the Mc Comb modification technique. Lower left: Immediate postoperative view of the nose. Lower right: Postoperative view after 3 years observing relapse of the nose

The most common poor outcome after primary cleft rhinoplasty is the nose deformity relapse. I do not agree with other authors who consider that relapse is due to cartilage memory because a significant number of our patients had a low rate of relapse. We personally believe that the relapse is mostly associated with deficiencies in the surgical procedure [14] (Fig. 10.22). In another study published by the author, we observed an increased rate of nose deformity relapse using conservative methods for primary cleft rhinoplasty, such as Mc Comb [28]. In a recent study published by the author, it is observed that 34.37% of total nostril symmetry and minor revisions were required in 56.26% of the studied patients [14] Yao and Mulliken reported that 65% of unilateral cleft patients underwent nasal revision after primary cleft nose repair, and Salyer observed a lower revision rate of 35% [29, 30].

Next, I present the poor outcomes associated with primary cleft rhinoplasty according to the affected anatomical segment.

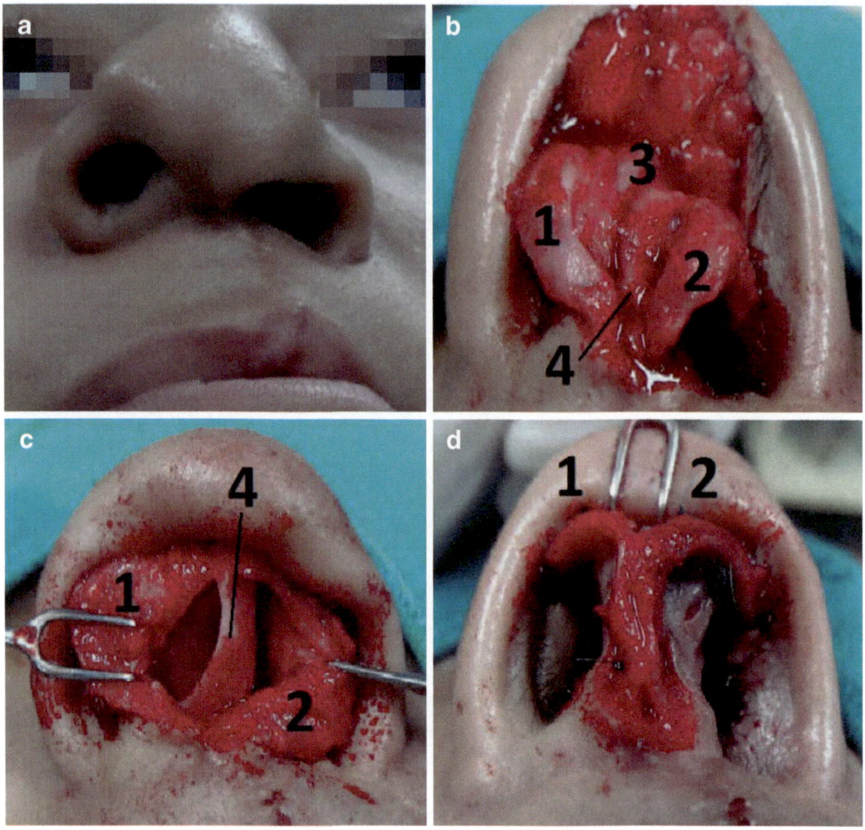

Fig. 10.23 Nasal tip asymmetry after primary cleft rhinoplasty. (**a**) Preoperative view illustrating the nasal tip asymmetry after primary repair. (**b**) Cartilaginous structure of the asymmetric nose: 1. Nasal septum. 2. Nasal dorsum. 3. Cleft side alar cartilage. 4. Noncleft side alar cartilage. (**c**) 1. Noncleft side alar cartilage. 2. Cleft side alar cartilage. 3. Nasal dorsum (nonvisible in this view). 4. Deviated nasal septum. (**d**) Appearance of cartilaginous structure after septoplasty. 1 and 2. Alar cartilages

Nasal Tip

Asymmetry, lack of tip projection, and a pinched nose are common bad outcomes after primary cleft rhinoplasty (Figs. 10.23, 10.24 and 10.25). Relapse of the nasal deformity occurs mostly due to surgical deficiency. The author addresses nasal tip asymmetries based on vestibular lengthening to prevent the scar contracture and deformity recurrence. Different surgical techniques used for treating secondary deformities are based on vestibular lengthening and alar cartilage repositioning, as well as the Potter's and Cronin's techniques [31, 32]. These methods allow the nasal cartilage to be repositioned, resulting in symmetry of the nasal tip. My personal technique is based on the combination of Potter's technique and Berkeley's lateral Z plasty in combination with septoplasty to improve respiratory obstruction [31, 33]. This is the same method described by the author for primary cleft rhinoplasty

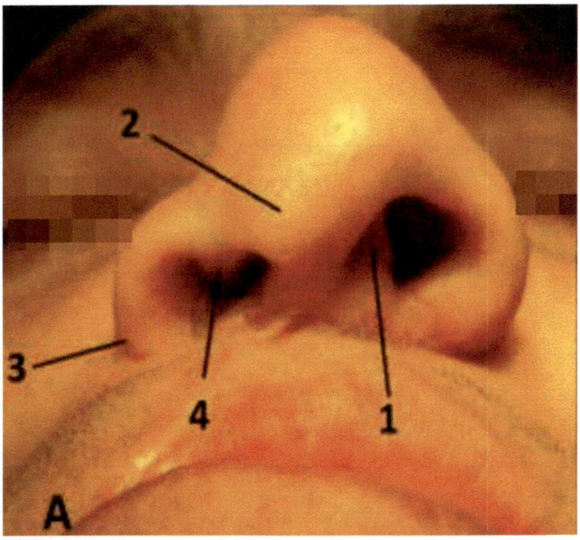

Fig. 10.24 Nasal tip asymmetry after unilateral primary cleft rhinoplasty. 1. Deviated nasal septum. 2. Nasal tip asymmetry. 3. Alae. 4. Nostril

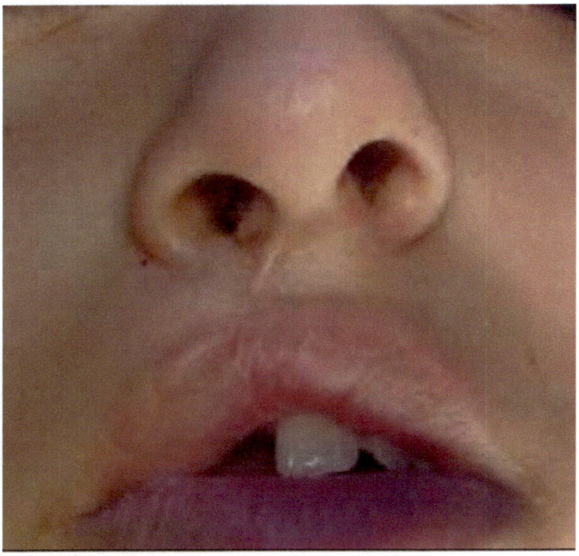

Fig. 10.25 Nasal tip asymmetry after primary cleft rhinoplasty

[13]. Cartilaginous grafts are used to reinforce the area from which the alar cartilage has been displaced medially using the V-Y technique. The surgical approach is left to the surgeon's preference and can be performed openly or closed. Open rhinoplasty has the advantage of allowing direct access to the septum after dissection between both medial crura. Minor deformities can be corrected using the rotational composite flap technique, which is another method that the author describes initially in the correction of primary incomplete cleft lip nasal deformities. Another technique used by the author is the Nakajima's vestibular Z plasty which is described for the treatment of secondary deformities [34] (Fig. 10.26). Recently the author

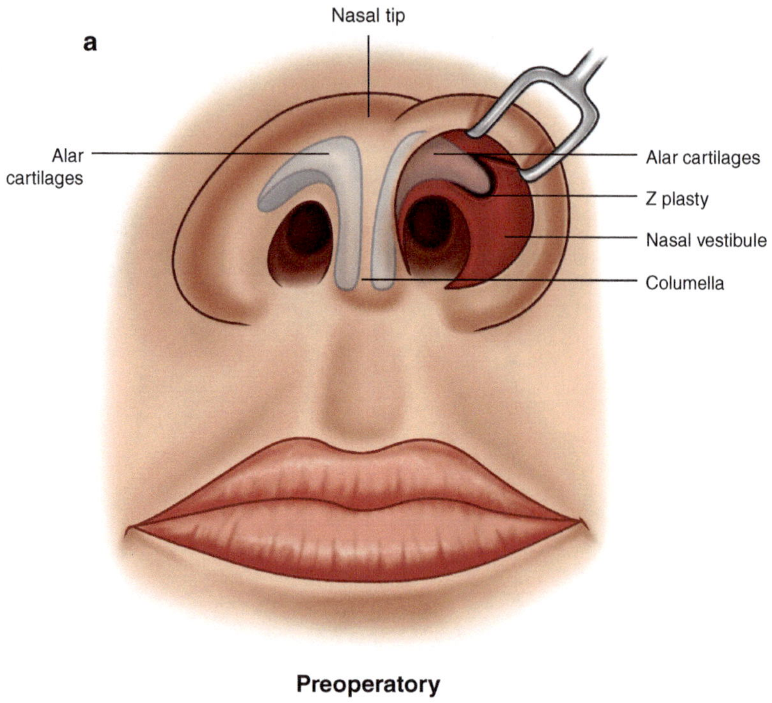

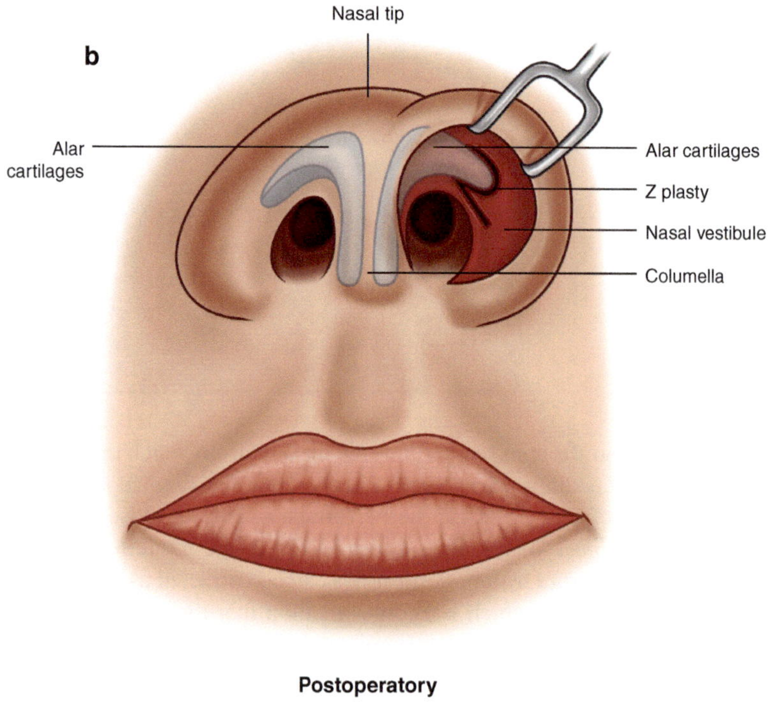

Fig. 10.26 (**a**, **b**) Nakajima technique for secondary cleft nasal deformity

(P.R.P) published an innovative method resecting small portion of vestibular skin for minor secondary deformities (Figs. 10.27, 10.28, 10.29 and 10.30).

The pinched nose is another poor outcome and this is associated with a lack of structural support. It is a permanent sinking of the vestibular wall, obstructing the nostril and creating an alar groove. Removal or medial displacement of the alar cartilage may produce this outcome. Surgical techniques such as VYZ rhinoplasty used the medial displacement of the alar cartilage and when this procedure is performed aggressively. It requires surgical treatment, and it is based on cartilage grafts placed below the nasal skin at the level of the donor site of the displaced alar cartilage.

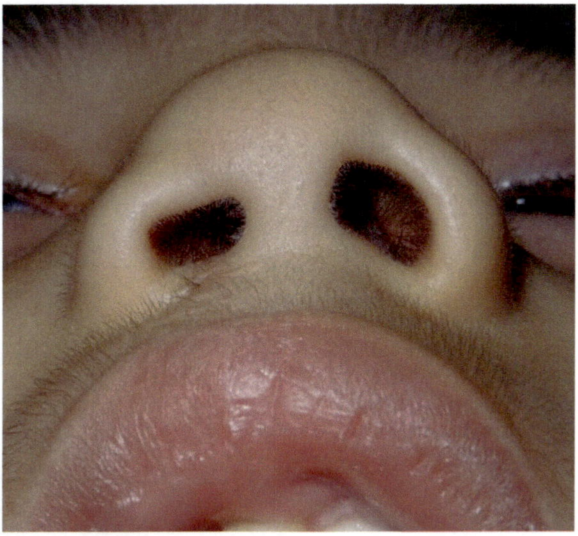

Fig. 10.27 A 5-year-old male patient with nasal tip asymmetry after unilateral primary cleft rhinoplasty

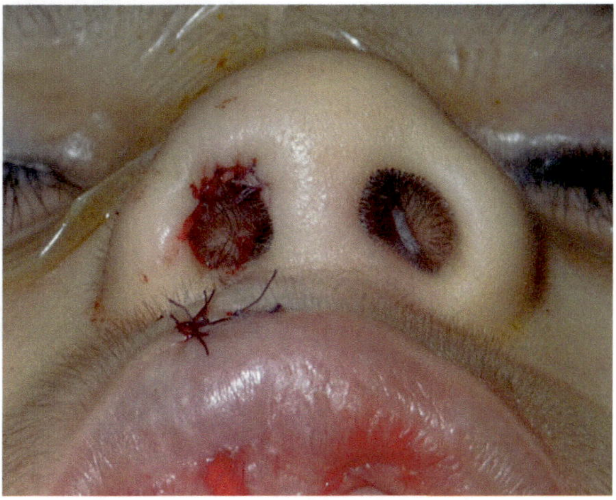

Fig. 10.28 Immediate postoperative after nasal tip correction using the semilunar vestibular skin resection method

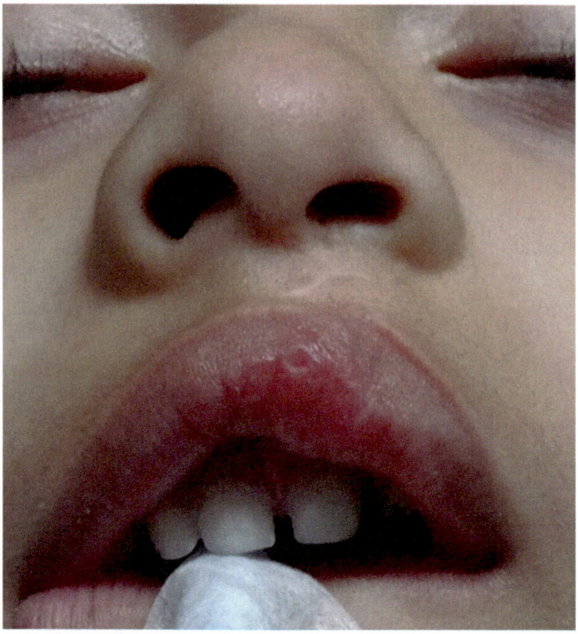

Fig. 10.29 Mild nasal tip asymmetry after primary cleft rhinoplasty in a patient with incomplete cleft lip

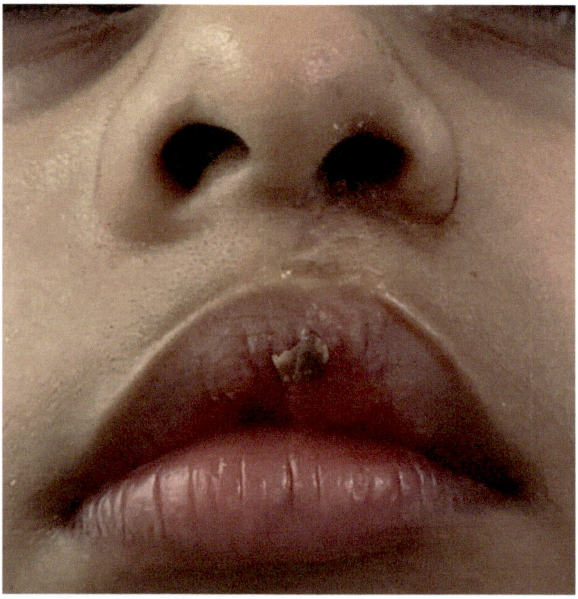

Fig. 10.30 Mild nasal tip asymmetry in a patient with incomplete cleft lip after correction using the vestibular marginal skin excision

Nasal Ala

Most likely, it is the most common component associated with bad outcomes after primary cleft rhinoplasty. The asymmetry of the ala is observed due to its position (lower, higher, or shortened). This nondesirable outcome can be prevented performing an adequate preoperative lip marking, preserving the integrity and location of the base of the ala. Sometimes, the subnasal sulcus is not clearly visible; its location can be easily located by flexion of the ala during preoperative marking. The diagnosis is made through careful physical examination of the lip, and the difference between the position of the cleft and noncleft alar bases will determine the diagnosis and the degree of malposition.

Nasal Ala in the Lower Position

Frequently, this outcome has been considered an expected result after primary cheilorhinoplasty and has been explained as a consequence of the absence of bony support (alveolar cleft). However, this is not true, and the bad outcome is related to a deficiency of the surgical procedure to provide adequate support to the alar base (Figs. 10.31, 10.32 and 10.33). A study published by the author studying a group of unilateral cleft lip patients followed for 5 years after primary cleft rhinoplasty revealed a well-positioned alar base using oral muscles to provide structural support [35]. Common causes include curved or straight line primary cheiloplasty, surgical marking deficiency, and deficient repair of the labial muscles. The linear incision methods for unilateral cleft lip repair may produce this outcome because the position of the ala is used to compensate the lip height deficiency. Therefore, adequate lip markings before the procedure are important, and the subnasal sulcus (sometimes

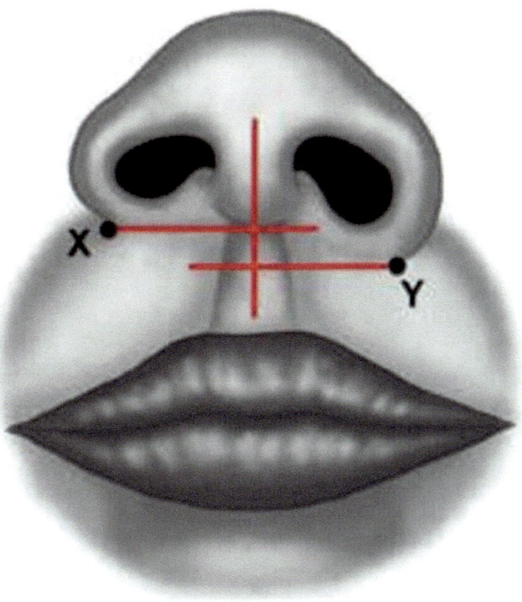

Fig. 10.31 Nasal ala in the lower position. Diagram illustrating the outcome after nose asymmetry correction

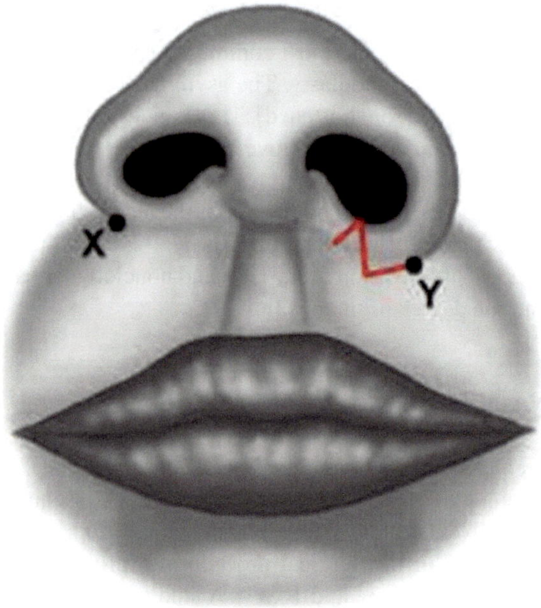

Fig. 10.32 Nasal ala in the lower position. Diagram illustrating the surgical technique used for its correction

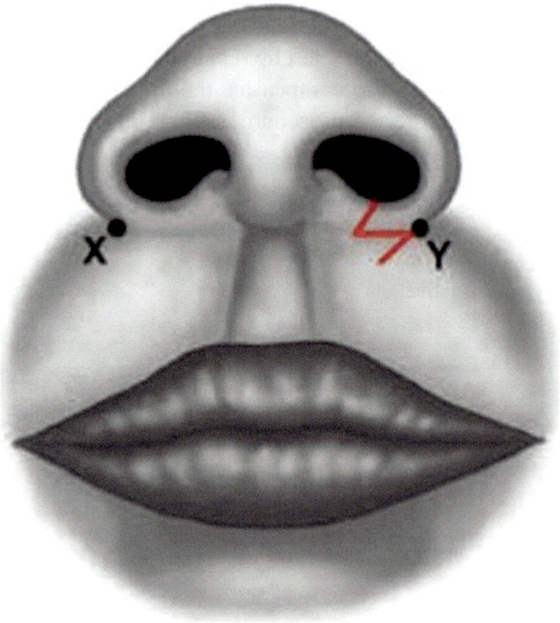

Fig. 10.33 Nasal ala in the lower position. Diagram illustrating the nose asymmetry associated with right ala in lower position

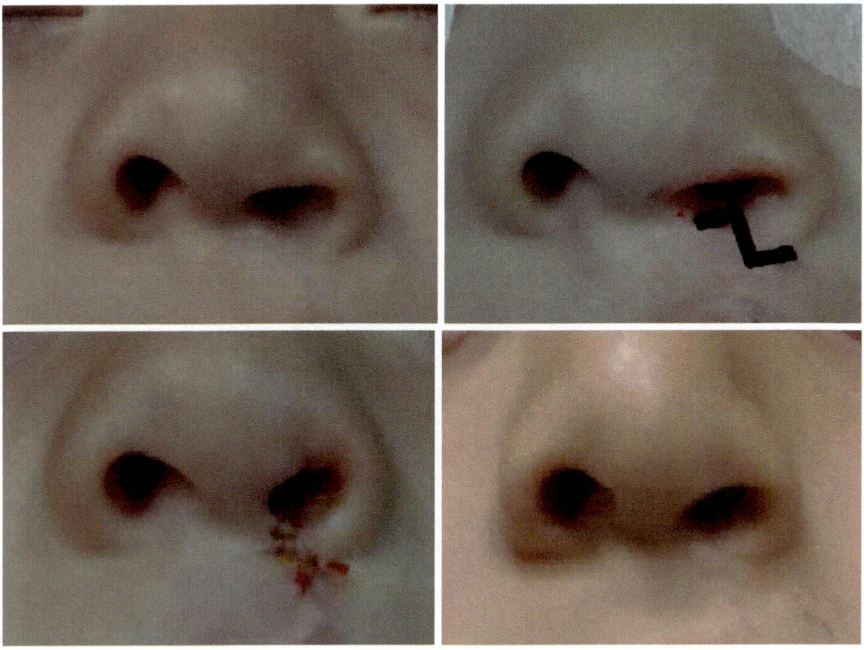

Fig. 10.34 A 3-year-old male patient born with unilateral cleft lip who developed nose asymmetry after primary cleft rhinoplasty. Secondary deformity is treated using a Z plasty

difficult to identify) should be located and preserved in a good position at the end of the surgery. Another cause of this bad outcome is deficient repair of the labial muscles. The upper lip muscles can support the alar base even in the presence of a wide alveolar cleft and lack of skeletal support. The alar fascicle of the levator labii superioris alaeque nasi muscle provides support through insertion at the level of the base of the caudal septum during lip repair. This bad outcome can be corrected performing a secondary muscular reconstruction or using an asymmetric Z plasty (Fig. 10.34).

Nasal Ala in Upper Position

This bad outcome is observed as a result of inadequate muscular repair of the lip.

To prevent this problem, the subnasal sulcus should be identified preoperatively and marked. For its diagnosis, a comparison between cleft and noncleft side alar base positions should be done as I mentioned before. The observed difference will allow the design of the skin area to be corrected for proper repositioning of the alar base.

Alar Nose Shortening (Figs. 10.35, 10.36, 10.37 and 10.38)

Two events are associated with this poor outcome, inadequate surgical technique higher placement of the subnasal incision (related to the rotation advancement

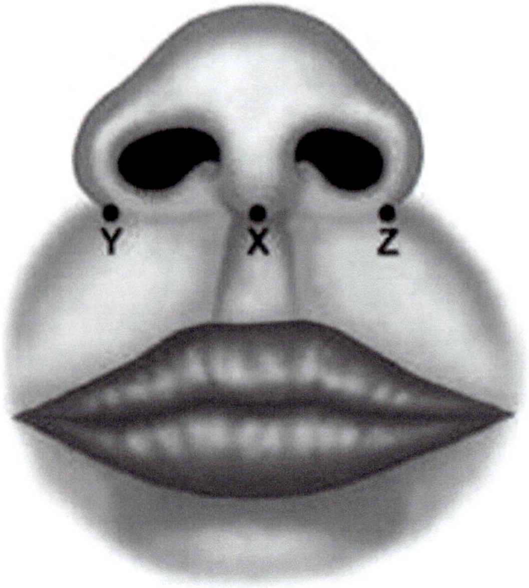

Fig. 10.35 Alar nose shortening. Diagram illustrating the nose asymmetry associated with short left ala position

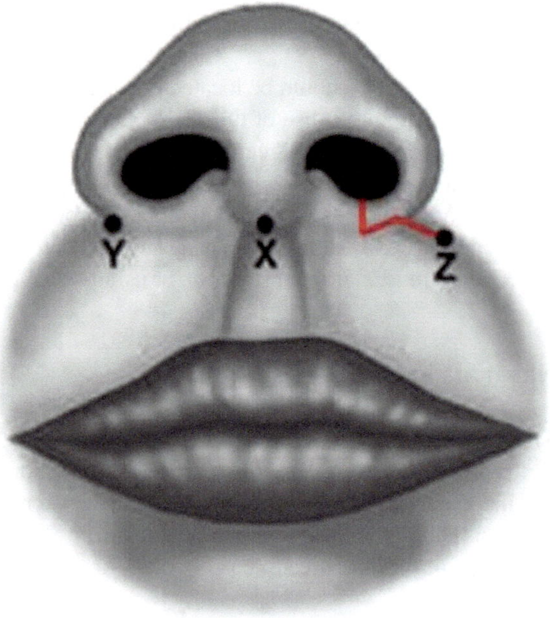

Fig. 10.36 Alar nose shortening. Diagram illustrating the surgical technique used for its correction

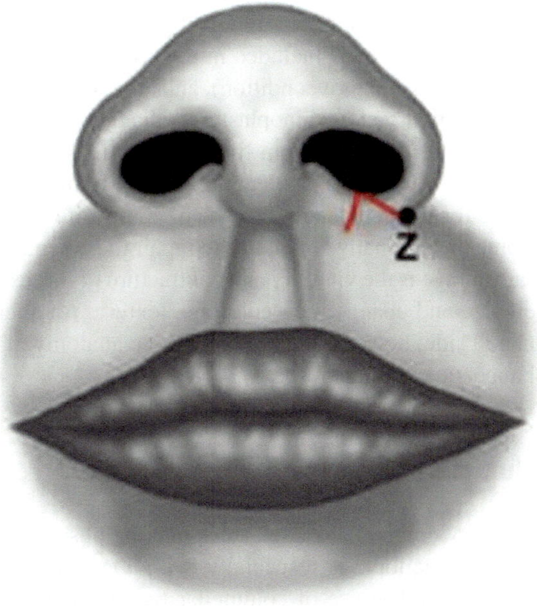

Fig. 10.37 Alar nose shortening. Diagram illustrating the outcome after nose asymmetry correction

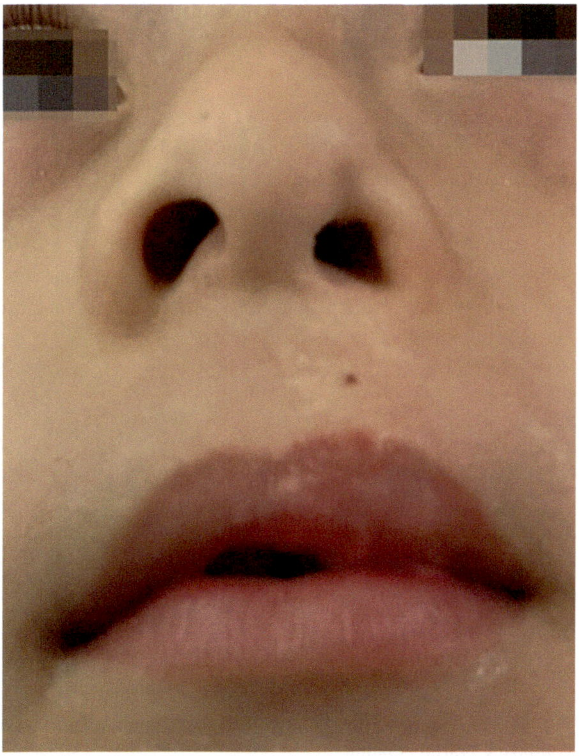

Fig. 10.38 A 5-year-old male patient born with unilateral cleft lip who developed nose asymmetry characterized by alar shortening after primary cleft rhinoplasty

method) and congenital hypoplasia of the ala. If the subnasal incision is not properly located and it is placed higher, then the surgeon leaves a short nasal ala because part of the nasal ala is included in the lip. The second event is the congenital hypoplasia of the ala (a rare condition), and another associated problem is the alar necrosis after primary cleft rhinoplasty. Its diagnosis is made by carefully observing the alar's length measured from the alar base to the nasal tip and comparing the two sides. Its correction is challenging since it requires the addition of tissues to compensate for the deficiency. The use of composite grafts from the auricular helix has become the alternative of choice to repair these sequelae (Fig. 10.39) [36]. The main disadvantage is the viability and contracture of these composite grafts, which reduce their size and change their color and texture. An alternative is the reduction of the noncleft side; however, this is altering the anatomy of the ala and affecting the natural appearance of the nose.

Columella

Secondary columellar deficiencies may be observed in association with the use of Mohler's cheiloplasty especially with the extended modification published by Cutting [37]. The use of columellar tissue for lip repair reduces the width of the columellar region and leaves a visible scar. Sometimes, the defect is minor and does not require any revision. The indication for surgery depends on surgeon's criteria and patient's expectation.

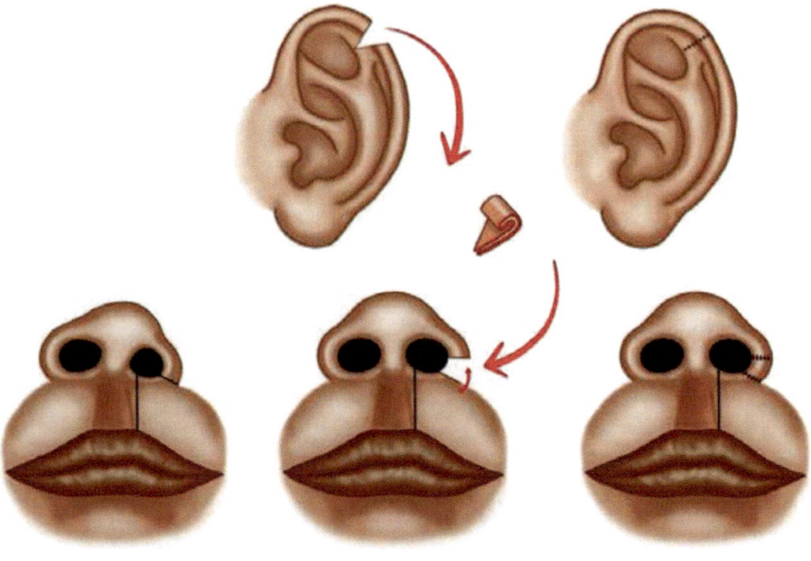

Fig. 10.39 Diagram illustrating the surgical technique used for alar shortening based on auricular composite graft technique

Nasal Sill: Wider Nasal Sill

This is a common nondesirable outcome after cleft lip repair and has been reported by different authors. This outcome is observed as a result of deficient surgical technique considering also the pulling action of the facial muscles or by hypertrophy of the lip scar. This problem is easier to correct by skin resection and the amount is determined by establishing the differences between cleft and noncleft alar base widths. This bad outcome is often associated with nasoalveolar fistulas (Figs. 10.40, 10.41, 10.42, 10.43 and 10.44).

Narrower Nasal Sill

Alar tissue may be hypoplastic; therefore, it could explain this bad outcome; however, this is mostly due to bad planning and execution of the primary surgical correction, and scar contracture may also be associated with this bad outcome too. The overcorrection technique, a surgical method popularized by centers such as Chang Gung University Craniofacial center from Taiwan, uses the nostril and nasal base overcorrection during primary cleft rhinoplasty. I do not agree with this concept because the nose may be overcorrected after long term and its repair is more difficult [38]. Its diagnostic is made similar to that of the previous case, in which the position of the alar bases is located and their diameter differences are established. A

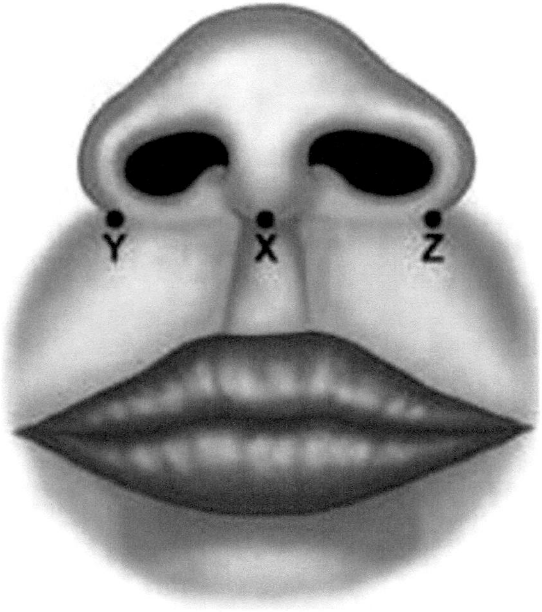

Fig. 10.40 Wider nasal floor. Diagram illustrating the nose asymmetry associated with right widening alar

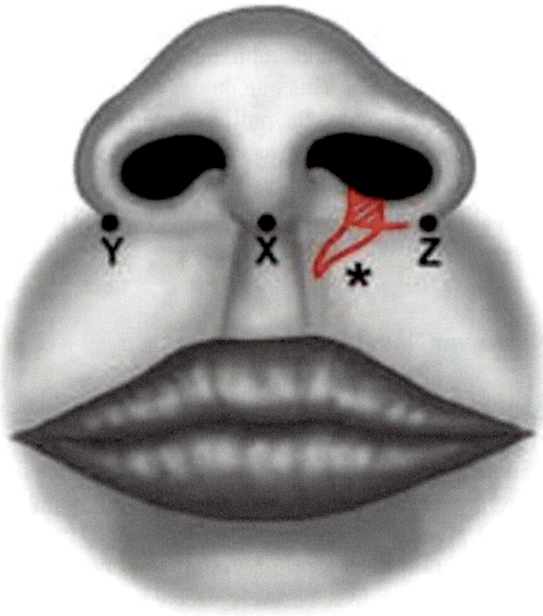

Fig. 10.41 Wider nasal floor. Diagram illustrating the surgical technique used for its correction

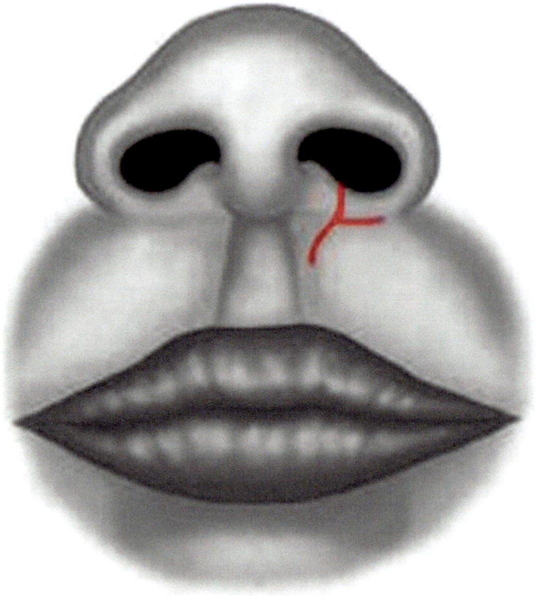

Fig. 10.42 Wider nasal floor. Diagram illustrating the outcome after nose asymmetry correction

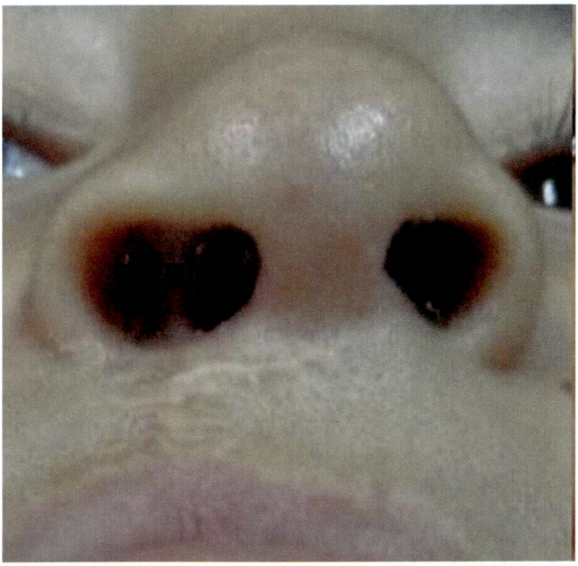

Fig. 10.43 A 6-year-old female patient born with unilateral cleft lip who developed nose asymmetry characterized by alar widening after primary cleft rhinoplasty

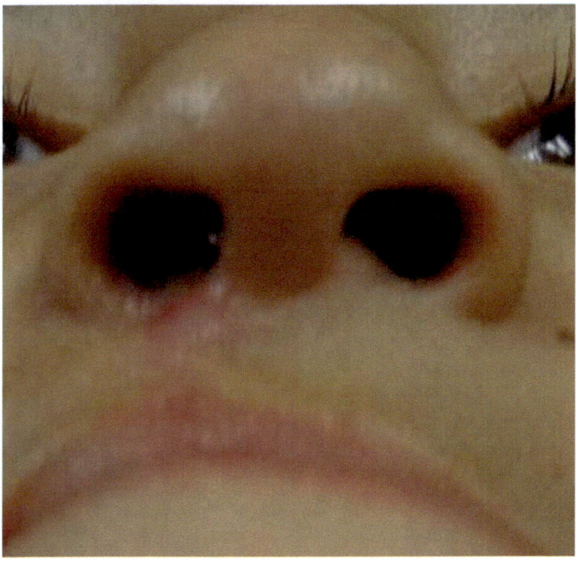

Fig. 10.44 Postoperative view after 1 year of the patient presented in Fig. 10.40

lateral flap from the cheek can be used to correct this secondary deformity, and the flap diameter is equal to the difference between the two alar bases.

The nasal floor is an anatomical structure made up of three anatomical segments: the nasal vestibule and the hard and soft palates. The anterior segment of the nasal floor (vestibular segment) is repaired during primary repair using three flaps: lateral (nasal ala), medial (base of the columella), and posterior (mucosal flap raised from the lips) flaps.

Nasal Vestibule

The vestibule is an important functional area of the nose, and its involvement during primary cleft rhinoplasty may affect breathing. Thus, the incisions made in this anatomical segment may produce scar retractions or synechiae, and this is the reason why the use of nasal conformers is recommended after primary cleft rhinoplasty. They can be associated with patient idiosyncrasy but also with the use of extended incisions through the nasal vestibule during primary cleft rhinoplasty (i.e., VYZ cleft rhinoplasty). Its diagnosis is made through the physical examination and airway obstruction symptoms (Figs. 10.45, 10.46, 10.47 and 10.48). Treatment of these conditions is challenging for the reconstructive surgeons, and recurrence is a common problem. Management is surgical, and different techniques are used for

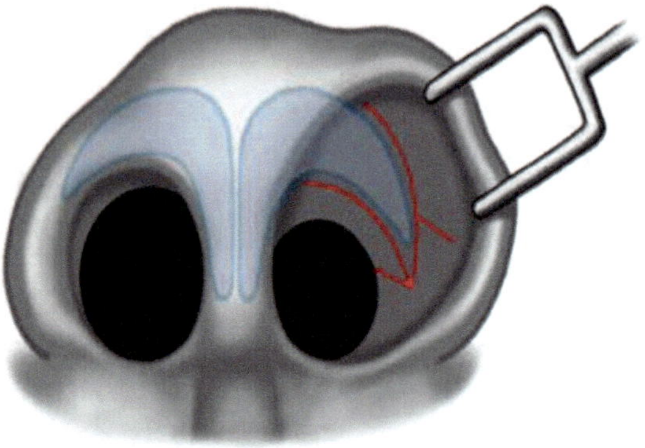

Fig. 10.45 Contracture of the nasal vestibule scar. Diagram illustrating the surgical technique markings used for correction of the nose vestibular scar contracture

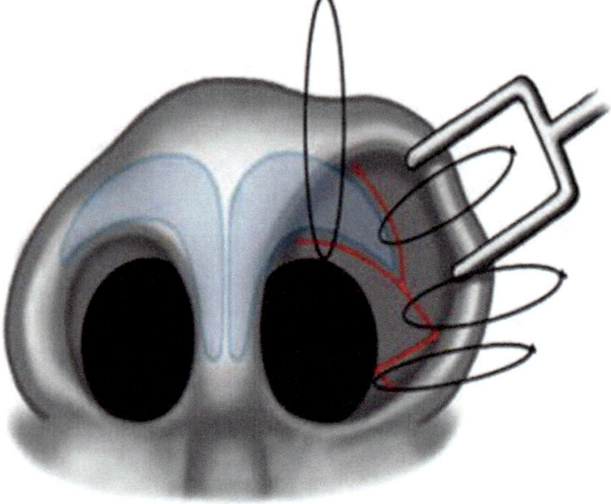

Fig. 10.46 Contracture of the nasal vestibule scar. Postoperative diagram illustrating the correction of the vestibular scar contracture using the VYZ method

this purpose, ranging from skin grafts to local flaps. The conservative use of steroid infiltration seems to help although only in the early stages and should be used in combination with nasal stents. In a recent study, we observed a reduced rate of this bad outcome after using these devices [39]. The proposed surgical technique for its correction is the V-Y composite flap plus lateral Z plasty in combination with postoperative nasal conformers. In addition, due to the increased rate of recurrence, the use of postoperative nasal stents for at least 6 months is recommended. The purpose of this technique is to lengthen the nasal vestibule while the scar contracture is breaking.

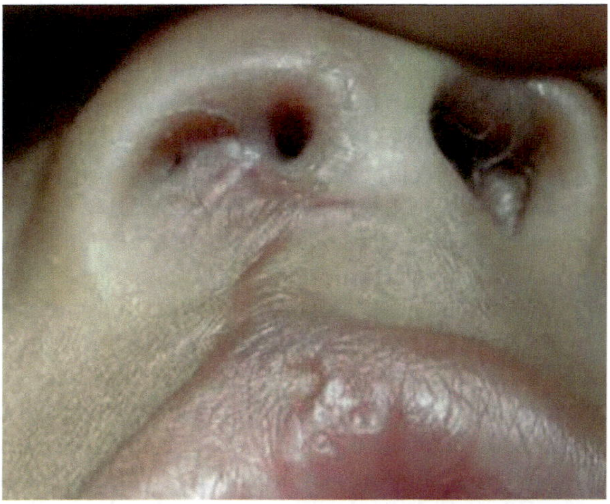

Fig. 10.47 A 10-year-old patient who developed a severe scar contracture of the nose after primary cleft rhinoplasty

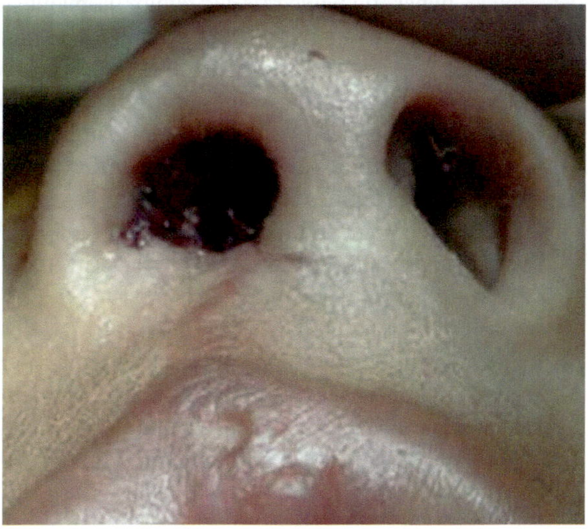

Fig. 10.48 Immediate postoperative view of the patient presented in Fig. 10.47 illustrating scar contracture release after correction using the VYZ method

Poor Outcomes Associated with Bilateral Primary Cleft Rhinoplasty

Compared with unilateral cleft lip, the bilateral cleft lip is more frequently associated with bad outcome and complications [1]. Brown described the nature of the bilateral cleft lip and palate as follows: "twice as difficult to repair compared to the unilateral cleft lips with outcomes that were half as good" [40]. Sir Harold Gillies, pioneer of reconstructive surgery, noted "the skeleton first," highlighting the importance of rebuilding the skeletal structure first in craniofacial reconstruction [40]. During primary lip and nose repair, the soft tissues are corrected before the skeleton which explains many of the bad outcomes observed after bilateral cleft lip surgery. Asymmetries, hypertrophic scars, and dental skeletal sequelae are commonly observed after primary bilateral cleft lip surgery due to the unrepaired skeleton. Another important factor is that due to the low incidence of bilateral cases (compared to unilateral cases), it takes more time for surgeons to acquire the necessary experience to treat them. Bad outcomes are often observed after bilateral cleft lip surgery, mostly in severe cases, and practiced by inexperienced surgeons. Based on the author's classification, a severe bilateral cleft lip and palate is one that has an alveolar cleft wider than 1 cm [1]. The author described the clock diagram, a practical scheme to illustrate this pathology in a better way [41]. An effective and timely interdisciplinary team management is essential to prevent these nondesirable outcomes. The use of presurgical treatment helps to improve the quality of the results but should be provided early (during the first weeks of life). These devices mobilize the cleft segments and premaxilla in a more anatomical position facilitating the primary surgical repair and preventing sequelae, and they are indicated for severe cases. When the lip and nose are repaired under tension, there are increased rates of dehiscence, hypertrophic scarring, premaxilla malpositioning, and nasal sequelae. Presurgical nasal molding combined with alveolar molding (known as NAM) was developed by the University of New York based on Matsuo's findings and is an alternative for facilitating nasal surgery; however, there is a lack of scientific evidence supporting its long-term effect, and similar outcomes can be achieved by using primary cleft rhinoplasty alone [42]. Different publications show a significant improvement in outcomes for bilateral nasal deformity after primary repair minimizing the psychological impact of patients [43, 44].

The secondary nasal deformity of bilateral cleft lip presented the following characteristics:

- Bad alar cartilage positioning and lack of projection of the nasal tip.
- Absent or short nasal columella. "Short" columella resulting from lateral displacement of the alar cartilage. In fact, this is not short; it is "hidden in the nose," as Mulliken pointed out for bilateral cleft lips.

- Obtuse labial columellar angle
- Wide nasal floor
- Ectopic insertion of nasal muscles
- Different degrees of maxillary hypoplasia

Some surgical technique shortcomings described in the literature are the use of banked fork flaps using lip tissues for nose repair which results in an unnatural outcome (Millard), skin resection from the soft triangle of the nose proposed by Tajima and Mulliken bringing a turned-up appearance of the nose and visible scars affecting vestibular function, and the Mc Comb's method which is associated with a high rate of nasal deformity relapse [28].

The author's philosophy for the secondary correction of the bilateral cleft lip nose deformity is based on the following principles:

- Any severe bilateral cleft lip form (alveolar gap greater than 1 cm) should receive presurgical treatment at an early age before primary cleft rhinoplasty. Older patients may be treated by vomer osteotomy and setback of the premaxilla.
- Columellar lengthening is based on alar cartilage reposition and vestibular lengthening, via the VYZ technique [13].
- Compared with unilateral clefts, the need for septal correction is less frequent, and this is mostly used for nonsymmetrical bilateral cleft lips.
- Any severe aesthetic or functional condition should be treated at an early age; this is before school age, preventing the psychosocial and functional impact of the patient. Any minor sequela can be corrected later in adulthood.

Careful physical examination and photographic documentation are recommended to address aesthetic and functional problems to be treated.

The anatomical areas to be analyzed include the nasal tip, columella, vestibule, alar bases, and septum.

Nasal Tip

The lateral displacement of alar cartilages in bilateral cleft lip is the reason for the lack of projection and definition. The proposed surgical technique for secondary nasal tip correction is based on medial repositioning of the alar cartilages which allows lengthening of the columella and nasal tip projection and lengthening of the nasal vestibule.

The technique used is a combination of V-Y (Potter's concept) and lateral Z plasty (Berkeley's concept), and it is indicated for complete bilateral cleft lips [31, 33]. By lengthening the nasal vestibule, it is possible to reposition the alar cartilages improving the nasal tip projection, and the lateral Z plasty prevents scar contracture of the lateral incisions. The surgical approach can be performed in an open or closed manner. Cartilaginous grafts are required to reinforce the area of the nasal vestibule that remains without cartilaginous reinforcement after medial displacement of the alar cartilages. An alternative for bilateral incomplete cleft lip cases is the rotational composite flap technique. This is based on the medial displacement of the composite flap through rotation, but really the alar cartilage is displaced in three dimensions (vectors) as medial, vertical, and posterior movements (Fig. 10.49). In case of minor deformities, the vestibular marginal skin excision is a good alternative providing long-term nasal symmetry [45] (Figs. 10.50, 10.51 and 10.52).

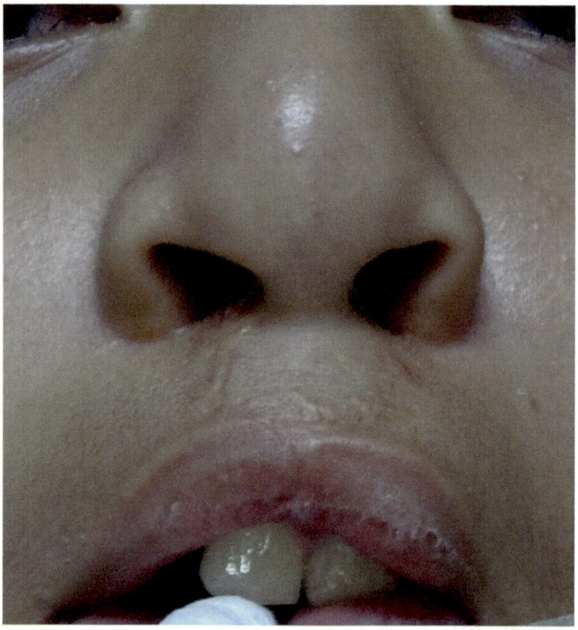

Fig. 10.49 Lack of tip projection in a patient with bilateral cleft lip after primary cleft rhinoplasty

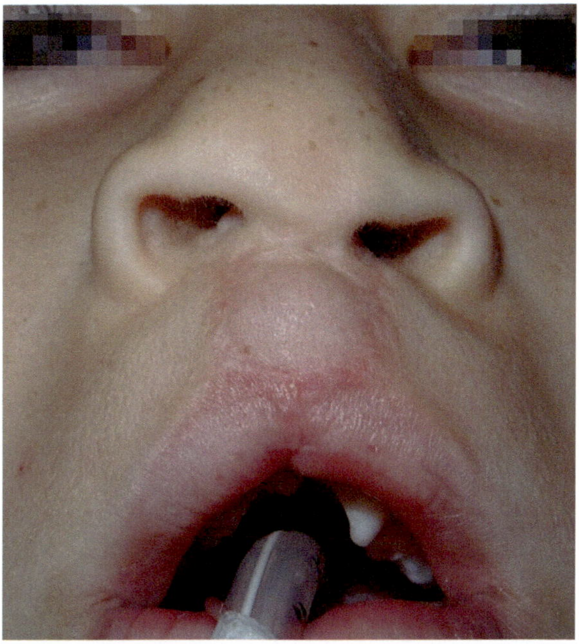

Fig. 10.50 Nasal ala asymmetry in a patient with bilateral cleft lip after primary cleft rhinoplasty

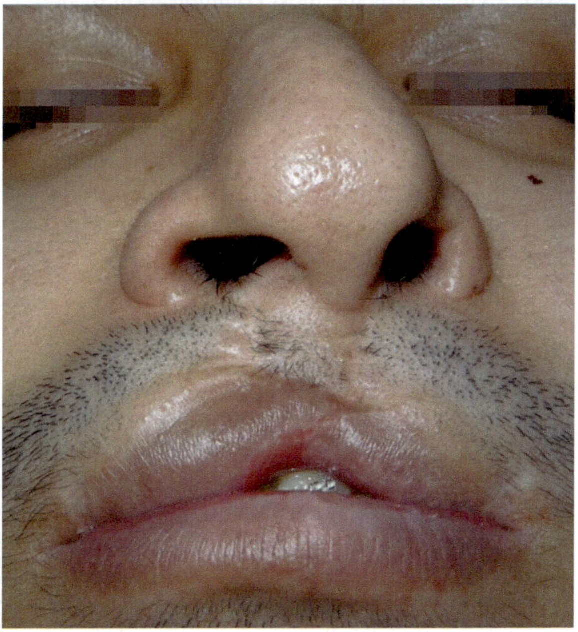

Fig. 10.51 Nasal ala asymmetry in a patient with bilateral cleft lip after primary cleft rhinoplasty

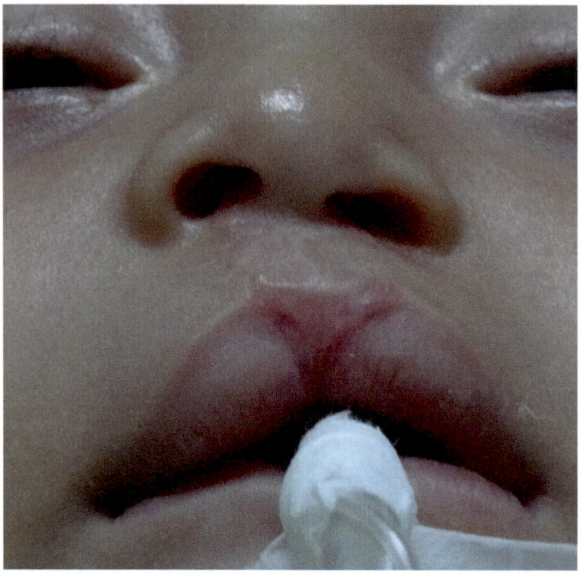

Fig. 10.52 Nasal ala asymmetry in a patient with bilateral cleft lip after primary cleft rhinoplasty

Nasal Ala

Nose asymmetry is the most common form of presentation of bad outcomes after primary cleft rhinoplasty. The nasal ala may be in wider, higher, or lower position when they are compared to the opposite side. It is important to be considered that all bilateral cleft lips are mostly asymmetric and the objective of the primary surgery is to create a symmetric lip and nose. The surgical alternatives for their treatment are similar than those presented for unilateral secondary deformities. The diagnosis is made through careful physical examination of the lip, and the difference between the position of the right and left alar bases will determine the diagnosis and the degree of malposition.

Nasal Ala Asymmetry

This complication may be observed on one or both sides and is considered an expected result after primary cheilorhinoplasty as a consequence of the absence of bony support. The muscular hypoplasia observed in cleft segments of the bilateral forms does not allow the surgeon to provide an adequate support of the alar bases in comparison with unilateral cleft lips. In addition, the skeletal discrepancy between the premaxilla and cleft segments does not help to position the alar bases properly (Figs. 10.50, 10.51 and 10.52). Common causes are Manchester type of primary cheiloplasty, skeletal discrepancy, and deficient repair of the labial muscles. The Manchester technique for bilateral cleft lip repair may develop a lower position of the ala because the oral muscles are not repaired and a lack of support for the alar base may exist [46]. The skeletal discrepancy creates a deficient support for the nasal ala because of the hypoplasia of the lateral cleft segments. This bad outcome can be corrected using secondary muscular repair and an asymmetric Z plasty or a combination of both procedures for severe cases.

Alar Nose Shortening

A short alar nose is not common and is associated with congenital hypoplasia of the ala, surgical technique deficiencies, or complications such as alar necrosis (rare). Its diagnosis is made by comparing the alar's length measured from the alar base to the nasal tip between both sides. Its correction is challenging since it requires the addition of tissues to compensate for the deficiency. The use of composite grafts from the auricular helix has become the alternative to repair these sequelae [36]. The main disadvantage is the viability and contracture of these composite grafts, which reduce their size and change color and texture. An alternative is a combined method in which one cleft side is reduced and the other is grafted; however, this method also alters the anatomy of the ala and affects the natural appearance of the nose.

Columella

Secondary columellar deficiencies are common after primary bilateral cleft rhinoplasty and short or absent columella are frequently observed. The most frequent sequelae observed after primary reconstruction of the nasal columella in patients with bilateral cleft lips are short, wide columella and outcomes after repair using regional flaps or grafts.

Short Columella

This sequel is related to the absence of primary nasal surgery or poor reconstruction (Figs. 10.53, 10.54 and 10.55). The objective for secondary surgery of nasal columella in adults is lengthening of the columella by 1 cm, on average, but we have to consider the height of the columella. The anthropometric parameters vary depending on the patient's age and race (Farkas) [47]. The surgical treatment for short columella is based on vestibular lengthening, which was previously described in detail in Chap. 6. This method has been described in the literature by the author as the V-Y-Z method. In addition, the use of the rotational composite flap method may be effective for incomplete bilateral cleft lips [13, 48].

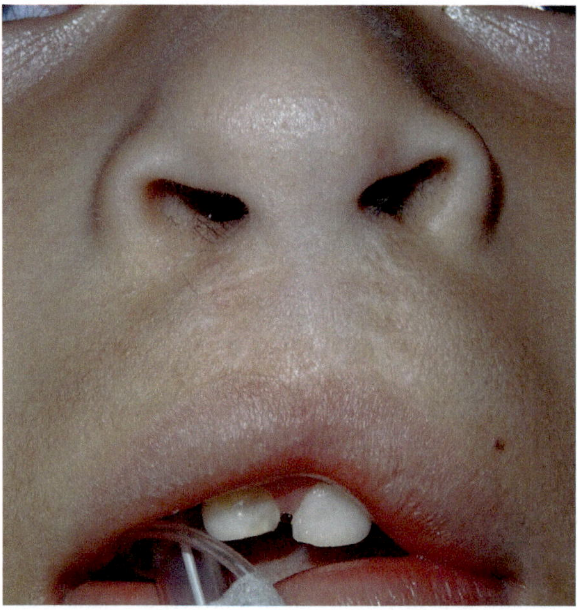

Fig. 10.53 Short columella in a patient with bilateral cleft lip after primary cleft rhinoplasty

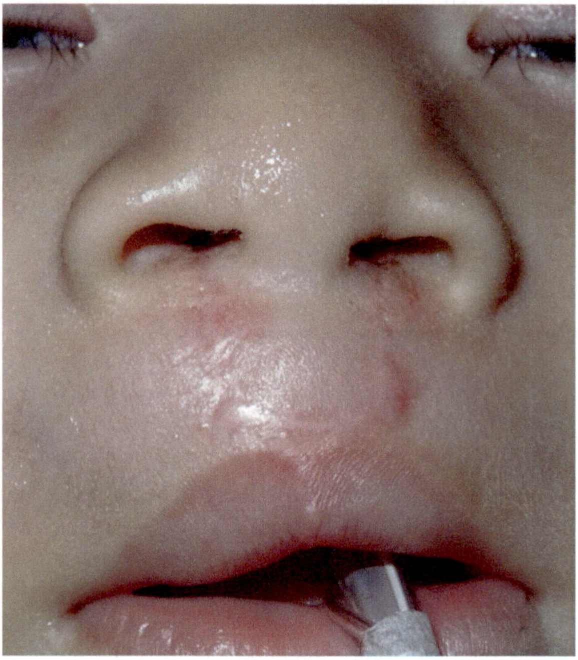

Fig. 10.54 Short columella in a patient with bilateral cleft lip after primary cleft rhinoplasty

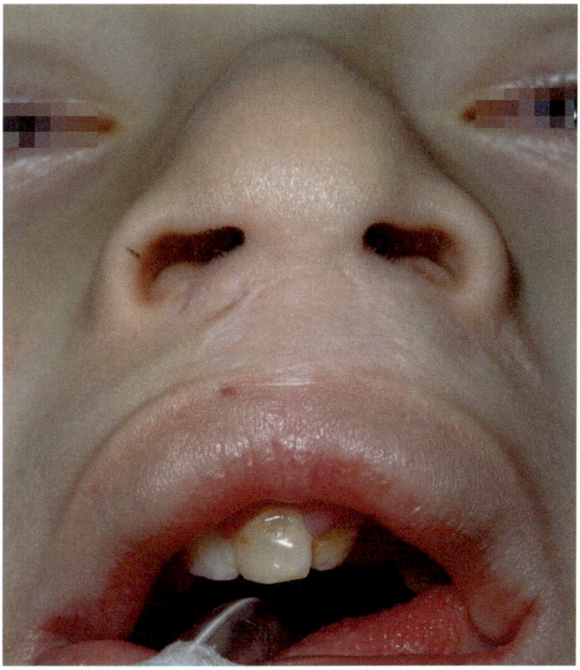

Fig. 10.55 Short columella in a patient with bilateral cleft lip after primary cleft rhinoplasty

Wide Columella

It is characterized by the presence of a wide columella and is usually accompanied by a wide philtrum, which is probably due to tissue expansion and scar retraction of the nostrils. It is also associated with congenital defects of the nasal pyramid with widening of the nasocolumellar area, as observed in syndromic patients (Fig. 10.56). Its diagnosis is established through physical examination, and correction is performed by resection of the excess skin and plication of the cartilaginous structures giving the columella a more natural appearance.

Nasal Sill: Wider Nasal Sill

This is a common nondesirable outcome after cleft lip repair that has been reported by different authors and is more frequently observed in bilateral cleft lip surgery. This outcome is observed as a result of deficient surgical technique considering also the pulling action of the facial muscles or by hypertrophy of the lip scar. This bad outcome is often associated with nasoalveolar fistulas (Figs. 10.57, 10.58 and 10.59). This problem is easier to correct by skin resection, and the amount is established by determining the differences between both alar base widths. The technique used for its correction is based on resection of the excess of the skin of the wider alar base (or both if necessary) considering the anthropometric parameters. Based on this concept, the length of the alar base should be equal to the vertical length of the philtrum; therefore, the first step is determining the desired lip height according to

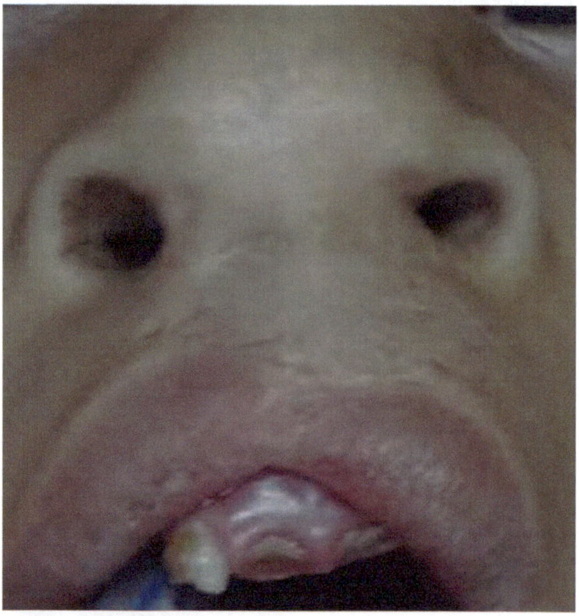

Fig. 10.56 Wide columella in a patient with bilateral cleft lip after primary cleft rhinoplasty

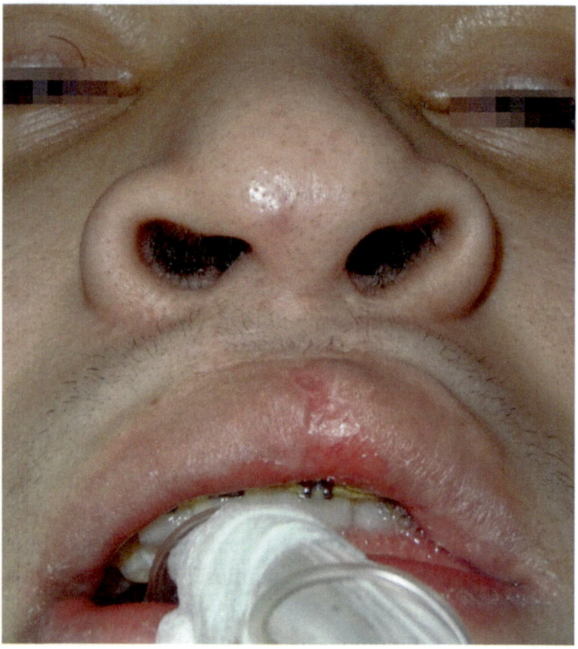

Fig. 10.57 Wider nasal sill in a patient with bilateral cleft lip after primary cleft rhinoplasty

the width of the largest lateral segment. If the lip height is greater than the estimated width, it is better to reduce it; otherwise, it will be a disproportionate and longer lip. In contrast, if the labial height is less than the largest lateral segment, this height should be taken as the desired lip height. It is important to understand that the

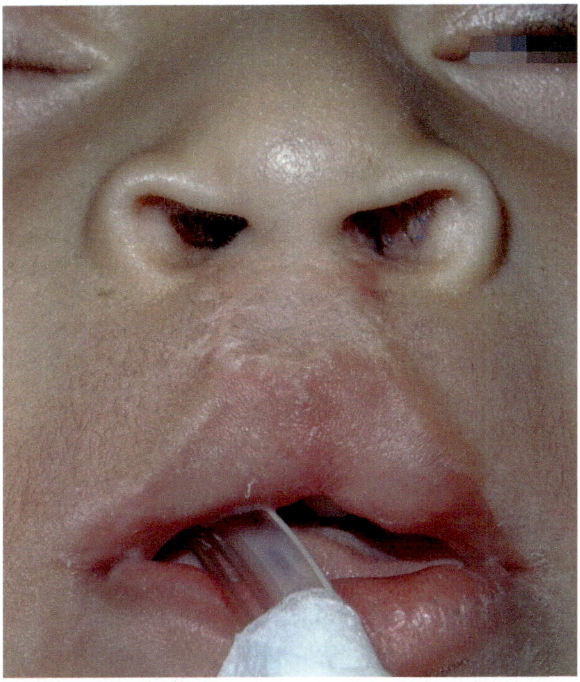

Fig. 10.58 Wider nasal sill in a patient with bilateral cleft lip after primary cleft rhinoplasty

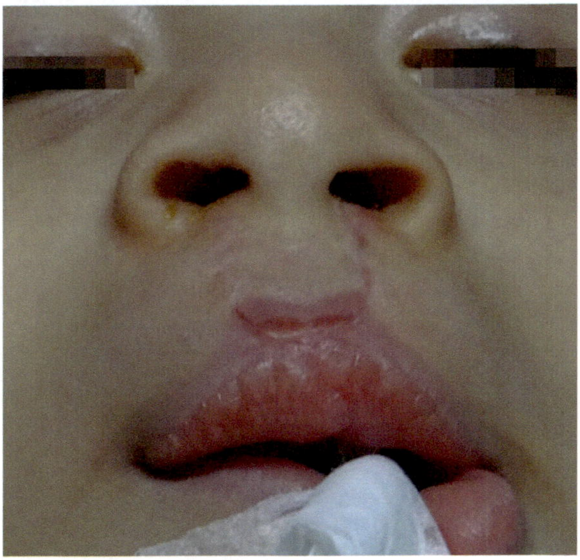

Fig. 10.59 Wider nasal sill in a patient with bilateral cleft lip after primary cleft rhinoplasty

objective in the reconstruction of the secondary bilateral cleft lip deformity is the lip symmetry and better proportions of the anatomical subunits. After estimation of the desired lip height, the alar bases can be shortened and positioned considering that the alar diameter is equal to the lip height. This correction can be performed by resecting a skin lozenge as necessary to ensure symmetry.

Narrower Nasal Sill

Alar tissue may be hypoplastic and therefore could explain this bad outcome; however this is mostly due to poor planning of the primary surgical correction and scar contracture. Overcorrection is a well-known method developed to prevent nose deformity relapse and was popularized by centers such as Chang Gung University in Taiwan [38]. Soft tissue resection may cause permanent long-term deficiency and its repair is more difficult. Oversized nostrils and narrower nasal floors are consequences of these techniques. Its diagnosis is similar to that of the previous case, in which the width of the nasal floor on both sides was measured and the differences in the nasal floor diameter were determined. A lateral flap from the cheek can be used to correct this secondary deformity, and the flap diameter is equal to the difference between the two nasal floor widths.

Nasal Vestibule

The nasal vestibule is a functional area of the nose and under the point of view of cleft lip nose repair is critical. This anatomical area is frequently affected by the development of scar contractures (Fig. 10.60). Nasal breathing may be severely affected by scar contractures and synechia of the vestibule of the nose. Any primary cleft rhinoplasty based on vestibular incisions should consider the complementary use of nasal stents postoperatively during for at least 6 months to prevent these adverse outcomes [49, 50].

A recent study published by us observed that the group of patients operated using postoperative nasal stents had lower rate of these postoperative complications [39].

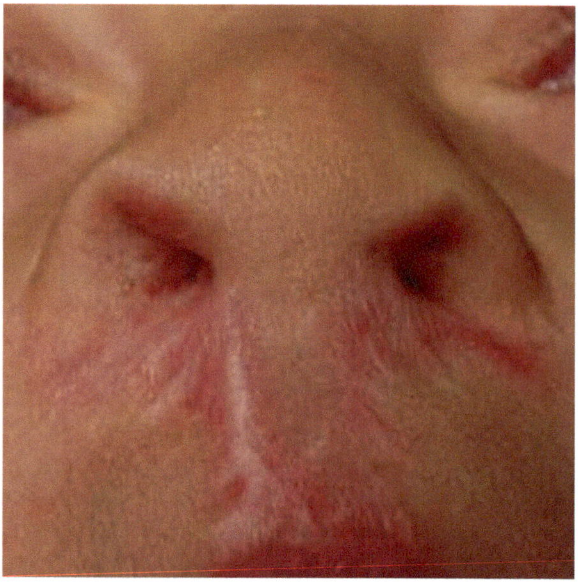

Fig. 10.60 Bilateral Nasal vestibule scar contracture

The diagnosis is made through the physical examination of the airway and patient's symptoms. Its treatment is surgical after initial conservative management including corticoid injection from skin grafts to local flaps in combination with postoperative nasal stents at least during 6 months.

The conservative use of corticoid infiltration seems to help although only in early time; however, it is difficult to apply when children are awake. If the conservative treatment is not successful, the surgical treatment is needed. The technique used for these sequelae is the V-Y-Z method in combination with postoperative nasal stents (orthonostric devices) for at least 6 months (Figs. 10.61, 10.62 and 10.63).

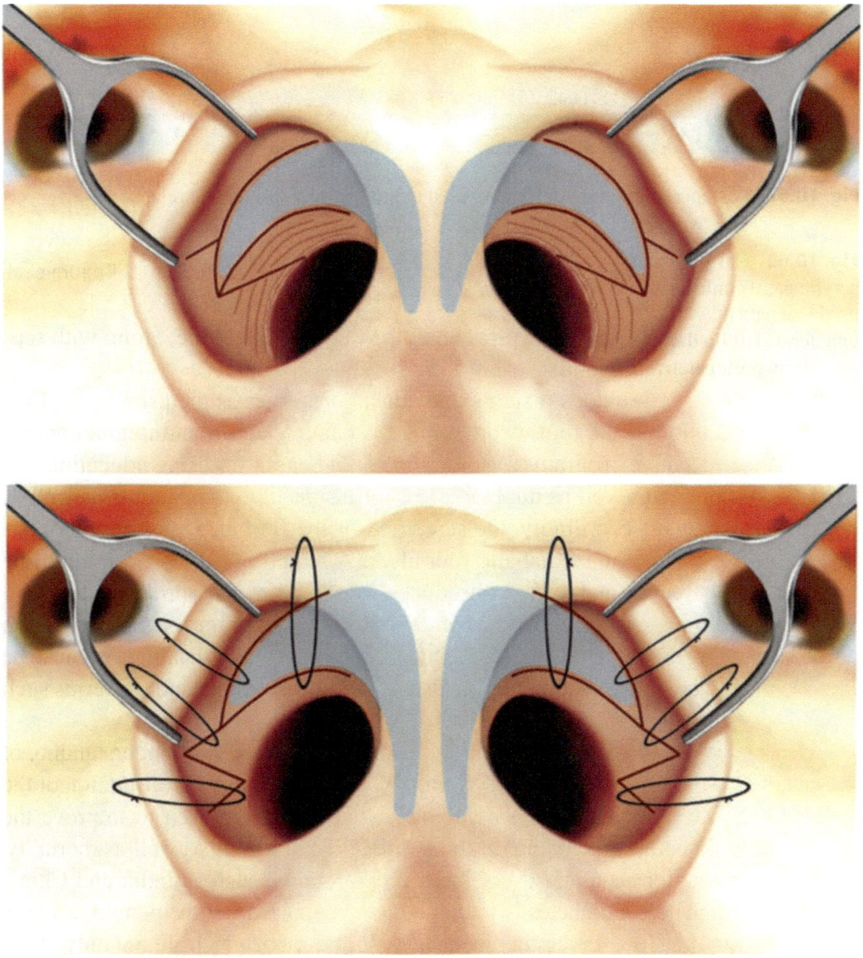

Fig. 10.61 VYZ surgical technique for treatment of bilateral nasal vestibule scar contracture. Upper: Surgical markings. Lower: VY advancement and lateral Z plasty for scar release and vestibular lengthening

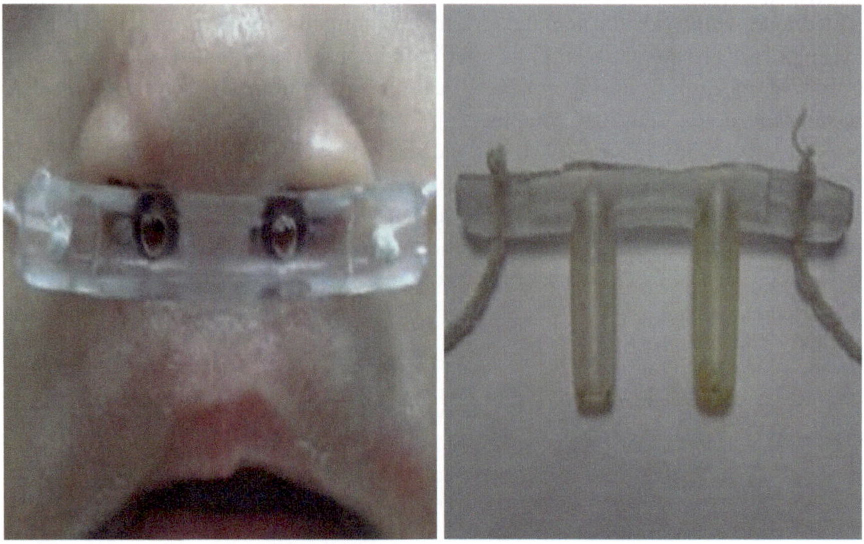

Fig. 10.62 Postoperative nasal conformers used to prevent scar contracture relapse

Fig. 10.63 Custom-made acrylic nasal conformer used in a patient with unilateral cleft lip during short-term postoperative period

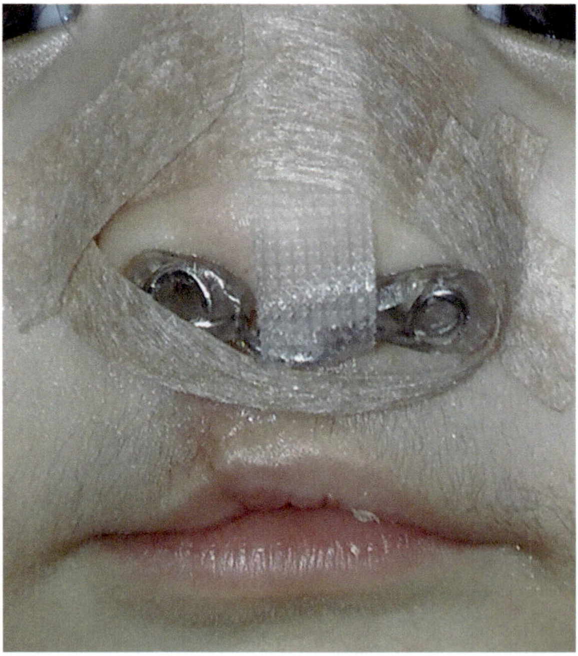

In case of more severe contractures and synechia, the use of auricular composite grafts is an alternative. The graft should be larger than the defect because of the secondary contracture of the graft.

Finally, for more detailed description of bad outcome treatment, the reader may revise the author's textbook: *Atlas of Non-desirable Outcomes in Cleft Lip and Palate* [51].

References

1. Rossell-Perry P. Atlas of non-desirable outcomes in cleft lip and palate surgery. Cham: Springer Ed; 2022.
2. Rossell-Perry P, Segura E, Salas-Bustinza L, Cotrina-Rabanal O. Comparison of two models of surgical care for patients with cleft lip and palate in resource-challenged settings. World J Surg. 2015;39(1):47–53.
3. Rossell-Perry P. Primary cleft rhinoplasty: surgical outcomes and complications using three techniques for unilateral cleft lip nose repair. J Craniofac Surg. 2020;31(6):1521–5.
4. Grayson BH, Santiago PE, Brecht LE, Cutting CB. Presurgical nasoalveolar molding in infants with cleft lip and palate. Cleft Palate Craniofac J. 1999;36(6):486–98.
5. Zheng J, He H, Kuang W, Yuan W. Presurgical nasoalveolar molding with 3D printing for a patient with unilateral cleft lip, alveolus, and palate. Am J Orthod Dentofacial Orthop. 2019;156(3):412–9.
6. Fillies T, Homann C, Meyer U, Reich A, Joos U, Werkmeister R. Perioperative complications in infant cleft repair. Head Face Med. 2007;3:9.
7. Levy Bercowski D, Abreu A, DeLeon E, Looney S, Stockstill J, Weiler M. Santiago complications and solutions in presurgical nasoalveolar molding therapy. Cleft Palate Craniofac J. 2009;46(5):521–8.
8. Yilmaz H, Hatipoglu S, Erdem B, Can B, Kadir T. Adherence frequency of candida albicans on nasoalveolar molding appliances. J Stomatol Oral Maxillofac Surg. 2020;121(5):473–7.
9. Yilmaz HN, Hatipoglu S, Erdem B, Can B, Kadir T. Adherence frequency of candida albicans on nasoalveolar molding appliances. J Stomatol Oral Maxillofac Surg. 2020;121(5):473–7.
10. Doyle E, Hudson I. Anesthesia for primary repair of cleft lip and cleft palate: a review of 244 procedures. Pediatr Anaesth. 1992;2:139–45.
11. Liu D, Pan L, Gao Y, Liu J, Li F, Li X, Quan J, Huang C, Lian C. Efficaciousness of dexmedetomidine in children undergoing cleft lip and palate repair: a systematic review and meta-analysis. BMJ Open. 2021;11(8):e046798.
12. Marston AP, Costello MS, Farhood Z, Brandstetter KA, Murphey AW, Nguyen SA, Discolo CM, Patel KG. Association of pediatric patient demographic factors and scar anatomic features with scar outcomes after surgical repair of cleft lip. JAMA Facial Plast Surg. 2019;21(5):452–7.
13. Rossell-Perry P. Primary unilateral cleft lip nasal deformity repair using V-Y-Z plasty: an anthropometric study. Indian J Plast Surg. 2017;50(2):180–6.
14. Rossell-Perry P, Gavino-Gutierrez A. Mixed dentition period follow-up of primary unilateral cleft nose deformity repair. Plast Reconstr Surg Glob Open. 2023;11(10):e5313.
15. Alef M, Irvin C, Smith D, Loose J. Nasal tip complication of primary cleft nasoplasty. J Craniofac Surg. 2009;20(5):1327–33.
16. Gopalakrishna A, Agrawal K. A status report on management of cleft lip and palate in India. Indian J Plast Surg. 2010;43(1):66–75.
17. Nagy K, Mommaerts M. Postoperative wound management after cleft lip surgery. Cleft Palate Craniofac J. 2011;48(5):584–6.
18. Marshall D, Slattery P. Intracranial complications of rhinoplasty. Br J Plast Surg. 1983;36(3):342–4.
19. Chuo CB, Timmons MJ. The bacteriology of children before primary cleft lip and palate surgery. Cleft Palate Craniofac J. 2005;42(3):272–6.
20. Stevens D, Bisno A, Chambers H, Dellinger E, et al. Practice guidelines for the diagnosis and management of skin and soft tissue infections. Clin Infect Dis. 2014;59(2):147–59.

21. Mankowski P, Cherukupalli A, Slater K, Carr N. Antibiotic prophylaxis in plastic surgery correlation between practice and evidence. Plast Surg (Oakv). 2021;29(2):132–8.
22. Olawoye O, Michael A, Olusanya A. A perioperative antibiotic therapy in orofacial cleft surgery. What is the consensus? Ann Ib Postgrad Med. 2020;18(1):S51–7.
23. Richardson C, Mattison A, Olusanya A. The optimal duration of antibiotic prophylaxis in plastic surgery: a meta analysis of 32 publications running head. Health Sci J. 2016;10(2):24–9.
24. Adams D. The granulomatous inflammatory response: a review. Am J Pathol. 1976;84(1):164.
25. Agarwal R, Chandra R. Alar web in cleft lip nose deformity: study in adult unilateral clefts. J Craniofac Surg. 2012;23(5):1349–54.
26. Patel KB, Mulliken JB. Correction of the vestibular web during primary repair of unilateral cleft lip. Plast Reconstr Surg. 2014;134(4):600e–7e.
27. Cho BC. Correction of unilateral cleft lip nasal deformity in preschool and school-aged children with refined reverse-U incision and V-Y plasty: long term follow-up results. Plast Reconstr Surg. 2007;119:267–75.
28. McComb HK, Coghlan BA. Primary repair of the unilateral cleft lip nose: completion of a longitudinal study. Cleft Palate Craniofac J. 1996;33(1):23–30.
29. Yao C, Mulliken J. The unilateral cleft lip nasal deformity: revisions within 20 years after primary correction. Plast Reconstr Surg. 2021;147:1379–87.
30. Salyer K, Genecov E, Genecov D. Unilateral cleft lip nose repair: a 33 year experience. J Craniofac Surg. 2003;14:549–58.
31. Potter J. Some nasal tip deformities due to alar cartilage abnormalities. Plast Reconstr Surg. 1954;13:358–66.
32. Cronin TD, Denkler KA. Correction of the unilateral cleft lip nose. Plast Reconstr Surg. 1988;82(3):419–32.
33. Berkeley W. The cleft lip nose. Plast Reconstr Surg. 1959;23:567.
34. Nakajima T, Yoshimura Y. Secondary repair of unilateral cleft lip nose deformity with bilateral reverse-U access incision. Br J Plast Surg. 1998;51:176–80.
35. Rossell-Perry P. The surgical nasoalveolar molding: a rational treatment for unilateral cleft lip nose deformity and literature review. Plast Reconstr Surg Glob Open. 2020;8(8):e3044.
36. Rossell-Perry P, Romero-Narvaez C. Evaluation of the use of auricular composite graft for secondary unilateral cleft lip nasal alar deformity repair. Plast Surg Int. 2014;2014:270285.
37. Cutting CB, Dayan JH. Lip height and lip width after extended Mohler unilateral cleft lip repair. Plast Reconstr Surg. 2003;111(1):17–23.
38. Lonic D, Morris DE, Lo LJ. Primary overcorrection of the unilateral cleft nasal deformity: quantifying the results. Ann Plast Surg. 2016;77(Suppl 1):S25–9.
39. Rossell-Perry P, Romero-Narvaez C, Gavino-Gutierrez A, Figallo-Hudtwalcker O. Postoperative nasal conformers in cleft rhinoplasty: are they efficacious? J Craniofac Surg. 2023;34(5):1416–9.
40. Millard R Jr. The cleft craft. The evolution of its surgery. 1st ed. Boston: Little Brown Ed.
41. Rossell-Perry P. New diagram for cleft lip and palate description: the clock diagram. Cleft Palate Craniofac J. 2009;46(3):305–13.
42. Rossell-Perry P, Olivencia-Flores C, Delgado-Jimenez MP. Ormeño-Aquino surgical Nasoalveolar molding: a rational treatment for bilateral cleft lip nose and systematic review. Plast Reconstr Surg Glob Open. 2020;8(9):e3082.
43. Hunt O, Burden D, Hepper P, Johnston C. The psychosocial effects of cleft lip and palate: a systematic review. Eur J Orthod. 2005;27(3):274–85.
44. Ardouin K, Hare J, Stock N. Emotional well-being in adults born with cleft lip and/or palate: a whole of life survey in the United Kingdom. Cleft Palate Craniofac J. 2020;57(7):877–85.
45. Rossell-Perry P. The vestibular marginal excision technique for secondary correction of nasal deformities in cleft lip. J Craniofac Surg 2024. ISSN: 1536-3732 https://doi.org/10.1097/SCS.0000000000010714.
46. Manchester WM. The repair of bilateral cleft lip and palate. Br J Surg. 1965;52(11):878–82.

47. Farkas LG, Hajnis K, Posnick JC. Anthropometric and anthroposcopic findings of the nasal and facial region in cleft patients before and after primary lip and palate repair. Cleft Palate Craniofac J. 1993;30(1):1–12.
48. Rossell-Perry P. Rotational composite flap technique for primary incomplete cleft nose deformity. Plast Reconstr Surg Glob Open. 2020;8(6):e2870.
49. Yeow V, Chen P, Chen Y, Noordhoof S. The use of nasal splints in the primary management of unilateral cleft nasal deformity. Plast Reconstr Surg J. 1999;103(5):1347–54.
50. Mendez R, Lopez-Cedrun J, Tellado M, Somoza I, et al. Nostril retainers in the primary cleft rhinoplasty. Cir Pediatr. 2005;18(4):200–3.
51. Rossell-Perry P. Atlas of non-desirable outcomes in cleft lip and palate. Cham: Springer; 2022.

Index

P. Rossell-Perry (ed.), *Atlas of Primary Cleft Rhinoplasty*,
https://doi.org/10.1007/978-3-031-68012-0

GPSR Compliance

The European Union's (EU) General Product Safety Regulation (GPSR) is a set of rules that requires consumer products to be safe and our obligations to ensure this.

If you have any concerns about our products, you can contact us on ProductSafety@springernature.com

In case Publisher is established outside the EU, the EU authorized representative is:

Springer Nature Customer Service Center GmbH
Europaplatz 3
69115 Heidelberg, Germany

Batch number: 10726133

Printed by Printforce, the Netherlands